DIVINING WITHOUT SEEDS

A volume in the series
The Culture and Politics of Health Care Work
edited by Suzanne Gordon and Sioban Nelson

A list of titles in this series is available at
www.cornellpress.cornell.edu.

DIVINING WITHOUT SEEDS

The Case for Strengthening
Laboratory Medicine in Africa

Iruka N. Okeke

**ILR PRESS
AN IMPRINT OF
CORNELL UNIVERSITY PRESS
ITHACA AND LONDON**

First published 2011 by Cornell University Press

Printed in the United States of America

Library of Congress Cataloging-in-Publication Data
Okeke, Iruka N., 1970–
   Divining without seeds : the case for strengthening laboratory medicine in
Africa / Iruka N. Okeke.
         p. cm. — (The culture and politics of health care work)
   Includes bibliographical references and index.
   ISBN 978-0-8014-4941-3 (cloth : alk. paper)
   1. Diagnosis, Laboratory—Africa, Sub-Saharan.   2. Medical laboratories—
Africa, Sub-Saharan.   3. Clinical medicine—Africa, Sub-Saharan.   I. Title.
II. Series: Culture and politics of health care work.
   RB37.O44   2011
   616.07'50967—dc22   2010037178

Cornell University Press strives to use environmentally responsible suppliers and
materials to the fullest extent possible in the publishing of its books. Such materials
include vegetable-based, low-VOC inks and acid-free papers that are recycled,
totally chlorine-free, or partly composed of nonwood fibers. For further information, visit our website at www.cornellpress.cornell.edu.

Cloth printing   10 9 8 7 6 5 4 3 2 1

For Chiji, Uche, and Ebele

Contents

Preface

I am privileged to spend much of my time teaching and performing research in one of America's foremost liberal arts colleges. I work with some of the brightest young students and some of the most talented biologists in the world. Much of my work is molecular biology, and I am amazed at how many times I get asked about the relevance of my work to health, particularly in Africa, where I visit and work very regularly. Nonscientists easily appreciate that there are connections between physics and engineering, and even between chemistry and the pharmaceutical sciences. The applications of biology to conservation science and agriculture or anatomy to medicine are frequently highlighted, but many people underestimate how much and how quickly microbial and molecular biology have changed how we prevent and treat disease. Microbiology, cell pathology, clinical chemistry, and molecular biology make it possible for medicine to deliver today's miracle cures. Unveiling the strong connections between science and modern medicine is a principal objective of this work.

When I completed high school at Queen's College, Lagos, in 1985, I would have returned to Europe, the continent of my birth, only if I had not secured admission into one of Nigeria's premier universities. By the following year, I was an undergraduate at West Africa's premier school of pharmacy and over the next twenty years, first as a student, then as a faculty member and finally as a visiting scientist, I have watched the ivory tower tarnish in the face of "structural adjustment" at the national level and noticed, in particular, the material decline of science education. By the 1990s, most of the biology papers in the foremost scientific journals, such as *Science, Nature,* and *Cell,* were unintelligible to Nigerian graduate students like myself. A few years later, students were blissfully unaware of these deficiencies because libraries could no longer stock the journals.

I was nonetheless privileged to take an elective class in advanced microbial genetics as a graduate student at Obafemi Awolowo University in Nigeria, taught by the late Professor Shonukan. The course introduced me to today's biomedical science, and, in researching my own project on childhood diarrhea in western Nigeria, I was startled to see how little of this "new" knowledge was being applied to such a pertinent problem. I chose to pursue a multinational program of graduate study and to seek postdoctoral training in molecular science abroad. By the time I had completed my training, I had gained expertise in molecular microbiology that would be invaluable in infectious disease research, but no Nigerian university was then equipped to do this type of science. Furthermore, as a young investigator, I was then ineligible for many international research grants that might have supported me in setting up my own lab.

I reconciled these paradoxes by refusing to choose between categories. Consequently, I am both a Western and a West African scientist. I spend the academic year in the United States but also devote a few weeks each year to working at my alma mater or elsewhere in Africa. Here, too, I work with some of the brightest young students and some of the most talented biologists in the world. African molecular biologists know that we cannot but build capacity in this area. Some are skeptical about feasibility and sustainability but almost everyone seems to understand that we are losing something without it. Although I was initially uncomfortable with my decision to train and then work outside Nigeria, it is easy for me and others to observe that I currently contribute more to African science than I might have done if I had stayed. This is not the pat on the back or assuagement of guilt that it might appear to be. Instead, it is the admission that a bicontinental existence currently contributes more than a full-time scientific employment in Nigeria and that this in itself is a reflection of the many shortfalls of laboratory science in that country and elsewhere. It is not a way of working that I pioneered. I know many other African scientists who have straddled two continents, making the most of the increased "networkedness" of science today.

Before I pursued graduate training in microbiology, I was a pharmacist at a university health center as well as in an urban secondary care hospital in Nigeria. My scientific research later took me to primary health care centers where I collaborated with doctors, nurse practitioners, and community health workers. The shortfalls in (and often complete dearth of) laboratory science I encountered in the clinic were significantly worse than those I met in education and research, in that they affected people's lives and health. However, I did not come to consider the true significance of these deficits until a decade later. Before then, as a hospital pharmacist and later a researcher who had a wonderfully close relationship with idealistic physicians, I found it difficult to see how modest investments in laboratory sciences might have greatly assisted us in pursuing our aims. To be entirely frank, we were all so busy that we had no time to think about it.

Thus, although on the one hand it appears somewhat presumptuous for one who does not practice medicine in Africa to criticize diagnostic protocols that help thousands of patients, on the other hand constructive criticism very often comes from the outside. Long after I had transformed myself from a pharmacist to the microbiologist I am now, I realized that laboratory shortfalls did more than just inhibit my own scientific curiosity. The realization came from straightforward and just criticism of one of my own papers. My colleagues and I had written about bacteria that cause diarrhea in one of the few papers that used molecular epidemiology to study the problem in Nigeria. A critique of our paper pointed out that the "standard" methods we had used to test for nonbacterial parasites were outdated and imprecise. In researching our response to this published critique, I became palpably aware and considerably demoralized by the sheer and overwhelming scope of the diagnostic gaps across sub-Saharan Africa.

In the last six years, as I researched this book, I began to visit other countries in Africa. I was curious to see whether the problem was similar there, as the literature seemed to indicate. My observations, most of them made in admittedly short visits, appeared to suggest that, for the most part, this was indeed the case. I heard the concerns of underresourced health workers, who would have liked to deliver more, and I also spoke with those who work at model sites and fear that what they have might erode. Thus, this story of diagnostic insufficiency is not mine. It is a story of those who are too busy saving lives to tell it themselves. Some are so busy that they have not noticed the story unfold around them and struggle in their attempt to deliver care in the absence of appropriate laboratory services. My combination of a background in science and in health care, proximity to health services in Africa, access to the global medical research literature and nonindexed African periodicals, as well as the time and space to write is unusual. This is my only explanation for why, even though the problem I describe is a pervasive and long-standing one, no one has articulated it cohesively before.

It has been important to sketch the problem comprehensively but in as few words as possible. I hope I do not convey the impression that there are no diagnostic facilities in Africa. Capabilities vary considerably within and among different countries. I have interacted with scientists from Nigeria, Ghana, and The Gambia who are struggling to secure an "in" into the world of molecular biology. I have also interacted with scientists from Nigeria, Ghana, and The Gambia who are leaders in the field. I have visited tertiary centers of excellence with modern equipment and first-rate scientists. I have even seen a few rural and suburban health centers that offer an admirable suite of diagnostic services in remote places. Thus, it is important to emphasize that the scale and scope of the problem described in this book is heterogeneous. Indeed, the few scientists who perform state-of-the-art research and diagnostic medicine on the continent point to the feasibility of laboratory development. The argument I try to make here is that every African patient should have appropriate diagnostic access and most currently do not. Perhaps most encouraging is the simple fact that things have improved on the diagnostic front since I began to write. The direction is a good one, but the pace is still far too slow.

Another unsettling personal truth I have had to come to terms with over the course of my career is that individuals and small groups engaged in a myriad of scientific activities can make great discoveries but in practical terms accomplish very little. This is a hard pill to swallow for a "lab rat" like myself, who lives for nothing but experimentation and analyses. Every drop in the ocean is of course important, but in the face of major diagnostic roadblocks, real impact requires a more widespread awareness of the problem and a concerted attempt to address it at multi-institutional, regional, and even global levels. The tools for controlling smallpox were invented by individual researchers, but until there was global buy-in, the disease could not be eradicated. Thus, I considered that it might be more important to communicate the magnitude and importance of laboratory deficits in general, and diagnostic shortfalls in particular, than to continue to chip away at these problems myself, or within small collaborative groups. The conscious decision to take some time away from my lab to write this manuscript is my response to this realization. However, as I am less directly interfaced with sick patients in want of a diagnosis, I am probably well placed to do this.

Iruka N. Okeke

Ile-Ife, January 2010

Acknowledgments

As my ideas took so long to crystallize into a book, it is impossible to acknowledge everyone whose comments, work, questions, and criticisms helped to produce the manuscript. I cannot but begin by thanking the health workers and scientists who are devoted to addressing infectious diseases in Africa. Many I know personally, some I have even cited, still more I know by reputation alone, and many others I will never encounter. It is my sincere hope that all will see that increasing diagnostic infrastructure will increase the impact of their contributions severalfold. I also hope that they will consider their story well told.

I am grateful to have had mentors who were less concerned with my scientific "output" than they were with the quality of my development. My graduate and postdoctoral advisers, Adebayo Lamikanra and James B. Kaper, were true teacher-scholars. They allowed me to think outside the box, and thereby come to the realization that there was more to what I do than the Petri dishes and scientific journals that I love. I have no natural talent for writing, I simply persevere. But by the end of my training, I had achieved clarity and attention to detail because "Lami-K," Jim, Robert Edelman, and a few other informal mentors also taught me to write, patiently reading draft after draft of many of the theses and scientific papers that preceded this book.

The recent award of a five-year Branco Weiss Fellowship from the Society-in-Science was a life-changing opportunity, for which I am sincerely grateful. It not only encouraged me to continue to explore connections between my work and society, but also gave me the means to establish research and scientific development activities in parts of Africa during the years that the book was written.

An important close-to-final polish of this work came from Ebenezer Obadare and other social scientist friends, as well as from my editor, Grey Osterud, who retaught me to write, this time for the nonscientist. They are the reason why the audience for this work will extend beyond what Ebenezer has referred to as my "narrow *E. coli* audience." I am also grateful for Cristina Fuller who volunteered to proofread, and punctuate, the final manuscript.

Over the last six years, as I transformed this work from pages of notes into a book, a number of individuals have given me tidbits and ideas that have sharpened my argument, honed the manuscript, and increased its rigor. Others patiently explained to me how an idea becomes a book. A partial list includes Oladiipo Aboderin (Nigeria), Ike Achebe (Nigeria, USA), Martin Antonio (The Gambia), Michael Bate (UK), Fiona Cooke (UK), Gordon Dougan (UK), Toyin Falola (USA), Martha Gyansa-Lutterodt (Ghana), Shannon Hader (Zimbabwe, USA), Maryke Henton (South Africa), Dominic Johnson (USA, UK), Keith Klugman (South Africa, USA), Andreas Krasse (Germany), Helen Lee (USA, UK), James Mwansa (Zambia), Ebenezer Obadare (Nigeria, UK, USA), Ike Okonta (Nigeria, UK), Japheth Opintan (Ghana), Thomas Pfieffer (USA), Mel Santer (USA), Megan Vaughan (UK) and John Wain (UK). I must also thank the academic communities in which I have freely tossed around ideas and received thoughtful feedback. They include Haverford College and the institutions with which we share an African Studies program, where I have had the opportunity to learn from students as well as faculty to become a more rounded and "liberal" scholar; the Society-in-Science and the talented set of "fellow fellows" selected with me, who encouraged me to be bold in seeking expertise from other disciplines; as well as a number of policy-driven working groups, which have helped me to make connections between microbiology and public health.

In the course of my research for this work, I interviewed a number of health workers and scientists and was graciously hosted at many laboratories, clinics, and hospitals. I am grateful to a number of individuals for sharing their lives and jobs with me, particularly 'Diipo Aboderin (Nigeria), Kwabena Bosompem (Ghana), Eric Böttger (Switzerland), Abdoulaye Djimde (Mali), Gordon Dougan (UK), 'Peju Esimai (Nigeria), Oliver Hazemba (Zambia), Kayode "IKT" Ijadunola (Nigeria), Helen Lee (UK), Aniete Moses (Nigeria), John Mwaba (Zambia), Flora Okeke (Nigeria, UK), 'Segun Ojo (Nigeria), Japheth Opintan (Ghana) 'Laja Osoniyi (Nigeria), as well as other staff of Addenbrookes Hospital (Cambridge, UK), Enuwa Primary Health care centre (Ile-Ife, Nigeria), Medical Research Council laboratories (Fagara, The Gambia), Obafemi Awolowo University Teaching Hospitals Complex (Ile-Ife and Ilesa, Nigeria), Obafemi Awolowo University health centre (Ile-Ife, Nigeria), Our Lady of Lourdes Catholic Mission Hospital (Ipetu-Modu, Nigeria), the Royal Victoria Teaching Hospital (Banjul, The Gambia),

Sulayman Jungkung Hospital (Bwiam, The Gambia), the University of Ghana Medical School and Korle Bu Teaching Hospital (Accra, Ghana), University Teaching Hospital (Lusaka, Zambia), and the Wellcome Trust Sanger Institute (Cambridge, UK).

I am grateful to family, friends, and loved ones, many of whom admit that they have "no idea" what I do, but who give me the space to spend almost all my time doing it, to their general neglect. I especially hope that, through this book, they might come to a better understanding of what happened to those we lost, or almost did, because we did not secure a diagnosis in time.

Abbreviations

ACT	artemisinin combination therapy
AIDS	acquired immune deficiency syndrome
CCD	clinical case definition
CD4+	"cluster of differentiation 4"-positive (cells preferentially invaded by HIV)
CDC	United States Centers for Disease Control and Prevention
DALY	disability-adjusted life years
DOTS	directly observed therapy short course
DNA	deoxyribonucleic acid
Hib	*Haemophilus influenzae* type B
HIV	human immunodeficiency virus
MDR	multidrug-resistant
MIC	minimum inhibitory concentration
MRC	UK Medical Research Council
PCR	polymerase chain reaction
PfEMP1	*Plasmodium falciparum* erythrocyte membrane protein 1
RNA	ribonucleic acid
RT-PCR	reverse-transcriptase polymerase chain reaction
SARS	severe acute respiratory syndrome
TB	tuberculosis
UNICEF	United Nations Children's Fund
WHO	World Health Organization
XDR	exceedingly drug-resistant

INTRODUCTION

Ohne Diagnostik keine vernünftige Therapie. Erst untersuchen,
dann urtheilen, dann helfen. (Without diagnosis, there is no rational
treatment. Examination comes first, then judgment, and then one
can give help.)

—Carl Gerhadt, Würsburg, Germany, 1873

On a typical day at a health center in southwestern Nigeria, patients arrive long before the outpatient clinic opens. Most patients are infants or young children, strapped to the backs or held to the breasts of tired young mothers. Babies wear pretty cotton print outfits and rubber shoes or slippers, perhaps with white socks. A trip to the clinic is an important outing, even if the visiting child is precariously close to death. Hospital visits place patients and their guardians in close proximity to some of the most highly respected members of their community. Mothers wear traditional apparel that permits them to carry a sick child on their back and to secure a moneybag, often containing borrowed funds, close to the body. Each woman carries a large, tightly packed bag containing several different types of food, which have, typically, all been rejected by the sick child, empty medicine bottles, a blanket or shawl, and clean and soiled cloth diapers. Because there is often no running water at the hospital, mothers also carry a keg, bottle, or polythene bag of drinking water. Those who do not bring water may have to buy it. Mothers carrying these burdens along with their babies enter the hospital gates looking harried. They had worked hard the day before, had little sleep because of a sick child, and may have begun the journey to the hospital as early as 4 a.m. Many mothers have already spent more than a day's wages on travel, have no savings, and will earn nothing on this day. Most have other children for whose health and welfare they are similarly concerned.

When the outpatient clinic opens at about 8 a.m., patients have been waiting for as long as three hours. First-time visitors to the hospital line up to "buy cards," that is, pay a registration fee, and then move to the consultation queue, shepherded by aides or volunteers. Squabbles occasionally erupt along the lines, but mutual desperation promotes a community spirit that typically keeps these tiffs brief. Each child, in turn, is seated opposite a paramedic worker or nurse-aide, who takes a temperature and does a quick examination. Children with extremely high temperatures, who are unconscious or on the verge of losing consciousness, or who are severely dehydrated, see an emergency doctor or nurse practitioner. The rest wait their turn in the next slow-moving line, until finally the mother and her young patient are seated outside the door of a consulting room.

At last, perhaps four or six hours after their arrival, a nurse-aide carries a patient's file and guides the mother into the consulting room. The file contains a temperature chart, previous medical records, if any are available, and sometimes a prescription sheet with the patient's name and registration number already entered. The mother sits down and uncovers her child as the nurse-aide takes her place at the side of the table, ready to translate if the doctor does not understand the local language. The doctor asks what is wrong and scribbles rapidly. His pen bears the insignia of an expensive new pharmaceutical, which is not stocked in the hospital pharmacy. The mother replies: she is hot, she does not eat. As she speaks, she looks down at the doctor's old but polished shoes and his worn-out but clean socks that dangle around his ankles. The doctor glances at the child, who has stopped crying, perhaps from curiosity, perhaps from exhaustion. He glances at the temperature slip and asks if the child is breast-fed. How long has she been ill? Any diarrhea? He may lift the pretty but faded cotton clothing to palpate or examine the child's abdomen for rash. If the child has been coughing, he may apply the stethoscope briefly to her chest. If the child is hot to the touch, he writes a prescription for antimalarials and scribbles something in the file. But he does not write down a diagnosis. If this is an early patient and he was not on call the night before, he might smile and tell the mother not to worry, just to use the medicine he is recommending.

The mother curtseys as she receives the prescription; she is grateful whether or not he smiles. She picks up the large bag in one hand and holds her baby in the other. The cloth she used to tie the baby on her back is slung over her shoulder. There will be time enough to organize herself outside the consulting room; now she is anxious to ensure that the next person in line can enter the room quickly. The next patient's mother is approaching the chair she just vacated and untying a little boy who holds a piece of *akara*, or fried bean fritters, in his hand. The first mother has been in the room for between two and five minutes. She makes a mental note to find some *akara* for her child as she walks out of the consulting room. But first she must hurry to the next long line.

The mother visits the nurses' station for injections and the pharmacy for medicines. She uses precious resources to buy *akara* for her child, who squeezes the snack but will not eat it. So the woman nibbles squashed *akara* on the pharmacy queue. Then she turns the plastic bag in which the snack was sold inside out and uses it to store the hospital registration card. Eventually, in the mid-to-late afternoon, she walks away from the hospital, hopefully with her child asleep on her back and her bag heavier with medicine. She mumbles to herself as she leaves, memorizing the dosage regimen.

When she gets home, she is asked, "What did they give you at the hospital?" and perhaps "How much did it cost?" No one talks about what disease the patient has, just what medicine was received. More often than not, the prescription is appropriate for the illness, or the patient recovers anyway, and the tedious visit is forgotten after the debts incurred are repaid. Problems arise only if the medicine does not work and the patient does not get better. Then, the failure to make a diagnosis in the initial visit stands in the way of obtaining a timely and cost-effective cure. The consequences can be fatal.

This pattern of consultation and prescription experienced by many African patients makes it possible for understaffed, underresourced public hospitals and clinics to offer medical care to so many patients each day. They do so much good in an area of so much need that it is easy to overlook shortcomings. However, their mode of practice routinely violates the key principle articulated by René Laënnec, one of the founders of scientific medicine, and emphasized by Carl Gerhadt: that diagnosis is a prerequisite for effective treatment.[1] An inevitable consequence of treating without adequate diagnosis is that many patients do not receive the most beneficial therapies; indeed, the medications they are given may even be harmful. The standard approach to treating most infectious diseases in high-burden, low-income countries is inefficient and ineffective. In order to serve African patients, medical protocols must be altered to deal with the underlying problem of *diagnostic insufficiency.*

Diagnosis, Treatment, and Cure

This book focuses on failures in the prevention and treatment of infectious disease occasioned by the inadequate application of laboratory diagnosis—or what I call diagnostic insufficiency. It explores the deficit in an often-repeated sequence of events that begins with health-seeking, includes treatment, and aims to end in cure. The book argues that it is not enough to get patients to clinics and to administer medicines to them. A diagnosis must precede treatment—one that is rigorous and precise. For infectious diseases, particularly in parts of the world like sub-Saharan Africa, this includes laboratory examination of patient specimens in order to identify the cause of infection. A cure can then be selected that specifically eradicates the microorganism that is responsible for ill health in time to prevent permanent tissue damage or spread to other individuals. To treat infectious diseases without taking advantage of laboratory tests is akin to treating an orthopedic fracture without the benefit of X-rays or, to use an indigenous example, asking the Yoruba diviner to offer a cure without having seen the pattern of seeds thrown during the consultation.

The invention of the microscope enabled medical researchers and health care practitioners to *see* the biological agents that cause infectious diseases. Until that time, in most cultures, serious illnesses were thought to have supernatural origins, and the spread or containment of contagion was largely inexplicable. Patients' highly variable responses to customary treatments added to the mystery. Why an individual fell ill and whether the sufferer recovered or succumbed seemed out of human hands and was often attributed to a god or demon. Microscopes and subsequent advances in the biomedical sciences have thrown considerable light on the cause and nature of infection, separating the secular occupation of the physician from the sacred vocation of the spiritual healer. Magnifying lenses and experimental microbiology have revealed a specific microorganism associated with each infectious disease. Once microbial enemies could be visualized, cultured, and characterized, specific weapons could be found or designed to attack them. Some effective antimicrobials were in use before microbes were known, but their number and variety increased exponentially after the biological basis for infectious disease was defined. Scientific advances have led to the development of spectacular strategies for the prevention and cure of many previously deadly contagions.

Scientific knowledge has been translated into significant improvements in public health in the developed nations of the Northern Hemisphere, but less so in the developing nations of the South. The part of the world somewhat controversially referred to as sub-Saharan Africa has benefited the least from scientific innovations in health care. Although ecological and economic factors are involved in the relative neglect of public health on the continent, a profound want of application is central to the problem. Most observers admit that, if every African were provided with safe drinking water, the scourges of cholera, dysentery, river blindness, guinea worm infestation, and the myriad other waterborne diseases endemic to the continent would virtually disappear. Our understanding of the biological bases of disease gives us good reason to infer that insecticide-impregnated mosquito nets, exclusive breast-feeding, adequate and appropriate nutrition, and vaccine development and deployment could have equally significant benefits. Unfortunately, all of these preventive measures are inadequately applied in tropical Africa. When preventive strategies fail, or are never implemented, infected people require curative medicine, without which they would suffer or die. Curative measures, too, are not optimally applied. African patients seek care from a variety of sources, commonly starting with the most accessible and least expensive form of treatment. What is variously termed Western, scientific, or allopathic medicine is only one possible option.[2] More money and expertise are invested in Western medicine than in indigenous or other forms of healing, and the expectations it arouses are correspondingly high. Its failures deserve to be scrutinized.

Pathogens, Diseases, and Diagnosis

Most microorganisms are harmless or even beneficial to humans. The minority that can cause diseases are known as pathogens. Sometimes a pathogen produces a discernible signature in the infected host, such as a rash or discoloration of the skin. But, since there are thousands of pathogens and only a few visible symptoms, many different diseases produce similar conditions. Educated guesswork is sometimes possible, but direct observation, even when accompanied by a detailed medical history and careful clinical examination,[3] is usually insufficient to differentiate between potential causes of infection. Pathogens are distributed asymmetrically with respect to age, location, and season, so an observant clinician can often narrow the potential causes to a handful of likely suspects. But, the larger the array of common pathogens within the physician's sphere of practice, the longer will be the list of possible causes. With the assistance of a medical laboratory, a doctor can find out exactly which pathogen is the cause of each patient's distress and prescribe a specific cure. When the infectious agent is not identified with some degree of assurance, prescribed therapies may well be useless or harmful.

Clinical diagnosis only needs to be precise enough to permit selection of the most appropriate treatment available. When better diagnostic techniques are available but more specific treatments are not, in-depth diagnosis for every patient would not be justifiable. Indeed, medical historian David Wootton has argued that in Europe, when diagnostic advances outpaced curative ones, most medicine was useless or harmful.[4] Similarly, the use of potentially effective but highly specific medicines is ineffective and wasteful when not paired with a system for determining when they should be used. This situation exists in much of Africa today. Diagnostic shortfalls seriously impair the use of the most effective medicines, both by undermining patients' faith in them and by compromising the efficacy of the drugs themselves. Diagnostic insufficiency also exacerbates disease transmission. Taking these two factors together, diagnostic development could pay for its cost.

In most developing countries, the health care system is plagued by varying degrees of diagnostic insufficiency, and even in the richest nations the application of diagnostic tests is far from optimal. In most of Africa, this problem is particularly acute, and chronic inadequacies of the health care system amplify its consequences. The continent has the world's highest infectious disease burden and a very wide range of potential pathogens for each clinical syndrome. Too many endemic diseases have markedly similar early symptoms to be differentiated by clinical examination. What passes for diagnosis is commonly made by community health workers or other people with limited medical training, so it is more likely to be incorrect than if it were done by a physician or nurse practitioner. When disease-specific signs appear, such as the convulsions of cerebral malaria or the intestinal perforations associated with typhoid fever, tissue damage is already advanced and treatment is more complicated, less accessible, and more expensive—as well as less successful. In some cases, the possible life-threatening pathogens are so diverse as to make even late-stage diagnosis based on clinical signs and symptoms unreliable. Sub-Saharan Africa suffers, more than any other part of the world, from the secondary consequences of this high infectious disease burden, which include poverty and political instability. A "ratchet effect"[5] occurs when the poor incur great expense to fight illness and so remain poor and at risk of failing to recover or of acquiring new infections. Other features of contemporary African societies, such as close contact with animals, rapid deforestation and urbanization, and population growth without commensurate development in public health infrastructure and sanitation, combine to increase the risks of the transmission of endemic diseases and the emergence of new ones. Many pathogens in Africa are highly virulent, so that the potential of contracting a fatal or disabling infection is intolerably high. Misdiagnosis has serious consequences, which include a shortening of the useful life span of antimicrobial medicines due to drug resistance. Existing medicines must be used judiciously, as drug development for Africa's distinctive pathogens is slow and seldom profitable enough to attract private investment.

Sub-Saharan Africa suffers from a double burden: adequate diagnostic tests are least likely to be available for its most severe endemic or epidemic pathogens. The development and deployment of diagnostic tests for pathogens is incomplete for the same reasons that specific medications for treatment are often absent or unavailable. In some cases, the etiologic agents of a specific disease are yet to be discovered or defined; in others, a reliable means of accurately detecting its presence in patients does not yet exist. The diagnostic tests for some diseases are so expensive or so sophisticated that they can be performed only in specialist laboratories and cannot be used routinely. In critiquing inadequate laboratory work, the absence of a suitable test must be distinguished from the failure to employ an existing and relatively reliable test. I use the phrase *diagnostic insufficiency* to describe a failure to apply existing and practicable technologies for the diagnosis of disease, and I extend the term to include those instances where a test is not presently available but the technology to develop one exists.

The scientific advances that have most significantly improved infectious disease control include differential diagnosis, medication and chemotherapy, immunization and vaccines, and information technology.[6] Although standard medications have been widely dispersed across the continent, vaccination programs are well under way, and information technology has been disseminated more recently, diagnosis has been the most systematically neglected aspect of health care in Africa. Too little is being done to address this problem; indeed, its existence is seldom acknowledged. Other potentially life-saving technologies, such as vaccines and antimicrobials, have limited effectiveness if they are inappropriately applied. In the introduction to his seminal collection on the history of medicine, Thomas Brock explains that microbiology began as an applied science: "microbiology developed to solve practical problems."[7] In most of Africa, it has barely been brought to bear upon them. This book highlights the consequences of diagnostic insufficiency in the region with the greatest need for simple, easily applied diagnostic tools. It argues that simple laboratory diagnostics for infectious diseases are needed more in Africa than in any other part of the world.

Because diagnostic needs and capabilities are often little understood by laypersons, however, chapter 1 begins with a brief overview of how scientists came to attribute diseases to specific pathogens and how this knowledge has revolutionized the control and treatment of infectious diseases. The second and third chapters examine fever, a key diagnostic quandary, and how, in endemic Africa, this symptom is often diagnosed or misdiagnosed as malaria without evidence. Chapter 4 focuses on drug resistance, the long-term and deleterious consequence of overusing antimalarial and antibacterial medicines. The next two chapters demonstrate that slow and inadequate diagnoses amplify epidemics of sexually transmitted diseases and incurable infections caused by viruses, including Ebola and HIV. Chapter 7 is focused on the importance of diagnostic certainty to disease eradication and control. While the six chapters that follow the introduction focus on the problem of diagnostic insufficiency, the last two chart a way forward. In chapter 8, I propose that today's diagnostic shortfalls are rooted in health systems built on a colonial model that neither sought to administer adequate care to Africans nor had a need to properly manage infections on the continent. Chapter 8 goes on to highlight, with specific examples, modern technology that could be used to overcome laboratory deficits in today's clinics. It leads into a conclusion that is entirely focused on the feasibility of diagnostic development and systematically debunks the arguments against investing in clinical laboratory infrastructure.

THE POWER OF SIGHT

It is no exaggeration to say that without the microscope doctors would never have acquired the capacity to defer death.

—David Wootton, 2006

Anyone who has lived in malaria-endemic Africa has probably been a victim of the febrile diagnostic quandary, whether they know it or not. Personally, I have only vague recollections of the month of my final examinations for the bachelor's degree at a Nigerian university. During reading period and exam weeks, my days began before dawn with frantic studying crammed in before the evening, when I was regularly felled by fever and headache. I had made three visits to the university health center in as many weeks. Each time, my temperature was taken, and I was examined by a medical doctor. At the end of each visit, I was prescribed the same antimalarial, chloroquine, which I took as prescribed. Nonetheless, my health continued to deteriorate. At the time, chloroquine was effective against most cases of malaria in Nigeria and was the drug of choice for managing the disease. Although the health center was equipped with a laboratory and affiliated with a tertiary care teaching hospital, only on my third visit were laboratory tests considered—and what the doctor ordered was a pregnancy test. In his opinion, pregnancy was the most likely cause of prolonged febrile illness in a female undergraduate. When the test came back negative, I was handed a third chloroquine prescription along with iron tablets to treat my worsening anemia. I took this course of medicine, but the mysterious illness—which, after the pregnancy test, my friends and I had dubbed "evening sickness"—began to eat away at me. As my classmates, too, were losing weight from the stress of exams, my appearance was no cause for concern to anyone but my mother, who stopped in to see me at the end of the third week of this ordeal.

My mother is a well-trained and experienced nurse. Although she studied at the University College Hospital Ibadan[1] and then took specialist training in Scotland and Birmingham in the United Kingdom, a large part of her valuable experience is not listed on her resumé. When she moved with her children back to Nigeria at the end of the 1970s, she ceased to practice in the hospital and began to practice at home. We four African children were immunologically British, so we were susceptible to everything that came our way. My mother passed out vitamin pills every morning, "Sunday-Sunday"[2] antimalarial pills every week, and deworming pills four times a year. We obliged her and took them, with the exception of my sister, who secretly planted them in the garden. As a result, during her first two years of school she made almost weekly visits to the clinic, returning with injections and more distasteful medicines, which my mother mashed into orange juice concentrate and force-fed her, only to retrieve them in a disgusting, regurgitated mess. My sister's regular, back-to-back illnesses were interspersed with occasional bouts of apparent malaria in my brothers and myself and with an occasional visit from an ailing relative. One of my brothers had a life-threatening case of infectious hepatitis. Growing up with three siblings and a number of visiting and live-in cousins, I remember the colds, coughs, cuts, abrasions, chicken pox, measles, mumps, and other childhood illnesses that are common everywhere. For me in Nigeria, these sicknesses pale in the face of the incessant fevers, malaria medicines, and injections that made our house a cross between a home and a clinic.

I recall chloroquine in much the same way that children born elsewhere think of cough syrup or cod-liver oil. A black and green box with a white cross stood on top of the refrigerator perpetually reeking of chloroquine. I came to associate the smell of chloroquine with that of medicine in general. In addition to our preventive medicine, we had mosquito netting on our windows and were not allowed to play outside after dusk or to sleep over at friends' houses. Our home was sprayed with insecticide every week by my parents and three times a year by professionals. There was no public water supply, but clean water was a priority in our house, so we had our own reservoir. We drank only boiled water and needed special permission to eat anywhere but home. We took our own lunch and water to school and were forbidden to eat the school meals. We had milk every day, even when austerity measures brought on by the structural adjustment program made milk more expensive than clothing. We grew and ate copious quantities of fruits and vegetables. The produce was grown in our enormous garden and hygienically processed in our kitchen. Yet, it seemed that someone was ill almost always.

My mother exchanged our surplus produce for milk at her cooperative society, patched holes in the window netting by hand, and saw that water was boiled and bottled daily. She took us to the clinic to see the doctor, brought our injections and other medicines home, administered them herself (making sure that we had only clean needles and received them on schedule), kept charts when required, and performed all manner of procedures to make sure that none of us ever had to be admitted to the hospital. Our family was small by contemporary Nigerian standards. I often wondered what it was like to live like my friends, who had six or even nine siblings. Perhaps, I imagined during my childhood, hospitals were designed to collect the overflow of the sick.

As I did not understand at the time, there was no basis for extrapolating our experience to larger families, and my own perceptions were distorted by having lived almost without illness throughout early childhood in England, prior to our relocation. The central role that disease played in our home was exacerbated by our nonimmune status. Nonetheless, it is illustrative of the high probability of infection among vulnerable subpopulations in present-day equatorial Africa. In addition to the tropical climate, which allows several pathogens and their vectors to thrive and be easily transmitted, preventive measures such as safe water, vector control, and improved sanitation and nutrition have been poorly implemented. It is these interventions that led to a decline in the infectious disease burden in Europe and North America, not the pharmaceuticals on which we were so dependent.

Medicines and home care are accepted facets of Nigerian life. In 2005, when I visited an aunt who had three children, I saw her handle one seriously ill and two slightly sick children with the same ease and familiarity as my mother. Since my aunt is not a nurse, we made daily trips along bumpy streets to a hospital several miles away for her daughter's injections. The young teenager was too sick to pay much attention to her surroundings, but from long habit the girl was able to pull together a hospital visit bag without difficulty, containing food, water, tissues, medicine bottles, and cover cloth to protect against mosquitoes in the waiting room. As I watched her get ready, I recalled my own early education in home nursing, which continued at boarding school even though it was not part of the formal curriculum. The Nigerian writer Sefi Attah's fictional description of life in a prestigious Nigerian girls' boarding school is uncannily similar to the secondary institution that I attended in Lagos: "At night we let down our mosquito nets and during the day we patched them up if they got ripped. If a girl had malaria, we covered her with blankets to sweat out her fever. I held girls through asthma attacks, shoved a teaspoon down the mouth of a girl who was convulsing, burst boils."[3] I also learned how to detect anemia, administer an antimalarial regimen, and determine when someone was unwell enough to warrant a visit to the sick bay. In addition to mathematics, history, science, geography, literature, needlework, nutrition, French, and home management, we learned these essential survival skills. When I graduated and left for university, I took with me my own thermometer and personal stock of malaria pills.

Four years later, during my final weeks as an undergraduate, my mother arrived for a visit. Even though what my supportive roommates referred to as "evening sickness" was not yet as serious as it became, my mother recognized at once that I was deathly ill and needed appropriate treatment immediately. She was dissatisfied with the care I had received at the health center, which had diagnosed "only malaria"[4] and ruled out only pregnancy. I persuaded her to go on to the funeral, but she returned immediately after my last exam and took me to Lagos. We went straight to a doctor friend's house. In spite of the history I recounted, the doctor was almost certain that I had malaria but admitted that typhoid fever was a remote possibility, particularly if malaria treatment had failed.

My mother was thought that typhoid fever might explain my illness, but she was not giving me chloramphenicol,[5] with its reported risk of blood cancers, unless she could be sure I needed it. So she took me to a private laboratory and asked that I be tested for typhoid. "Where is the doctor's order?" asked the laboratory technician. We were somewhat taken aback by his question. Pharmacists in Nigeria rarely insist on a doctor's prescription to dispense medication, and we did not expect a commercial laboratory to request a doctor's order. "I don't have a doctor's order, but I want her tested for typhoid," my mother said determinedly. "Which test do you want?" asked the technician, with a detectable edge of sarcasm in his voice. He only worked at the lab; he did not own it. Labs were few and far between, so that profits were assured regardless of how customers were treated. "There are many types, and they are all expensive." Apparently the need for a doctor's order could be bypassed if payment was assured.

My mother had no idea which test to ask for, but I recalled from my recent studies that the Widal test might be suitable. We paid in advance and the technician obligingly performed the test. "Does she have typhoid?" asked my mother. "Madam," said the indifferent technician, who was alone in the establishment, "I perform the tests, I do not read them. If you order a test then you should know how to read the results." As neither my mother nor I could interpret the results, we took the sheet back to our doctor friend, who cried, with some measure of shock and disbelief, "It is typhoid! It is typhoid! Come, let me write a prescription. She needs chloramphenicol and you must get it tonight. She has been sick for so long! She could have intestinal perforations soon!"

The doctor's anxiety was not misplaced. Intestinal perforation from protracted typhoid is a significant cause of surgical emergencies in Nigeria. In the pre-antibiotic era, up to 20 percent of patients with typhoid fever died of the disease, and mortality rates remain high among patients with perforations. I was fortunate: three weeks later after the degree results were released, recovered but still emaciated, I stepped onto the dais to be inducted into the pharmacy profession. I had scored at the top of the class, but a classmate had prepared to read the speech because no one could be sure that I would be there. Thus, in 1989, I almost died of an entirely curable illness, and lived only because of a mother's professional knowledge, experience, and persistence. In spite of our relative affluence, and having consulted multiple physicians, I, like so many others living in Africa, found it so difficult to access the benefits of modern medicine even though such benefits had been established almost a century before.

The Microbial Pathogen, a Microscopic Organism That Causes Disease

By the nineteenth century, Western medicine was more predictable and more effective than medical treatments that were based on customs and theories handed down from the past. From Hippocrates (ca. 460–377 BCE), widely recognized as the "father of medicine" in ancient Greece, well into the medieval period, a leading thesis in medical circles was that disease was caused by an imbalance of body fluids, or "humors," and that healing involved restoring the balance, often by bloodletting. Doctors studied their patients carefully, observing them over the long term if possible, but they understood only surface anatomy. Treatment was either extremely conservative—minor alterations in diet and honey-and-vinegar mixtures were often prescribed—or painfully aggressive, with purging or bleeding. A cure served to validate the diagnosis, and when treatment failed, the patient was often blamed.[6]

Only when dissections and vivisections were performed by careful physician-scientists did the actual workings of the body began to inform the practice of healing. Following this groundbreaking reconceptualization of medicine by anatomists and pathologists of the sixteenth through the eighteenth centuries,[7] great emphasis was placed on careful physical examination, clinical record-keeping, and autopsies. Physicians began to palpate their patients and listen to their chest and abdominal sounds; after René Laënnec invented the stethoscope, this instrument became medicine's signature diagnostic. Medical practitioners shifted the focus from the patient's feelings and behavior to his or her anatomy. With this shift came the idea of looking for commonalities among cases, producing scientific definitions for different pathologies.

Infectious or contagious diseases are caused by invaders that are too small to see. A scientific reconceptualization of contagious disease came later, in the face of experimental microbiology. First, microscopes had to be invented and used to examine specimens from patients. Roughly two hundred years elapsed between the first descriptions of bacteria, made by Dutch draper and microscopist Anton Leeuwenhoek in 1676, and the conviction, championed by Robert Koch (1843–1910), that the tubercule bacillus is the cause of tuberculosis.[8] Reaching the conclusion that infections were caused by microorganisms required overcoming two long-standing, erroneous beliefs: the assumption that microscopic life could be generated spontaneously, and the notion that fermentation, putrefaction, and infection were caused by noxious chemicals rather than by living things. Both assumptions were elegantly debunked by the French scientist Louis Pasteur, and shortly after, microorganisms were linked to disease.

When the role of microbes in infectious disease became known, infectious diseases were no longer categorized in an entirely symptom-based manner; description became based almost entirely on etiology, in terms of their microbial causative agents. For example, consumption came to be known as tuberculosis, and recurrent fevers were defined as malaria; the term hydrophobia, or "a fear of drinking fluids," was generally discarded in favor of the more specific term rabies. As Andrew Cunningham has observed, in its most extreme form, exemplified by the plague, the newly discovered causative organism *became* the disease: "Hitherto what had been named in Latin or Greek was the disease (pestis); henceforth it was the micro-organism....Its first name was *Bacterium pestis*, the bacterium of plague."[9] The process through which this reorientation in thinking took place demonstrates the centrality of laboratory science to the productive linkage of science and medicine, which I argue has been particularly pertinent for the treatment of infectious diseases.

Cell biologist Friedrich Gustav Jacob Henle pointed out in *The Formation of Pus and Mucus* (1838) that while microbes could be seen in diseased tissues, they were invariably absent in healthy ones. Henle had the right idea, but like many scientists of his day he was stumped by a significant chicken-and-egg problem. Did the microbes cause the infection, or did they grow in infected tissues *because* of the infection? Henle recognized that in order to infer causation, it would, at the very least, be necessary to transfer a microorganism from an infected individual to an uninfected one and observe for signs of the disease. But deliberately inducing an infection in humans as a scientific experiment was a clear violation of the sacred principle of medicine articulated in the Hippocratic Oath: *prinum non nocere*—first, do no harm.[10] If he had had the prescience and wherewithal to infect laboratory animals, Henle might have come up with the landmark postulates of Robert Koch. Many plant scientists, who did not suffer the same ethical constraints, did manage to infer causation, and Agostino Bassi had demonstrated that the silkworm muscardine disease was a fungal infection by 1844.[11] However, the disconnect between microbiological science and medicine made it impossible to transfer the concept to clinical practice at that time.

A second roadblock was technical. Experimental medicine could not address the question of causation until scientists had learned to delineate, manipulate, and separate bacteria. Indeed, Koch's postulates require that an organism suspected of causing a disease be grown, or cultured, away from the infected patient. Microorganisms are everywhere, and most of them are harmless. Most bacteria are tiny spheres or rods, and therefore telling different species apart requires more than simply magnification. Once bacteria could be differentially stained, it became possible to propose that specific microbial species produced certain disease manifestations, but differential staining was not specific enough to delineate closely related bacteria. An often understated scientific breakthrough that made it possible to attribute pathogenicity to specific microbes was the ability to allow a separate, single microbe to reproduce thousands of times until it produced a population of organisms identical to itself. The mass of microorganisms in resultant pure cultures is large enough to see with the naked eye, akin to viewing a city from the air when a single house might not be visible. The structure and properties of this microbial colony can be analyzed and differentiated from other microbial species.

A pure culture of an organism excludes all other forms of life. Pasteur and other early microbiologists grew bacteria in liquid broths. In theory, a pure broth culture could be produced if a single organism was used as a starter in a broth culture. Julius Oscar Brefeld showed that this could be done for fungi by beginning with a single spore, but single bacteria are too small to allow for such fine manipulation.[12] Many scientists put a lot of effort into diluting and dividing infected broths, a procedure referred to as fractional culture, to produce pure bacterial liquid cultures.[13] Not until Joseph Schroeter grew pigmented organisms on potato slices did laboratory scientists realize that isolation was much more practicable on solid media than in liquid broths. Schroeter discovered that by spreading the culture extremely thinly, single organisms would have a place on the slice from which they would generate numerous direct descendents by multiplication.[14] In this way, a colony of organisms could be generated from a single cell. Although individual bacteria can be seen only under a microscope that magnifies them four hundred times or more, bacterial colonies are visible to the naked eye and can be manipulated, stained, and visualized; they can also be subcultured onto solid as well as liquid media. Manipulating microorganisms in this manner is what is generally referred to as "culture" and with microscopy comprises the cardinal methodology for diagnosing infectious disease.

Robert Koch received the Nobel Prize in 1905 for his work on developing and validating principles and procedures for unequivocally attributing disease causation to specific microbial species or subspecies. In his laboratory, Koch examined specimens from animals with anthrax. He discovered a rod-shaped bacterium, *Bacillus anthracis,* and showed that the organism could form hardy spores. In the course of developing his postulates,[15] Koch demonstrated that *B. anthracis* caused anthrax and published the results in 1876. He went on to identify the etiologic agents of wound fever in 1878, tuberculosis in 1882, and cholera in 1883.[16] Koch's postulates were most instrumental in showing that tuberculosis was an infectious, rather than an inherited, disease, the common belief at the time.[17] Formally published in 1884, these postulates are so sound that they remain the gold standard for identifying specific pathogens that are implicated in disease causation.[18]

Koch advanced Schroeter's methods, using serum solidified by heating or broths solidified with gelatin to create media more conducive for the culture of human and animal pathogens.[19] Gelatin was not an ideal culture ingredient because it melts at high ambient temperatures and is digested by some bacteria. Fannie Hesse and Walter Hesse developed agar, a gelling agent from seaweed that allowed modern methods of culture to be applied to almost all bacteria. The invention of the Petri dish[20]—a flat, transparent, sterilizable, covered, and invertible plate—was the final essential component in modern bacteriology. Standard bacteriological technique involves the isolation of organisms by streaking or spreading specimens across a plate of media solidified with agar. Selective media, which inhibit the growth of confounding harmless and environmental organisms, have been developed for many pathogens. Diagnostic media contain reagents that produce different colors and morphologies in closely related organisms, permitting preliminary identification. The identity of pure cultures can be confirmed by determining which enzymatic activities are exhibited by the organism in question.

Protocols for isolating and identifying most major bacterial pathogens were worked out by scientists before laboratories contained sophisticated electronic equipment. They were used in the most basic of laboratories during the late nineteenth and early twentieth centuries and continue to be employed in clinical laboratories today. Additional techniques have since become available that supplement older methods. For example, specific antibodies can be used to detect subspecies or identify surface proteins on a microbe. Recently, molecular methods have been adapted to identify actual genes or proteins more rapidly and with greater precision.

Now that we know which microbial species causes almost every infection, doctors can prescribe therapies that specifically deal with the root cause of each infectious illness, if such therapies exist. Diagnostic laboratories are essential to detect previously unknown pathogens in infected patients as well as for routine identification of known agents of disease. As the physician and medical historian Sherwin Nuland has explained, causation and precise diagnosis lie at the heart of disease prevention and cure: "I proceed on the principle that a disease can be effectively treated only when I as a doctor understand its causes in that particular patient, its site of origin, the internal havoc it creates, and the course which the process is likely to take whether treated or not. With that knowledge, I can make a diagnosis, prescribe a program of treatment, and predict an outcome."[21]

Importation of Scientific Medicine to Africa

Modern allopathic methods for treating infectious disease assume a diagnostic precision that was absent from Western medicine before the mid-nineteenth century. Although some indigenous African schools of medical philosophy acknowledge infectious agents, many other types of indigenous medicine are more representative of a holistic approach to healing, in which illness is considered a departure from wellness that is not deconstructed. Nonholistic diagnosis can be considered its antithesis, seeking to pinpoint a single problem with apparent disregard of its context. The patient's physical as well as spiritual ills are treated by a prescription that typically involves herbal and spiritual remedies.[22] Western-trained physicians and medical researchers, including those trained in Africa with Western-derived curricula, have been taught to use modern, evidence-based methods. They often presume that indigenous medicine is necessarily unsound and ineffective because it is "unscientific," and that its lack of scientific precision lies primarily in its failure to diagnose the causative agents of specific illnesses.

There are scientific bases for much of the medicines used by indigenous people, which accounts for the relative success by drug developers who take cues from indigenous medicine. The clinical experiments that led to the discovery of these medicines have, to a large extent, been observational rather than hypothesis driven, the standard for today's "evidence-based" Western medicines. However, indigenous therapies are in some cases based on observations that have continued for decades or centuries. Although herbal cures are the most popular example of indigenous practices that have undergone some scientific evaluation, there are also good diagnostic examples. African indigenous practitioners use ants in a urinary sugar test to diagnose diabetes.[23] More allied to infectious disease is the recent discovery that the Navajo people of what is now the southwestern United States not only understood the deadly viral disease caused by Hantavirus but also had determined that the disease vector was the deer mouse and, by revering and avoiding contact with the mouse, devised a way to prevent infection. This indigenous knowledge came to general notice in the 1990s, when orthodox science identified the cause and life cycle of what was viewed as an emergent disease.[24] That European physicians Ignaz Semmelwiess and John Snow discovered the transmission routes for childbed fever and cholera, respectively, without ever seeing or knowing of the existence of the causative bacteria is further illustration of the power of deductive epidemiology. Unfortunately, deductive epidemiology and macroscopic diagnosis of specific infectious diseases is only sufficiently sensitive and specific when the disease has uncommon signs or symptoms, or when they occur in the face of an outbreak.

Given the conflicts in philosophy, particularly in what constitutes evidence of effectiveness, it is particularly perturbing to find that most Western-trained physicians practicing in sub-Saharan Africa offer treatment based on diagnoses made with insufficient evidence. The worst form of this practice is prescribing specific treatments for infectious diseases that have nonspecific clinical signs through signs and symptoms alone. This method is similar to that used by some indigenous practitioners but is problematic because the treatments offered by Western practitioners are effective only when diagnosis is precise. Although malaria cannot be accurately diagnosed clinically, in equatorial Africa the majority of patients with fever are presumed to have this disease and treated accordingly. This rapid and cheap diagnostic protocol is helpful to the majority who do have malaria fever but is life threatening to the significant, and growing, minority who do not. As Jerome Groopman has explained,[25] clinical judgment is subject to representative bias. In a malaria-endemic area, patients who present with illnesses that might not have been considered malaria in another part of the world are in danger of being lumped with the majority, even if they have subtle clinical signs that suggest otherwise. Without diagnostic support, clinicians cannot practice medicine according to the tenets they have been taught. Patients become the diagnostic test tubes, and they may have recovered or died before the diagnosis is confirmed.

If Western medical practice in much of Africa is a risky experiment, why do its practitioners continue to be held in esteem in African societies? The answer lies in the high infectious disease burden and restricted access to care; success rates for entirely curable diseases that approach 80 percent appear high. Postmortems are rarely conducted, so poor outcomes are not catalogued. In some parts of the world, a one in five treatment failure rate for a curable disease would give rise to medical malpractice suits. But medical expectations are based on their social context: most patients feel entitled to the quality of care that their neighbors receive. Health care of a higher quality is generally viewed as a privilege until it becomes widely accessible. Poor success rates may also be underrecognized because practitioners often apportion posttherapy credit or blame in an Aesculapian manner. In this practice, used extensively in ancient Greece and common among unsanctioned providers of Western medicine and faith healers in Africa today, the practitioner takes credit if the patient recovers, but if the patient remains ill or dies, he or she is blamed for failing to follow instructions or for lacking faith in the cure.[26] Finally, many maladies, including infectious ones, are self-resolving. As Lewis Thomas has put it, "most things get better by themselves."[27]

Patients and unsanctioned health providers in Africa can obtain the most useful Western medicines without a prescription. An accurate diagnosis, which for most endemic infections requires laboratory input, is presently the only thing that Western medicine could offer that indigenous medicine and unsanctioned practitioners cannot. When it is absent, the distinctions between health care alternatives become blurred, and patients' use of multiple providers and forms of care is justified. When delivery of Western medicine to Ghanaians was a relatively new development, Dr. P. C. Selwyn-Clark wrote to Governor Alexander Ransford Slater to argue in favor of retaining curative medical services at maternal and child preventive health care centers. He emphasized the need to gain the confidence of Africans in Western medical services and practice by offering "something tangible"—the cure of disease.[28] Western medicine still fails to put its best foot forward by neglecting diagnosis, diminishing the chance of a cure.

Western medicine's most impressive feature is its relatively recent evidence-based approach, which depends on attainable diagnostic precision. The failure of Western medicine to wrest diagnostic authority has limited its ability to displace other forms of medicine, in spite of a strong will to do so. Diagnostic insufficiency in Western-style clinics has also slowed the introduction of evidence-based methods into indigenous systems, many of which have incorporated other aspects of Western health care delivery. Unsanctioned providers of Western medicine have learned to exploit this deficiency by setting up practices that combine features of indigenous and Western systems. Some use traditional methods and treatments but practice within a modern environment that includes white lab coats, waiting rooms, and medical records. Others have introduced Western pharmaceuticals into their practice by either administering them overtly or covertly or referring patients to clinics and pharmacies for injections or antibiotics.[29] Most of the Western medical curriculum is focused on diagnosis. Quacks have successful and competitive practices because Western-trained doctors in Africa apply only a fraction of their hard-won knowledge to patient care. Precise diagnosis becomes even more pertinent for life-threatening disease. In contrast to most outpatients in Western countries, who have mild ailments, most patients visiting Western-trained prescribers in sub-Saharan Africa are infected with a pathogen that can cause disabling disease or death if left unchecked.

The chapters that follow emphasize the significant costs of adapting medical protocols that are designed for temperate environments to a different cultural milieu, an underresourced health system, and a distinct disease ecology in tropical Africa without including one of the most valuable components of these protocols: laboratory support. Prescribing medicines without ascertaining the probable cause of disease is akin to seeking a specific destination via an uncertain path and not asking for directions. In equatorial Africa, almost every individual is exposed to multiple potentially life-threatening pathogens. Failing to ask for directions can be fatal.

FEVER: IS IT MALARIA?

**The first prerequisite for learning anything is thus utterly lacking—
I mean, the knowledge that we do not know.**

— Gottlob Frege, 1884

The untimely death of Ogonim, the only child of the protagonist in Flora Nwapa's epic novel *Efuru*, illustrates the consequences of failing to intervene quickly
and effectively in fevers in malarious areas.[1] Set in an Ibo town close to the Niger
River in the early twentieth century, the text depicts the time when Western
medicine had arrived in Nigeria but was not yet widely available or trusted by
the populace. The characters in Nwapa's tale journey to distant hospitals in the
event of major or unusual illnesses, particularly for surgery, but they treat most
illnesses in the home or with indigenous medicines. Efuru, the entrepreneurial
heroine of the novel whose husband has left her for another woman, devotes all
her love and attention to her beloved daughter Ogonim and is very distressed
when the girl falls ill. Ogonim's illness begins with loss of appetite, constipation,
and a fever. The child's condition deteriorates rapidly, in spite of all the efforts
made to care for her, and eventually she goes into convulsions and dies. This
fictional account resembles the biographies of many children who died of fever
at a time when so-called scientific medicine had not yet become the predomi-
nant form of care in Ibo-land. No one can be sure what killed these children.
No doubt many died of malaria, but others succumbed to one of the numerous
other infectious diseases endemic in this region of Africa.

A visit to Aro-Ndizuogu, a small town located just to the east of Ogonim's fictional home, shows how little has changed in the health situation of people who
live in rural Nigeria despite the social changes that have transformed the region
over the past century. The Aros, a feisty Ibo clan,[2] migrated directly from their
place of origin, Arochukwu, to found this settlement. Prominent Aro-Ndizuogu

families have historically had ample landholdings and great material wealth. As the value of food crops declined and people migrated to the cities, the rural populace became increasingly impoverished and marginalized. In the 1980s, the Nigerian government decided to connect the market town of Onitsha by a new express road to another large city, Okigwe. The road was planned to run right through Obinetiti, a community at the center of Ndi-Aniche village in Aro-Ndizuogu. Villagers whose houses were marked with the fatal letters "ONOK," for Onitsha-to-Okigwe express road, were told that their homes would be demolished to make way for the roadway. Owners whose farmland and homes were eaten up by the road would be eligible for financial compensation. Typically, this sort of task requires wading through bureaucratic mire and expending personal resources to grease the palms of civil servants. Whatever compensation may be obtained is small compared to the value of the property appropriated. Without recompense, even more people would have no choice but to emigrate. The only benefits the road would bring the village were the potential for hawking farm produce and snacks to travelers and a more comfortable ride home for the holidays for the town's sons and daughters in the diaspora.

The graves of Charles Onwenu, an Aro-Ndizuogu politician who contributed to the fight for Nigeria's independence and to the nation's first republican government, and of his brother, a landowner of considerable wealth who bankrolled Onwenu's career, would be desecrated as the road was proposed to run right over them. As the time for construction approached, a popular journalist and Onwenu's daughter narrated a documentary about the unfairness of the road-building projects that was screened on national television.[3] Beyond the loss of village monuments, the road would inflict harm on the living. Not only would there be no sidewalk, but no one had thought to consider a footbridge or tunnel; children on one side of the wide, busy, and dangerous road would be left without a school, and other residents would lose access to the village stream, the principal source of household water at the time. At that time, no Obinetiti resident actually owned a vehicle that could travel on the expressway. In spite of these arguments, the plans could not be halted.

The construction of the road brought unprecedented destruction to Obinetiti. The dichromatic reddish brown and green village was defaced by bright white, crude brushstrokes on mud walls to mark where the road would go. This mark of death was splashed rudely to the left of the front door of an old, blind widow's house. Thankfully, concerns about her losing her bearings were ameliorated by another splash of paint a few weeks later. One morning, the intense orange sunrise over the red clay soil of Aro-Ndizuogu became unusually fiery. Gigantic yellow earthmoving machines tore through the village's narrow and bumpy paths, knocking over cocoa trees and smashing traps children had left to catch small forest animals that might spruce up dinner. Clouds of red dust rose into the air and coated everything; men in lorries spat out the red grit that collected between their teeth. Children lined the construction sites each day after school and had to be dragged home at dusk by irate mothers.

Young women on their way to the stream were beleaguered by the outsiders employed in road-making. Many local young men had migrated to the city, so village maidens were unaccustomed to male attention. The overworked and poorly paid foremen and laborers evidently regarded consorting with the golden-brown-complexioned Aro-Ndizuogu girls as compensation for their heavy toil in this remote location. Catcalls soon led to lunch-break conversations and then to escorts to the stream and other places. Unfortunately, the bride-price for many an Ibo girl in the 1980s was far in excess of what a laborer could afford, and the protracted negotiations surrounding an Ibo marriage take longer than it takes to build a road. Many young women who strolled too far were left with nothing but a "child of the road."

These disturbances were highlights in the lives of the three grandsons of the blind widow who, through last-minute cartographic revisions, lost the wall of her compound but not her home. In many ways, their childhood resembled that of children Nwapa describes in her novel. True, unlike children in the early 1900s, these boys were sent to school, in addition to doing chores, and they were almost always given Western medicines when they were ill. Their grandmother's house bordered the busy road, offering the boys a great vantage point from which to view the progress of construction. The boys' mother, on whose meager income the family was largely dependent, pampered all three of her sons, just as Efuru did Ogonim, but the second son, Emeka, received preferential treatment because, in her view, he earned it by doing well at school. The oldest son cut school altogether to watch the road-building and later descended to petty theft. The youngest boy was having difficulty selecting a role model; the appeal of his delinquent eldest brother's exciting and less demanding life seemed irresistible. But middle son Emeka was special. He was well mannered and polite; above all, he was a good student. When he gained admission and a scholarship to one of the federal government boarding schools, it seemed that it was only a matter of time before his family's poverty would be history. When the road was completed, it carried him away to a new life at a prestigious school and brought him home for the holidays. Villagers debated whether he would become a doctor, a lawyer, or an engineer.

One morning during the summer vacation after his third year at secondary school, Emeka's mother found him shivering on his mat with a raging fever. She thought carefully about where to seek help. The road that had promised to bring modern amenities to Aro-Ndizuogu and facilitate their travel to the city had not made health care more accessible. It was next to impossible to take him to the clinic in a neighboring town; bus fare for two was too expensive, and hitchhiking with a seriously ill fourteen year old was unlikely to succeed. Besides, primary care clinics were infamous for their long queues and scarce resources. Resorting to a traditional healer who used indigenous medicine was out of the question; one of the boy's distant aunts was a trained nurse, and practitioners of Western medicine frown on indigenous medicine. The mother considered consulting a nearby drug seller, but discounted this option because of the rumor she had heard recently that his tablets were not bitter, and therefore presumably ineffective. She decided to leave the child with his grandmother and visit the more reputable drug dispenser at the other end of the village.

At sunrise, the mother tied her savings in the corner of her wrapper and walked to the dispenser's shack. After describing his condition, she paid for a selection of his best pills containing the usual *iba*, or fever, medicine and memorized the directions by muttering them under her breath as she hurried home. Emeka, now a gangling, slightly underweight fourteen year old, was given more medicine than the last time he had fever. Like all mothers, she worried about her sick son even though, after nursing all three boys through countless bouts of fever, she knew that he would probably be better the next day. She had already lost one child, but her only daughter had died in infancy, as newborns are likely to do. In contrast to her friends, most of the children she had borne had survived that trying period. She knew she was fortunate. After all, one in twenty children in West Africa are estimated to die of malaria before they are five, and another sizable fraction is killed by diarrhea, respiratory infections, and other preventable diseases.[4] The loss of a day's pay here and there to nurse her son was a small price to pay for his survival. In the 1980s, Emeka's mother did not have to worry about compounding or cooking her son's medicine, a task that was incumbent upon mothers who lived in the early 1900s, when Efuru's tale was set, but which they learned to perform with skill and precision. All she had to do was buy standardized tablets and administer them at stated intervals.

It came as a shock that, despite the age-adjusted dose of antimalarials, the boy showed no improvement the next day and suffered a convulsion. Convulsions are not entirely unexpected in malaria but are usually only seen in very young children. The combination of therapeutic failure and convulsions made his mother suspicious. With a child of Emeka's promise, the actions of envious enemies who would work to keep the family down could not be ruled out. Such a stellar character with fine career prospects would be the ideal target for malevolents.[5] After a quick family conference attended predominantly by women with no formal schooling, the boy was carried to a nearby spiritualist church,[6] where he became the center of a night vigil with prayer and fasting.

In the small hours, prostrate on a pew, he had another convulsion and then breathed his last.

Fever Is Malaria, or Is It?

Emeka's illness and death mirrors that of the fictional Ogonim. Over the course of the twentieth century, in Africa as well as in the West, the understanding of fevers due to infectious disease and the repertoire of drugs that can be used to treat them have expanded considerably. Whereas Ogonim's relatives accepted her premature death as a painful fact of life, Emeka's relatives—especially those who were city dwellers—were both saddened and angered by what they saw as inappropriate care for a boy who, in their eyes, obviously had malaria. How could anyone be sure that he had received the correct medicine from an unsanctioned drug dispenser? What if the drugs were fake or the dose insufficient? When the medication did not bring relief, why was he taken to a local church instead of to a medical clinic? Yet, it is not clear that the small health center in the next town could have resolved the unanswered questions that surround his death. How was the mother to have known that she should have taken him to a hospital even further away?

Although Emeka's mother's choices were criticized after they proved ineffective, there is nothing to suggest that she did anything wrong during the early stages of her son's illness. In a part of the world where malaria is considered synonymous with fever, she had concluded that the signs and symptoms were consistent with *falciparum* malaria and, consistent with guidelines issued by the World Health Organization (WHO), had sought treatment close to home as quickly as possible.[7] The only relevant diagnostic tool at the nearest primary care center was a thermometer, but it didn't take a thermometer to detect his raging fever. At his initial visit to the clinic, Emeka probably would have been given first-line drugs to treat malaria. If the staff had found his condition particularly alarming, they might have referred him to a hospital. But it is uncertain that his mother, with the limited resources available to her, would have been able to get him there in the short time between his convulsion and his death. She did recognize the severity of his condition and the ineffectiveness of the initial treatment. With hindsight, we might argue that the health-seeking behavior of Emeka's mother was inimical to her child's best interest, but her choices are typical of those made by many Africans.[8] Medical pluralism flourishes on the continent, and the equal or higher weight given to both indigenous medicine and spiritual healing, which are today less patronized but have by no means disappeared in the West, is a function of the failure of the Western medical system to compete effectively with alternative systems of care.

The most important question, which neither the dispenser nor the primary care clinic could have answered, is whether Emeka had malaria at all. That was regarded as a foregone conclusion, which perhaps contributed to suspicions of a noninfectious diagnosis when antimalarials did not work. Other than the possibility that he was felled by a cruel curse cast by enemies, no alternate diagnosis was considered. Although malaria reputedly accounts for 31 percent of childhood deaths in Nigeria, there is a compelling need to consider other possible diagnoses. It is a well-established but little acknowledged fact that, even in areas where malaria is highly endemic, the disease can be diagnosed by clinical signs and symptoms alone in only about 50 percent to 80 percent of cases.[9] Malaria remains a likely cause of Emeka's illness and death, but emerging data from several locations within Africa suggests that there is at least a one-in-four chance that the youth had a bacterial infection that could have been treated successfully with antibacterial medications. Emeka was well above the age at which convulsions are most likely to accompany malaria, and he failed to respond to standard treatments for the disease. So the appropriateness of the treatment that he received remains questionable. Today, as with the deaths of children such as Ogonim so long ago, and in spite of unprecedented advances in health care over the intervening period, we can draw no definitive conclusion about the cause of this teenager's death. Even more seriously, it is not clear that his prognosis would have been any better had his mother taken him to a primary care center.

Standard Western treatment for severe malaria and similarly presenting severe infections is not ideal, but it is certainly better than no treatment at all. More critically, early treatment of malaria and diseases that present with similar symptoms prevents progression to the deadly central nervous system involvement that Emeka may have suffered on his final day. The intervention that would most likely have led to a different outcome for Emeka is consideration of an alternative diagnosis and the prompt administration of appropriate medicines. This course of action might have been undertaken at a hospital, but only if a bacterial infection could be diagnosed, if malaria could be ruled out, or ideally, both. If, on the day that he showed symptoms, Emeka's mother had been told that her child was seriously ill but did not have malaria, she might have got him to a hospital, albeit at great expense.

Fevers are so common in tropical Africa that many children die without precise diagnoses or effective treatments in spite of medical intervention. Emeka's story is representative of millions whose lives end prematurely in a feverish haze. Indeed, he fared better than many other children, who are unable to learn in school because fevers have interrupted or permanently damaged their cognitive development, or whose repeated illnesses so impoverish their families that they cannot then afford to educate them.[10] If Emeka had died of some obscure or emergent disease, his death might be more understandable, though equally un-bearable. What is paradoxical is the claim that the boy died of an age-old disease that is endemic in his hometown and is considered the leading childhood illness in Nigeria, and he died in spite of receiving what is generally accepted as ap-propriate initial treatment. Malaria has been described as "utterly treatable and highly preventable,"[11] largely because of scientific innovations that occurred a century ago. Dr. Ronald Ross of the University of Liverpool received the Nobel Prize in 1902 for "work on malaria, by which he has shown how it enters the organism and thereby has laid the foundation for successful research on this dis-ease and methods of combating it," a discovery made in 1897.[12] A hundred years later, a young boy treated with antimalarials died without anyone being able to say whether or not this parasite was present in his blood. In cases like Emeka's, why can malaria be neither confirmed nor ruled out?

Plasmodium falciparum

Malaria is an ancient disease that probably emerged along with agricultural settlements. Humans who began to congregate in residential communities con-stituted a pool of hosts, allowing the malaria parasite to propagate. Settlements were often located close to bodies of water and created stagnant pools in which the vector for this disease could breed. By the early nineteenth century, malaria was endemic in most populated places, particularly in tropical and subtropical regions. Early in the twentieth century, the disease was eliminated from the tem-perate zone as well as from subtropical parts of Western countries such as the United States and Italy. Presently, malaria is endemic only in equatorial Africa and parts of Asia and Latin America.[13] In 2005, 95 percent of recorded malaria cases worldwide occurred in African children, and malaria remains a principal cause of death in this vulnerable population. The most deadly form of the dis-ease, *falciparum* malaria, when promptly diagnosed and appropriately treated, usually has no long-term consequences. When episodes are protracted because of diagnostic failure or improper management, however, many patients—partic-ularly children—can die. Many more children survive multiple and protracted bouts of malaria but suffer from anemia and neurological damage that affects them for the rest of their lives.[14]

Malaria parasites, like frogs and insects, have several stages in their life cycles. Whereas insects metamorphose from egg to larva, larva to pupa, and then pupa to adult in two different habitats, each of the six main stages of the malaria para-site inhabits a different niche. These stages are all one celled and contain the same genetic code, but otherwise they have little or no resemblance to one another.

Malaria parasites, known as *Plasmodia* (sing. *Plasmodium*), enter the human body with saliva from an infected female Anopheline mosquito. As the mosquito finishes her blood meal, the sporozoite stage of the parasite wends its way to the liver of the newly infected host. The sporozoite bores into a liver cell, develops, multiplies, and emerges in about a week (for *Plasmodium falciparum*) or two (for other species) as hundreds of merozoites.[15] The merozoites spill out into the bloodstream, where they infect red blood cells. They grow and divide until the infected cell can no longer hold them and ruptures, spilling out over two dozen merozoites, which in turn infect new blood cells. The blood stage is repeated until the patient is cured or dies. During the cyclic blood stage, particularly when merozoites spew out and attack new targets, the patient becomes feverish and weak. Some merozoites produce sexual forms of the parasite, called gametocytes, which are sucked up with blood by biting mosquitoes. Gametocytes mate in the mosquito and develop into embryonic forms, the last of which burrow through the mosquito intestine and end up in the salivary gland as a sporozoite, completing the cycle. A susceptible host is infected during a future blood meal.

Many people can recognize a fever, and the majority of fevers are initially detected by laypeople, who then seek medical attention. In many parts of Africa, patients do not have access to clinics or hospitals, and even those who do typically commence antimalarial treatment at home before seeking professional care. As a matter of public health policy, home care must be supported because malaria can debilitate and kill very quickly. The WHO recommends immediate antimalarial treatment for feverish patients in endemic areas.[16] At the same time, it has clearly enunciated and recently reiterated that "the signs and symptoms of malaria are nonspecific."[17] For several decades (until 2006), WHO advocated presumptive treatment of febrile patients close to home, not because it is optimal, but because it is the only possible course of action in many places:

> The diagnosis of malaria is based on clinical criteria (clinical diagnosis) supplemented by the detection of parasites in the blood (parasitological or confirmatory diagnosis). Clinical diagnosis alone has very low specificity and in many areas parasitological diagnosis is not currently available. The decision to provide antimalarial treatment in these settings must be based on the prior probability of the illness being malaria. One needs to weigh the risk of withholding antimalarial treatment from a patient with malaria against the risk associated with antimalarial treatment when given to a patient who does not have malaria.[18]

That risk includes the failure to treat the patient's actual infection, which may also be life threatening and could be treatable.

In the vast majority of infectious conditions, even when the patient is acutely ill, his or her appearance and history are not enough for even an experienced clinician to make a definitive diagnosis. Circumstantial evidence, such as the patient's location and contacts, or the diseases endemic in the environment, can only inform an educated guess. Many people claim to "know" when they have malaria, and medical practitioners, who are under greater pressure to make definitive pronouncements, often claim to be able to diagnose the disease using clinical signs alone. In crowded hospitals, a temperature slip from a nurse is enough to prompt a clinician to begin scribbling a prescription for antimalarials for a shivering child before the patient and the mother have had time to take a seat in the consulting room. Contradicting the general confidence that prescribers have in their clinical diagnosis of malaria, scientific studies suggest that fever is little more than a clue that points to malaria as one of several possible diagnoses.[19]

The historical "success" of symptom-based diagnosis of malaria in Africa is linked to the high prevalence of the disease. If 80 percent of fevers in a locality are actually malaria, then anyone diagnosing all fevers as malaria will be right eight out of ten times. This outcome is fine for the lucky majority, but the prognosis for patients with other infections is grim. Using current methods to diagnose bacterial infection in all febrile infections would be expensive and slow. But a negative diagnosis for malaria could serve as a valuable prescreen that could improve these sick patients' survival chances either by short-listing patients for additional tests or by identifying those with a likely bacterial infection for empiric antibiotic treatment. Paul Farmer and others have criticized the developed world for turning its back on the infections that are prevalent among the poor.[20] Failing to diagnose impoverished patients ensures that the costs and benefits associated with their treatment are not even considered. At least 20 percent of febrile patients in areas with a high burden of malaria receive inappropriate treatment because their conditions are regarded as too expensive to diagnose.

One-in-five odds of misdiagnosis and ineffective treatment would be unacceptable to many Western practitioners and their patients, but in parts of Africa where as many as one in ten children die before they are five years old,[21] this level of imprecision continues to be accepted. As children grow older and develop some immunity to malaria, and as antimalarial interventions are implemented, the proportion of misdiagnosed fevers increases. Routine, nonsevere malaria infections typically present with a fever, headache, and weakness—symptoms of generalized malaise. If the infection is caused by certain species of *Plasmodium*, in which the merozoite or blood cycle is synchronized, symptoms appear at precise intervals of three or four days, which is of considerable diagnostic value.

With *Plasmodium falciparum*, the most prevalent species in Africa, there are no such rhythmic clues.

Diagnostic Tests for Malaria

To determine unequivocally whether a patient has malaria, it is necessary to examine stained blood smears for parasite blood stages.[22] A drop of blood collected by pinprick is spread thinly across a glass slide and stained with a dye (Field's or Giemsa stain). Using a microscope, technicians can see blood stages of parasites, if present, as well as the patient's blood cells. Conveniently, *Plasmodium falciparum* is the easiest malaria parasite to identify. The best way to diagnose malaria is to perform a crude count of parasites because most people in malarious areas carry a few parasites even when they are well. The density of parasites in the blood often, though not always, correlates with the severity of the disease. This enumeration is done by counting the parasites in a set volume of blood or comparing the parasite count to the number of white blood cells, which serves as a sample calibrator.[23] The laboratory needs only a microscope, slides and staining reagents, and a trained technician. The entire operation can be performed without electricity if a mirror is used to direct sunlight onto the microscope.[24] Compound light microscopes are expensive but, if well maintained, last for decades. A number of clinics that have offered this service in the past do not do so presently because they lack a properly trained microscopist. However, people with secondary or even elementary schooling can be trained to prepare and view blood smears for malaria parasites.[25] In some African countries, graduate professionals with expertise in microbiology and other biomedical sciences are forced to seek employment in other sectors because there are few biomedical laboratory positions.[26] Many more technicians and aides have experience in parasite microscopy but stopped providing the service because blood smear examination was considered a lower priority than other services, such as dispensing medicines.

Routine diagnosis by reliable blood smear microscopy offers considerable advantages. When adults with fever attending Kenyan health centers were appropriately tested, drug costs were 80 percent lower. Even when the microscopist's skills were not optimal, so that specificity and sensitivity dipped below 90 percent, drug costs still decreased by 50 percent.[27] The long-term savings from avoiding the detrimental overuse of antimalarials in these cases is incalculable. Appropriate diagnosis for malaria, in addition to ensuring that feverish patients who do not have the disease in endemic areas are considered for other diagnoses, can provide sufficient savings to pay for itself.

Blood smear microscopy is a powerful but imperfect tool. If the malaria parasite is present in a non-blood-stage form, for example as the dormant hypnozoites seen in *P. ovale* or *P. vivax,* or in another liver stage, it cannot be detected by microscopy. It takes at least an hour to prepare, stain, and examine slides, although they can be processed in batches. Some technical expertise is necessary. Even in the best situation, Emeka's mother could not have accessed this type of testing locally, but reliable diagnosis needs to be routinely available at every single health post in a malaria-endemic area. To get around the need for skilled parasitologists and microscopists, less technically demanding, less labor-intensive, more sensitive, and more rapid tests have recently been developed.[28] Some take advantage of new biomedical techniques, such as fluorescent microscopy and the polymerase chain reaction, but require additional equipment, special expertise, and expensive consumables, so they cannot readily be introduced when diagnostic infrastructure is poor. Others, however, are potentially well suited to African health centers, particularly the rapid diagnostic tests that are performed without equipment.[29]

Many rapid diagnostic tests for infectious diseases detect the host's response to infection, rather than the pathogen itself. For malaria, however, the host response is of little diagnostic value because of the difficulty in distinguishing between current and previous infection. Malaria rapid diagnostic tests use a parasite protein as the diagnostic target and search for it in much the same way the immune system does. The tests, which are sold in a card, cassette, or dipstick format, detect proteins on the outer surface of the parasite. Two of these, the parasite lactose dehydrogenase and aldolase, are expressed by all *Plasmodia*, and the other, histidine-rich protein-2, is present only in the deadly *P. falciparum* parasites.[30] The advantage of this type of test is that anyone who can draw a pinprick of blood can perform it successfully. No equipment is required, and a positive result is indicated by an easily discerned color mark, typically a line on the test strip. Interest in and use of rapid diagnostic tests for malaria has increased exponentially in the last four years, but their use is still significantly short of need. Far too many health practitioners in Africa have yet to see them, let alone use them to guide patient care. As at 2007, only 20 percent of patients with "malaria" were diagnosed by microscopy or rapid diagnostic test.[31]

Malaria rapid diagnostic tests are easy to perform, and results are ready in less than twenty minutes but three important challenges have been associated with their use. The first is cost: as each quality controlled, disposable stick or strip must be impregnated with test proteins and detection reagents, and can only be used once, rapid diagnostic testing is not cheap. OptiMAL, a dipstick-type test that detects *falciparum* and *vivax* malarias within fifteen minutes, cost over U.S. $3.00 per test in 2003, more than the cost of a course of most antimalarials in Africa at the time. By 2008, the cost of rapid diagnostic tests had fallen to $0.67 to $1.00 per test, below the $1.00–2.40 cost of recommended combination therapies for malaria, excluding subsidies.[32] Ideally, a malarial diagnostic should cost less than 40 cents per test, and similar subsidies would be applied to tests as to drugs. Although rapid diagnostic tests remain beyond the reach of many patients in most malaria-endemic countries, their price continues to fall as the market expands due to more widespread use. Thus, if proper diagnosis were integral to malarial care, testing would be much more affordable. Furthermore, savings from inappropriate antimalarial use could be funneled into the cost of diagnostics.

The second challenge associated with rapid diagnostic tests for malaria is test quality, which determines reliability. Following donor interest in diagnostics for malaria, the number of commercially available rapid diagnostic tests increased from zero in 1993 to over a hundred different brands fifteen years later. In addition to the general requirements for test production, manufacturers need to produce tests that work reproducibly under real conditions. Real patients might be infected with multiple pathogens, and storage and use temperatures are high in tropical Africa. Not all tests that were initially marketed were sufficiently robust to compel health policymakers to incorporate them into their malaria treatment programs. In 2009, WHO published its quality assessment of 120 brands, for the first time providing health systems with data that allows them to select brands that are cost effective and perform well.[33] In a sense, the technical resolution of a century-long malaria diagnostics problem—from test development to quality assurance—in as little as a decade illustrates how concerted interest in a disease, rigorous assessment of treatment protocols, and global leadership can lead to rapid and effective diagnostic development.

The final challenge associated with rapid diagnostic tests is getting clinicians in endemic Africa, who have for decades been educated to believe that "fever is malaria," to use the tests and pay heed to the results. Yoel Lubell and his colleagues recently investigated diagnostic testing in fifteen year olds—children who, had they lived in eastern Nigeria, might have been Emeka's classmates. They found that 60 percent of fevers were actually malaria but the tests were not cost effective because antimalarials were still prescribed for patients who tested negative.[34] It is probable that the clinicians trusted their judgment better than the tests, and the absence of tests to diagnose confounding infections may also have prompted the prescribers to offer antimalarials. Rapid diagnostic tests for malaria are an important first step, but they cannot be used in a vacuum. Health providers need support in making the transition and will be more likely to do so as the quality and reliability of diagnostic tests improves and the diagnostic and treatment protocols for other febrile diseases catch up with the recent progress for malaria.

On May 13, 1998, Gro Harlem Brundtland, the then WHO director general, initiated a new goal-oriented and sustained effort to "Roll Back Malaria." By 2010, this global effort was implemented by a consortium of over five hundred government, humanitarian, and scientific organizations with the intermediate goal of reversing the incidence of malaria by 2015 and a long term objective of eradication.[35] Zambia, a pioneer country in the effort to Roll Back Malaria, issued new treatment protocols in 2003. A strategy to use rigorous diagnostics to delineate patients who needed the new effective antimalarials was not issued until 2006, with a target date of 2008 for 80 percent implementation. The 2003 guidelines, which as of 2009 operated in many of the country's health institutions, advocate laboratory diagnosis through blood smears "if possible" at health centers and hospitals. These criteria are realistic, but the position illustrates long-standing official acceptance of extremely weak diagnostic criteria for a major killer, even when there is global interest in combating malaria. The pattern of policy adjustment is reflective of a general willingness to increase spending on drugs that typically does not extend to the diagnostics required to use them optimally.[36] These problems are not limited to Zambia. In Kenya, where malaria policy is just a step behind Zambia, treatment protocols were adjusted in 2004 but policy recommending diagnostic testing took two more years to emerge. It took three years to implement the 2004 drug changes at the grassroots and the shift required considerable health personnel training. By 2008, most patients were receiving the recommended new therapy, artemether-lumefantrine. However, by that time only 36 percent of the 193 health centers evaluated in one survey had any kind of testing available.[37]

Patients, health systems, and donors have traditionally been unwilling to foot the bill for diagnostic tests that cost more than available drugs.[38] The cost of the test in fact may be justifiable, but because many of the benefits accrue to the health care system rather than to the patient, the advantages are often not recognized. The new impetus to use diagnostic tests has been prompted by the emergence of resistance to affordable antimalarials, which have recently been replaced by artemisinin-based combination therapies (ACTs), such as artemether-lumefantrine used in Kenya. Since the cost of ACTs is high (up to U.S. $3.00 per course in 2004) rapid diagnostic tests (some costing about $0.60 in 2004) became easier to justify.[39]

The almost prohibitive cost of ACTs creates access problems and makes these life-saving medicines attractive to counterfeiters; a recent global effort has proposed that these drugs should be heavily subsidized through an Affordable Medicines Facility for Malaria.[40] An important omission from this program, however, is the partnering of drugs with diagnostics that are essential to assure appropriate use. Just before the inception of that program, about five billion antimalarial regimens were handed out each year, and at least a fifth of these may have been unnecessary in high-burden areas, that is African countries with endemic, stable transmission. The 2000 annual estimate was between 122 and 303 million malaria attacks in areas of high burden. Therefore, at least 25 million antimalarial regimens are consumed needlessly each year in these countries. In areas with lower endemicity or seasonal variation in malaria infection rates, more people without malaria may be being treated with precious antimalarials than individuals who actually have the disease. Based on data collated by Julie Thwing and her coworkers in Angola, this translates to between $500 million and $960 million per billion U.S. dollars in wasted funds donated for antimalarial treatment.[41]

When absolute and immediate cost-effectiveness is computed in settings where expensive ACTs are employed, malaria microscopy and rapid diagnostic tests are cost effective.[42] Analysis that takes accuracy into account greatly increases the cost-effectiveness of rapid diagnostic tests in areas where quality assurance for microscopy is weak. Factoring in indirect and long-term costs from avoidance of antimicrobial resistance, adverse effects from unnecessary medication, and diagnostic delay for other infections, the cost-effectiveness of malaria diagnostics at the population level is indisputable.

By comparison, policies of clinical diagnosis are uniformly unsuccessful and the WHO's recently altered malaria diagnostic recommendations insist on parasite, rather than clinically based, diagnosis.[43] Improving access to, and the sensitivity and specificity of, testing can best be achieved with rapid diagnostic tests, even though a few technical challenges associated with their use remain. Currently, rapid diagnostic tests work well when performed by laboratory technicians or health workers.[44] The yet-to-be-developed but ideal home-based or village health worker rapid diagnostic test would require urine or saliva instead of blood, and would detect only high levels parasitemia that are associated with malaria. Village health workers could instruct patients who test negative to go to a health center for alternate diagnosis. In health centers, tests need to be specific enough to detect low-level parasitemia and at least a few of the other causes of fever. Testing rubrics should be enhanced, and the variety of tests available for the etiologic agents of febrile disease should be increased, to provide prescribers with clear directions for treating malaria test-negative patients.

"The billion-dollar malaria effort is flying blind"

Malaria researchers are aware that development and deployment of diagnostics is a priority, and health policymakers acknowledge that the current state of diagnostic testing for malaria is below par.[45] However, diagnostic development and deployment is frequently low on the list of priorities for malaria control. The current scarcity of functioning diagnostic laboratories continues to cow decision makers into accepting that laboratory diagnostics are beyond the means of African health systems. A report on the 2005 Multilateral Initiative on Malaria conference held in Yaoundé, Cameroon, entitled "What Are the Priorities in Malaria Research?" and published in January 2006, summarized ten "crucial issues," including new directions in drug and vaccine development as well as improving the delivery of interventions. More recent expert discourse has emphasized diagnostics, but the list emanating from that pivotal meeting lacked any reference to diagnostic development, either in terms of new technologies or promoting the more effective use and simple availability of existing ones.[46] The consequences of underprioritizing diagnostics are visible. Zambia, a front-runner in the effort to Roll Back Malaria across Africa, has shown phenomenal progress in halting transmission due to successful use of insecticide-treated bed nets and indoor residual insecticide spraying and treatment programs, but parasite-based diagnosis has lagged. The 2008 World Malaria Report noted similar progress, and the same diagnostic slowdown, in other African countries and inadequate uptake or scale up of interventions in some countries because of the difficulty in measuring the impact of different interventions due to underuse of diagnostics.[47]

In 2006, the newly appointed director of WHO's malaria program, Arata Kochi, declared that until science addresses the problem of malaria diagnosis, malaria control strategies will be "like religion, based on faith."[48] Modern malaria control interventions, such as insecticide-impregnated bed nets, targeted insecticide use, and new antimalarial drugs, are largely chemical interventions. When used without epidemiological monitoring, chemical strategies for disease control have always been rendered ineffective by drug or insecticide resistance—this is why an earlier attempt to eradicate malaria failed.[49] The effective use of both existing and new therapies depends on the routine deployment of diagnostic tests for malaria.

Toward the end of the twentieth century, as other infectious diseases were brought under control, the unruliness of malaria became more evident, more intolerable, and more embarrassing. *Plasmodium falciparum* is responsible for many of Africa's ills and erroneously blamed for many others, forcing individuals, organizations, and countries that only a few decades ago were barely aware of the devastation from malaria to support a global effort to tackle the disease head-on. WHO's Roll Back Malaria program's target was to halve malaria deaths by 2010, and halting the upward trend in the number of malaria infections is a 2015 Millennium Development Goal.[50] Plans and budgets for reaching these targets have been drawn up, donors have been wooed, and the hopes of affected people in Africa and other malaria-endemic areas have been raised. Funding support for malaria reportedly increased tenfold between 1998 and 2006, and African governments have announced "rolling back malaria" as national and regional priorities.[51]

In 2005, when the global effort to roll back malaria was under way, although behind schedule, Oxford malariologist Bob Snow and his co-workers suggested that previous World Health Organization estimates of how many people actually had malaria each year were all wrong. From South America and Asia, the disease is underreported, and in Africa, where 79 percent of malaria infections occur, researchers handicapped by "a notoriously weak system of reporting infectious diseases"[52] derive uncertain estimates by extrapolating from sometimes biased research data. The Snow group suggested a 2002 estimate of 515 million (range 300–600 million), which is much greater than the WHO's figures of 213 and 273 million in 1990 and 1998. Malaria epidemiologists and policy makers have debated the accuracy of various estimates; they agree only that "it is preferable to present any malaria incidence estimate as a range."[53] The differences between the upper and lower limits of this range typically approach two hundred million people.

Inaccurate estimates of the true prevalence of malaria in Africa means that those who are sickened and impoverished by the disease do not have an effective voice. But knowledge of the true burden of malaria is of more than humanitarian and academic value: it would help public health planners to define at-risk populations, to distribute resources rationally, and to evaluate and refine intervention programs. Only reliable methods of estimating malaria cases will give the world the capacity to detect any gains that may result from current initiatives. A case in point is Mto wa Mbu or the "River of Mosquitoes" area in Tanzania, historically rampant with malaria. In 2009, the entomological infection rate, or chance of being bitten by a malaria-infected mosquito, was less than one: malaria had gone from being very common to rare. However, based on data from 1981, 40 percent of outpatients in 2006–2007 were still receiving expensive antimalarials.[54] On a global scale, any intervention that leads to a decline of fifty million cases per year or less would have a valuable but potentially undetectable effect on malaria worldwide simply because such effects can only be measured if diagnosis is parasite-based. Snow, who is working continuously to improve malaria estimates, correctly concludes: "Inadequate descriptions of the global distribution of disease risk make it impossible to determine priorities and advise funding agencies appropriately. Redressing these deficiencies with robust data must be a priority if international agencies are to understand the size of the challenge set by their targets over the next ten years."[55] Progress has been made: some countries, such as Zambia and Tanzania, are noticing declines in the incidence of all fevers, and declines in pediatric admissions due to malaria ranging between 28 percent and 63 percent were recently reported from three coastal hospitals in Kenya.[56] Given the questionable quality of available reliable data that is dependent on routine testing, progress will be difficult to quantify.[57]

Disease control programs typically find it easiest to recruit support at the beginning of a campaign, when millions are sickened or killed. But it is the endgame that is most crucial and ensures that the health and economic gains of a successful program are not lost. The endgame can be compromised by "donor fatigue." In the upcoming decade, as malaria control improves, better data that makes it easier to showcase progress could convince results-oriented donors to stay on board.

As more malaria cases are prevented, the proportion of febrile illnesses caused by other pathogens will rise. The possible range of confounders is tremendous. In addition to bacteria and hemorrhagic viruses, there are hundreds of well-known possible causes of fever in malaria-endemic areas. Some causes are underrecognized; for example, a serological screen of Gabonese schoolchildren recently pointed to influenza as one of them. In the absence of diagnostic tests for the major confounders, alternate causes of fever are essentially invisible.[58] If today's interventions against malaria are effective, clinical diagnosis of fevers will become even more imprecise because only a minority of febrile illnesses will actually be malaria. In order to increase, or even maintain the effectiveness of care, laboratory diagnostics will have to be employed more intensively.

Between 15 percent and 83 percent of parents of ill children in different parts of Africa procure medicine for their sick children from a local dispensing point or shop, typically staffed by a semitrained village health worker or an untrained dispenser.[59] Therefore, malaria diagnosis needs to be possible at or close to the home-based level. Only then might a child like Emeka, with a sudden high temperature and chills, receive appropriate therapy in time to save his life.

FEVER: BEYOND MALARIA

I confess myself unable to differentiate certain cases of malarial remittent from typhoid fever, without the blood examination.

—William Osler, 1892

In 1844, in *Zeitschrift für rationelle mediz,* a treatise exhorting physicians to apply scientific thought and methods to medicine, Jacob Henle wrote:

> Only in medicine are there causes that have hundreds of consequences or that can, on arbitrary occasions, remain entirely without effect. Only in medicine can the same effect flow from the most varied possible sources. One need only glance at the chapters on etiology in handbooks or monographs. For almost every disease, after a specific cause or the admission that such a cause is not yet known, one finds the same horde of harmful influences—poor housing and clothing, liquor and sex, hunger and anxiety. This is just as scientific as if a physicist were to teach that bodies fall because boards or beams are removed, because ropes or cables break, or because of openings, and so forth.[1]

Over a century and a half later, Henle's eloquent description of the problem of confounding causes with effects remains applicable to the case of fevers in Africa. Despite scientific advances in the understanding of specific febrile illnesses, the treatment of fever continues to be based on empirical symptoms rather than laboratory diagnosis—with consequences that are often fatal to individuals and devastating for whole societies.

In tropical Africa, malaria exerts a heavy burden by sickening up to half of the population in highly endemic areas each year. Most malaria attacks manifest as a brief but debilitating fever, but the more severe forms of the disease account for most of the deaths. In severe malaria, parasite-infected red blood cells stick to each other, to uninfected cells, and to the lining of blood vessels. This clumping reduces the number of red blood cells available to deliver oxygen to vital organs and occludes blood vessels. In the worst cases, red blood cells stick within the brain and, in the case of pregnant women, the placenta. *Plasmodium falciparum,* the parasite form that causes severe malaria, produces these effects through a specific and deadly mechanism. Red blood cells are converted from oxygen couriers for the host into parasite factories. Channels created on the red cell's surface serve as ports for nutrients, and many blood cell proteins are digested to provide fodder for the developing merozoites. New parasite proteins are mounted on the outside of the red blood cells, forming unsightly knobs that can be seen with an electron microscope. A key component of these knobs is a recently described protein called PfEMP1 (*Plasmodium falciparum* erythrocyte membrane protein 1), which is encoded by *var* genes, so named because of their ability to shuffle, ensuring that the precise nature of PfEMP1 varies constantly. Each strain of *P. falciparum* boasts about sixty different *var* genes, providing a large repertoire of potential cassettes that can be used to vary the part of PfEMP1 that is recognized by the host immune system. Although some iterations of PfEMP1 are probably more effective, and therefore more deadly, than others, by and large the variable regions are interspersed with the functional regions so that the structure of these proteins changes only ever so slightly but strategically. This variation allows the parasite to prevent the immune system from learning how to identify and remove infected cells. It also makes it difficult to make vaccines that protect against severe malaria.

Mounting proteins on the host cell membrane is an extremely effective tactic. Even more ingenious is endowing these knob proteins with the ability to make the infected cell sticky. Unlike normal red blood cells, PfEMP1-coated red blood cells fail to slip through capillary blood vessels. They stick to the sides of capillaries and to each other, providing a cozy cocoon for forms of the parasite that do not live in cells, including the sexual forms, gametocytes, which are sucked up with blood by mosquitoes in order to infect new hosts. The infected patient's blood vessels are soon dotted with sticky clumps, known as rosettes. Uninfected red cells become trapped in rosettes made by infected ones, making it easier for newly emerged parasites to find a target host cell without being destroyed by armies of protective white blood cells. The formation of rosettes ultimately leads to blood vessel clogging, and, depending on their location, convulsions, potentially fatal coma, or organ failure in the same manner that internal blood clots cause strokes. As more blood cells are pulled from circulation or ruptured by escaping parasites, patients become acutely anemic; not enough oxygen is conveyed to the body's cells, leading to further complications. Four of the many *Plasmodium* species can cause disease in humans, but only *P. falciparum,* the

predominantly African species, produces the deadly PfEMP1. PfEMP1 has pre-
ferred binding sites on human cells, and variation in the distribution and location of host proteins could account for some of the interindividual variation in
the predisposition to severe malaria. Severe malaria is therefore a syndrome with
a very specific cause: a protein produced by the pathogen. The action of this protein and many other virulence factors, most of which remain unknown, make it
vital that *falciparum* malaria is diagnosed promptly and treated appropriately.

The severe malaria that was presumed to have killed fourteen-year-old Emeka
is the cause of almost two million deaths each year, mostly very young children
in Africa.[2] Typically, the central nervous system is involved, causing convulsions,
and severe malaria is often fatal, even when patients are taken to the hospital.
The shocking truth is that the optimal way to intervene in this deadly course
is not known. As many as 15 to 20 percent of patients admitted to the hospital
with severe malaria die, even if they are given antimalarials and supportive care.
Patients in a *P. falciparum*–endemic area with fever who also show anemia and
convulsions or impaired consciousness are presumed to have severe malaria.[3] Diagnosis depends on a combination of clinical examination and relatively simple
laboratory testing. The syndrome is defined by both a lowered hemoglobin level
and an elevated parasite count, making it one of many conditions common in
Africa in which definition of the disease assumes a laboratory diagnosis even
though one is rarely implemented. The syndrome's inordinately high parasite
counts can readily be determined by microscopy, while hemoglobin levels can
be estimated with the most rudimentary of centrifuges or with a more recently
devised portable testing system. Fortunately, many secondary care and some
primary care institutions can perform these tests, since these patients urgently
need transfusion. However, some facilities lack the capacity to screen blood, so
transfusions carry the risk of transmitting an even more deadly disease such as
HIV or hepatitis.

That so many of these patients do not survive is attributed to the poor response of the severe malaria syndrome to available therapies, which do not affect the deadly cascade of blood clumping and central nervous system damage.
This attribution in turn depends on the presumption that clinical diagnosis of
severe malaria is reliable. In many parts of Africa, *falciparum* malaria is so highly
endemic that many patients with these symptoms do have the syndrome. But
the symptoms of severe malaria resemble those of life-threatening systemic bacterial infections, which respond well to timely medical intervention. Blood is a
nutritious medium, and a wide variety of organisms will thrive there. Although
malaria parasites have the edge of an injecting vector, the mosquito, bacteria,
viruses, and other parasites also can cause bloodstream infections. Many of these
infections are treatable, provided they are identified in time.

Recent reports from multiple African sites have observed that clinical diagnosis of severe malaria is often imprecise. Doctors in a teaching hospital in Kumasi, Ghana, found that the clinical signs and symptoms were insufficient to distinguish patients with severe malaria from those with life-threatening bacteremia. According to Jennifer A. Evans and her co-workers, 182 of 251 patients (72.5%) were shown to have malaria, but 11.1 percent of patients—who without laboratory workup would have been diagnosed as having malaria—were negative for malaria parasites and actually had a bacterial bloodstream infection, that is, bacteremia. The other twenty-three patients (9.2%) were infected with both plasmodia and bacteria. Indeed, the severe presentation of many children with bloodstream infections arose from misdiagnosis at an earlier stage in their illness. In 2000, 42 percent of all illnesses and 32 percent of all deaths in Tanzania were attributed to malaria, but when clinical scientists attempted to verify malaria diagnoses in the laboratory, only 46 percent of patients diagnosed with malaria actually had the disease. Doctors in Kilifi, Kenya, like their colleagues in Ghana and Tanzania, noticed a high mortality rate among children admitted with high fever. When they processed blood cultures in the lab for every child admitted between August 1998 and July 2002, much to their surprise they found that bacteremia was a leading cause of death in children, responsible for one in three infant deaths and a quarter of deaths in older children. The most common bacteria identified were *Streptococcus pneumoniae* and *Haemophilus influenzae*, both of which also cause respiratory and ear infections, as well as nontyphoidal *Salmonella*, that is, those strains that do not produce typhoid fever. In a fourth example from Malawi, clinical signs alone had an acceptable predictive accuracy for bloodstream infections caused by *Mycobacterium tuberculosis* or *Streptococcus pneumoniae*, but they were unable to differentiate bacteremia caused by nontyphoidal *Salmonella* from malaria. In 2007, a group in Tanzania found that severe infections in young children were more commonly bacterial than malarial and that severe bacterial bloodstream infections were a leading cause of death at the Muhimbili National Hospital in Dar es Salaam.[4]

Blood culture by first principles, which is still the most common approach used in the African laboratories that provide this service, is challenging but possible on a small budget, provided that a skilled and dedicated microbiologist performs the procedure. Because blood culture directly informs treatment for the most deadly infections, the expense, time, and effort that must be invested is worthwhile. Culturing pathogens from blood specimens is fraught with technical difficulties for laboratories in developing countries. Blood is a supremely nutritious medium, and some organisms that infect blood are very demanding to culture outside the body. First, blood must be collected from the patient, taking care to avoid contamination of the sample from the patient's skin or the environment. A liquid broth culture is prepared by adding 3–5ml of blood to media in large bottles. Some patients are too ill to spare enough blood for the test. Blood culture bottles are expensive and, because of their large size, difficult to ship, an important consideration in a continent where virtually all laboratory materials are imported from abroad.

If bacteria grow in the primary culture medium, the causative organism is subcultured on plates of solid media, isolated, and identified. To recover some of the most common isolates from children, including *Streptococcus pneumoniae,* clean blood must be added to media as a supplement. Many African laboratories are forced to use expired human blood obtained from blood banks. If the blood contains antibodies against the causative organism being cultured, growth will be inhibited; if the blood donor had recently taken antimicrobials before donating the sample, these too might inhibit target organisms. Western laboratories use commercially available sheep or horse blood. There is little incentive for companies to produce blood culture bottles or sheep blood in many parts of Africa because so few institutions use the products. Many more things can go wrong in this process, making the isolation rate of many diagnostic laboratories low and sometimes confounded by contamination. When common, but fastidious, organisms such as *Strep. pneumoniae* are missed, physicians lose confidence in the laboratory. Thus diagnostic development must be implemented to the highest standards of quality. Western laboratories overcome many of the difficulties associated with blood culture by using automated systems. Although these are costly, because of the challenges associated with blood culture by traditional methods, they are cost effective, particularly if many specimens must be processed. This is true even in Africa, and automated systems, though few and far between, are the best option for reference laboratories and large hospitals and have even been used successfully in rural hospitals.[5] In the Kilifi, Kenya, and 2007 Dar es Salaam studies, basic blood culture conditions were close to ideal, and a very high yield of bacterial cultures was reported, although in both cases the authors observe that it is likely that some cases were missed. Accurate results from blood cultures can improve cure rates considerably. Given the case-fatality rates for bacteremia, particularly in young children, investment in at least some form of blood culture is justified by the results.

Parsing "Typhomalaria"

In addition to septicemia, Lyme disease and a number of viral infections, including influenza, produce symptoms that are similar to malaria.[6] In 1989, I was diagnosed with typhoid fever after four medical consultations. In parts of Africa that are hyperendemic for malaria, such as Nigeria, typhoid and other bacterial infections are commonly suspected only when malaria medicines do not work. Typhoid fever is caused by the human-adapted Typhi variety of the bacterium *Salmonella enteritidis.* People become infected with the organism by ingesting contaminated food or water. Most non-Typhi *Salmonella* cause uncomplicated diarrhea, but typhoid fever, sometimes called enteric fever, is a systemic illness characterized by a fever that is clinically indistinguishable from malaria. A few other *Salmonella* serovars, Paratyphi A, B and C, can also produce an enteric fever, but it is sometimes milder than that caused by the typhoid bacillus. The typhoid bacillus is the worst of its cousins: prolonged infection can result in death from intestinal perforation.

The ease of typhoid transmission in many parts of the world and the significant fatality rates associated with the infection make early and accurate diagnosis imperative. The only reliable means of diagnosing typhoid fever is by culturing the organisms—that is, by growing and then identifying them. A culture is produced by spreading bacteria, or a specimen containing them, onto a Petri dish containing nutrients and a gelling agent called agar. To grow *Salmonella,* nutrients for growth and chemicals, which inhibit many other bacteria, are added to the agar. Indicators are also added, which produce different colors with different bacteria. The plate is incubated at human body temperature (37°C). The next day, if bacteria are present, they will be visible to the naked eye. Each bacterium laid down the night before will produce a small circular colony a few millimeters in diameter. If the colonies have an appearance consistent with that of *Salmonella* and test positive in confirmatory tests, the laboratory technician then screens for capsule, gooey carbohydrate material on the outside of the bacteria, and flagella, the whiplike structures that bacteria use to move. If the capsule and flagella types are those of Typhi and the patient has a febrile illness, then a diagnosis of typhoid fever can be made. It is possible to test the bacterial culture for susceptibility to different antibiotics. Such susceptibility testing can provide the patient's prescriber with valuable information about which drugs can be used to clear the infection.

Culture is slow and is difficult in poorly equipped laboratories. And the results are not always definitive for typhoid fever. At certain stages of the illness, patients who actually have typhoid may be culture-negative: 75 percent of those infected are culture-positive in the first ten days, but by twenty-one days, the proportion of infections that can be identified by blood culture falls to about 30 percent.[7] In the case of my own probable typhoid infection, at the time I was tested I had been ill for at least a month, so I probably would have been culture-negative. As it is, culture was never attempted on my behalf. To overcome the limitations of culture, serological methods, such as those used in my case, which detect antityphoidal antibodies in blood, have become prominent for diagnosing typhoid and related infections.

The pioneer in serological diagnosis of typhoid was Georges-Fernand-Isidor Widal. In 1896, he developed the classic test that bears his name after observing that a clumping reaction occurs when serum (blood from which the blood cells have been removed) from people who have, or have had, typhoid is mixed with S. Typhi. The clumping reaction is indicative of an immune system that has learned to fight the typhoid bacillus. In the Widal test, the serum is serially diluted, or titered, to determine the greatest dilution that can still produce a clumping reaction. The more dilute the titer, the more antityphoid antibody in the serum of the patient, and therefore the greater opportunity the patient's body has had to respond to typhoid bacteria. A presumptive diagnosis of typhoid is made when antibody titer is shown to rise over two successive and appropriately spaced tests. Three-quarters of typhoid patients will show a twofold to threefold increase in the second of two titers measured during the first week of infection.

Although the theoretical basis for the Widal test is sound and has become the basis for other diagnostic protocols, the Widal test itself is insufficiently sensitive and problematic. Like all diagnostic tests, the Widal test is most reliable when performed by a properly trained technician and the reagents have been appropriately stored. Serological reagents are notoriously unrobust. Different Salmonella Typhi bacteria have different capsule and flagella types. Each type must be tested, making the test rather complex to set up and perform, and therefore prone to error. Unlike blood cultures, the Widal test provides no opportunity to determine antimicrobial susceptibility, which is becoming increasingly important as drug resistance becomes more common. The Widal test is nonspecific. It is possible to get a significant titer for one or more of the typhoid antigens, and consequently a false-positive result, when a patient does not have typhoid fever but instead has dysentery, malaria, tuberculosis, hepatitis, cirrhosis, tularemia, rheumatoid arthritis, immunological disorders, infectious mononucleosis, or a recent vaccination against typhoid or cholera. As many of these conditions are common in Africa, depending on a single Widal test for the diagnosis of Salmonella infection is highly unreliable. When a negative result is obtained, the patient may not have typhoid, may be a typhoid carrier, may have a low-grade infection, or may be a poor responder—if they are not the victim of a test error from damaged reagents.[8] In my own case, described in chapter 1, the combination of early malaria chemotherapy failure, a single Widal test, and the signs and symptoms of my disease and recovery following chloramphenicol therapy—not to mention the wisdom of my nurse-mother—suggest that I had typhoid fever, but I might have had one of many other bacterial infections.

Culture, with all its attendant shortfalls, remains the gold standard for typhoid diagnosis. When the Widal test is properly performed and the results carefully evaluated, it is of some value in the diagnosis of *Salmonella* infection. Unfortunately, patients screened by the Widal test in many parts of Africa are rarely tested more than once, because testing is costly relative to medicine and access to laboratories is limited. Because of the confounding from other antigens, Widal tests are most useful when they detect a rise in titers over time. A properly performed Widal test would evaluate *Salmonella* somatic (O) and flagellar (H) antigen levels in blood at initial presentation and then a few days later. A fourfold increase in titers measured over a week apart, but particularly the somatic O titer, is diagnostic for typhoid fever. About 85 percent of typhoid patients exhibit such a rise in titers across the first month of infection. In my own case, and in those of the few others who get tested, however, a diagnosis is based on a single test reading.

The test is not misused in this way from lack of knowledge. As Michael O. Ibadin and A. Ogbimi explain, "In most tropical countries, saddled with enormous burden from the disease, recourse is often made to other methods because modern facilities are lacking. Thus despite acknowledged shortcomings the single Widal test on serum samples collected during active phase of the illness is commonly used in these countries, including Nigeria."[9] Hypothesizing that cross-reactivity from malaria was a potential cause of overdiagnosis of typhoid, they demonstrated that agglutination reactions with several of the Widal antigens, particularly anti-D agglutination, were significantly greater in patients with malaria parasitemia than in controls. Patients with malaria are more likely to generate a single false-positive Widal test result.

Distinguishing malaria and typhoid is an old problem. During the late nineteenth century, Sir William Osler, a renowned physician and one of the most knowledgeable typhoid specialists of his time, was concerned about the high rates of typhoid fever in the United States as well as by the failure of many doctors of his time to distinguish malaria from typhoid.[10] Many of his contemporaries made a diagnosis of "typhomalaria" because of their inability to delineate these two infections. Although he did not have access to diagnostic tools that could unequivocally differentiate these two fevers, Osler knew that by observing the trends in temperature charts it was possible to distinguish the ups and downs of benign (non-*falciparum*) malaria from the smooth waves of typhoid fever. Osler proposed that a single consultation with a patient was an insufficient basis for a diagnosis. Clinical monitoring of patients is impossible in many parts of present-day Africa, where physicians and hospital beds are few and death from fever can come swiftly. Nor would temperature charts distinguish typhoid fever from the *falciparum* malaria that is most common in Africa. But the high level of background noise from confounding infections endemic in the region compromises the Widal test. To make matters worse, at the other end of the spectrum researchers in Cameroon blame the Widal test for large-scale and long-standing *over*diagnosis of typhoid fever.[11]

At the Korle-Bu Teaching Hospital, in Accra, Ghana, where diagnostic capabilities exceed what is available in most of Africa, physicians concluded that the Widal test adds little to clinical diagnosis:

> From the foregoing [data] it is recommended that typhoid fever should be diagnosed by culture of blood samples. The Widal test is non-specific, poorly standardized and often confusing and difficult to interpret. In our opinion, the Widal test should not be used in isolation as a diagnostic procedure for *S. typhi,* but as an additional aid. If culture facilities are not available a strong clinical suspicion, rather than the Widal test, warrants therapeutic intervention.[12]

A standard test that cannot return a result that is any more accurate than "strong clinical suspicion" is difficult to justify and may contribute to the perception that laboratory testing is not cost effective. Why does the uninformative Widal test remain the mainstay for laboratory diagnosis of typhoid fever in Africa? As diagnostic tests go, it is relatively inexpensive even though it is prone to error. It requires no sophisticated equipment and can be performed by a minimally trained technician. But mere convenience is not enough to advocate the routine use of a test, even when there is no alternative. Zurich-based medical microbiologist Eric Böttger observes that funds expended on Widal tests, which yield equivocal results, could be funneled into malaria diagnosis because clinical signs combined with a negative malaria test are almost as predictive as a positive Widal test for typhoid fever, or at least bacterial infection, in highly endemic areas. The Widal test may be inexpensive, but it is cost ineffective.

A reliable, single-point spot test for typhoid fever would have inestimable value, not only in Africa but also in Asia, where typhoid fever is highly endemic. Unfortunately, sensitive and suitable methods of testing for typhoid that could be used in remote, resource-constrained parts of the world do not yet exist. Only a few attempts have been made to replace currently available but highly problematic tests. Returning from a meeting of typhoid researchers in November 2005, Gordon "Doog" Dougan, a microbiologist who has devoted his life to the study of typhoid pathogenesis and vaccine development, described typhoid diagnosis as "an absolute mess. It's in the dark ages."[13] His frustration is well founded. He is developing vaccines for which field testing will be problematic if it is impossible to say who has and who does not have typhoid.

Salmonella Typhi's disease cycle and progression are among the more complex for bacteria. There are reasonably effective vaccines in use and in development. It is more complicated to develop a typhoid vaccine than a diagnostic test, ruling out scientific roadblocks as the principal reason why the disease poses such a formidable diagnostic challenge. In fact, after the threat from typhoid in Europe and North America waned with improved sanitation, the impetus to develop new tests diminished. Widal's outdated test, which represented the cutting edge of infectious disease diagnosis almost a century ago, has yet to be replaced. By contrast, cancer and HIV testing have evolved considerably in the last three decades, becoming more specific, more sensitive, and simpler to execute. Similar strides in typhoid fever diagnosis have not been made, or even attempted, even though more people are infected with this disease each year than with HIV. Current scientific technology has not yet been rigorously applied to typhoid fever diagnosis. Molecular technologies for the detection of specific bacterial antigens in urine seem promising, but much needs to be done before such tests are available, particularly in African clinics.

In 2008, the Ugandan Ministry of Health noticed an unusually high rate of hospital admissions due to intestinal perforations. A collaborative investigation by the Ministry of Health and the U.S. Centers for Disease Control uncovered an epidemic of typhoid fever. Typically, 2–3 percent of patients with untreated typhoid fever will succumb to perforations of the small intestine, but in this epidemic, an estimated 50 percent suffered this life-threatening condition, which requires emergency surgery. The reason for the unusually high rate of complications is still under investigation, but the scientists that investigated the epidemic agree that it is due to one of three possibilities: an extraordinarily virulent strain of Typhi bacteria, underreporting of mild infections, or delays in treatment.[14] The last two possibilities would arise directly from diagnostic shortfalls.

Typhoid may be one of the more prevalent and serious infectious diseases that are often confounded with malaria, but many other bacterial infections are commonly misdiagnosed as malaria. Existing diagnostics for bacterial bloodstream infections are too slow, too expensive, or too unreliable. The absence of cheap and easily applicable tests for invasive bacterial infections is undermining the introduction of routine rapid diagnostics for malaria as well. In several pilot studies, it was found that health workers were consistently prescribing antimalarials for patients who tested negatively for malaria parasitemia. Perhaps they did not trust the new tests, many of which needed to be evaluated further at the time, but they also had no diagnostic protocol for febrile patients who do not have malaria. Ideally, multiplex diagnostic tests would allow point-of-care diagnosis of malaria and its most common confounders. But simple and reliable tests for many common bacterial and viral diseases have yet to be developed. The technology to develop them does exist. For example, a rapid diagnostic test for *Yersinia pestis,* the causative agent of plague, was developed and tested in Madagascar and successfully applied in an Algerian epidemic.[15] Similar methods could be used to design blood tests for other bacteria.

Diagnosis and surveillance are better in South Asia, where vaccines have been piloted, than they are in Africa. In the last decade, the introduction of a new Vi vaccine in many parts of Asia has led to a significant fall in the number of typhoid fevers. Unfortunately, this drop was followed by a rise in the number of enteric fevers caused by *Salmonella* Paratyphi.[16] The distinction is important: Typhi serovar causes typhoid fever, and Paratyphi serovar causes paratyphoid fever. Collectively, these systemic diseases are referred to as enteric fever. Although paratyphoid fever is reputed to be less lethal than typhoid, it still is a critical illness. There are some indications that Paratyphi strains currently circulating in Asia are just as virulent as Typhi. It is not clear whether the apparent rise in paratyphoid fever is due to better case detection or to a true resurgence of the disease to fill the niche recently vacated by typhoid fever. Had a similar event been seen in Africa, where typhoid fever is rarely differentiated from paratyphoid or other infectious fevers, it is likely that the vaccine would have been deemed ineffective. Without appropriate diagnostic tests, the number of enteric fevers would seem to have remained unchanged after vaccination. (Even more likely, enteric fevers would have been entirely overlooked by clinically diagnosed "malaria"). The rationale for vaccination would not have been evident and its cost would have been regarded as unjustified. This observation could have resulted in the withdrawal of an effective intervention and would have blinded health policymakers to the need for a paratyphoid vaccine. Indeed, one of the reasons why typhoid vaccines are not used routinely in Africa is because diagnostic shortfalls mean that their value has never been estimated.[17]

A few people infected with Typhi have no symptoms but carry the infectious bacteria in their gall bladders. These carriers shed the bacterium and can infect others. The best-known typhoid carrier was "Typhoid Mary" Mallon, a food preparer who infected forty-seven people in New York City between 1900 and 1915.[18] Mary was repeatedly asked to pursue an alternate career, and her refusal to do so eventually led to her incarceration on public health grounds after the deaths of three people she had infected. The prospects faced by food handlers are much less bleak today. Carriers can be treated and the bacillus eradicated. Since they are asymptomatic, however, carriers must be identified through laboratory testing. Many countries require or recommend that food handlers be tested for the typhoid bacillus, particularly if they are working in highly endemic areas. In Kumasi, Ghana, 2.3 percent of food handlers tested by one research group were identified as typhoid carriers. Similar rates are found in The Gambia,[19] but most

African food handlers have never been tested. Eating food prepared in restaurants or by street vendors is commonplace; so is communal cooking in family compounds. As long as testing is unavailable, hundreds of incognizant people are at risk of contracting typhoid. A good many are likely to be misdiagnosed as having malaria. Clearly, reliable and practicable diagnoses for typhoid fever and typhoid carriers need to be developed and applied. The technology exists to develop them, but they presumably are a low priority.

In addition to developing and deploying typhoid diagnostics and vaccines in Africa, priority should be placed on tests and vaccines for nontyphoidal salmonellosis. The spread of multiresistant strains of nontyphoidal *Salmonella* in Africa has made the need for a vaccine more pressing. Enteric fevers caused by *Salmonella* not belonging to the highly virulent Typhi and Paratypi sero-vars are generally rare. Most people with nontyphoidal *Salmonella* infections do not suffer more than a mild to moderate, self-resolving diarrhea. Malnutrition, the AIDS epidemic, and possibly malaria endemicity, however, have made some patients, notably African children, vulnerable to diseases that resemble typhoid but are caused by its less virulent cousins. This "new" illness is increasingly being documented in laboratories in Kenya and Malawi and presents yet another diagnostic challenge.[20] Before vaccines that protect against one or more deadly forms of *Salmonella* are effectively piloted, adequate monitoring protocols must be developed and implemented. These protocols will also be valuable in diagnosing the disease, identifying outbreaks, and caring for patients. In truth, they should have been in place years ago.

DRUG RESISTANCE

Many have become concerned that laboratory services are the "Achilles heel" in global efforts to combat HIV, tuberculosis, and malaria and the antimicrobial resistance that accompanies them.
— Ruth Berkelman et al. 2006

Between 1990 and 2000, childhood deaths from malaria rose across Africa. Substantial advances in the treatment and prevention of other major killers of children, particularly oral rehydration therapy for diarrhea and vaccination against pneumonia bacteria,[1] were offset by increases in malaria mortality. Although the failure to identify and properly implement key preventive interventions has contributed to the continuing prevalence of this disease, malaria parasites do not appear to have become more virulent. The rise in childhood mortality was largely attributable to the emergence and spread of resistance to antimalarial drugs. Resistance to chloroquine, sulfadoxine-pyrimethamine (Fansidar), and newer antimalarials appeared first in Asia and over the last three decades has spread throughout malaria-endemic parts of the world.[2] In Africa, where up to 30 percent of young children, adults without previous exposure, and pregnant women with *falciparum* malaria are at risk of dying if they do not receive effective treatment, resistance is exceptionally costly.[3]

Drug-resistant malaria is representative of a fundamental problem in twentieth-century approaches to treating infectious disease. Virtually any drug or chemical used to attack specific microbial organisms will eventually be compromised by the emergence of drug resistance. The process is a normal consequence of biological evolution. Susceptible microbes randomly accumulate errors in their genetic material (DNA) as it is copied, or by acquiring new genes from another source. Most DNA miscopies are deleterious to microbes, but a few confer a selective advantage upon those exposed to life-threatening conditions such as an antimicrobial drug.[4] When an antimicrobial drug is used, susceptible strains are eradicated and resistant organisms multiply. *Selective pressure* from antimicrobial drug use engenders resistance. The process can be significantly slowed by the judicious use of antimicrobials, or overcome by introducing new ones, but it cannot be stopped. The evolutionary processes of genetic change and selective pressure are the mechanisms by which most organisms of clinical significance have become resistant to the drugs commonly used to treat infection.[5]

The discovery of several antibiotics early in the twentieth century, along with concomitant improvements in vaccine development and public health, convinced many Westerners that the age-old threat from infections could be vanquished. As a 1954 book titled *The Miracle Drugs* put it:

> The goal is simply *to live in a world without menacing microbes;* to have all disease-producing microbes rendered harmless and domesticated; to see infectious diseases vanish from the earth, or at least be easily controlled; to make this planet free from the dangers of death from infectious diseases, so that the common cold, pneumonia, plague, meningitis and other dread ailments may be as rare phenomena as dangerous wild beasts are.... Will such a world exist? We believe so.[6]

Antimicrobials, which were commonly referred to as "magic bullets," quickly became a mainstay in human and veterinary medicine. Within a few decades, however, new infectious diseases began to emerge, drug resistance by old pathogens became evident, and optimism about a future free from communicable diseases dissipated. Had the "bullets" been aimed at specific targets, they would have retained their utility longer, even though the hoped-for miracle was impossible to achieve.[7]

The term "magic bullet" was coined in 1909 by Paul Ehrlich, who is considered the pioneer of antimicrobial chemotherapy, although he himself was unable to develop an ideal antimicrobial drug. Ehrlich proposed the basic principle for treating infections that is still employed today: the use of chemicals with selective toxicity, that is, drugs that attack an invading pathogen without harming its host. He thought that selective toxicity could form the basis for effective but safe drug treatment, which he called *chemotherapy*.[8] By the first decade of the twentieth century, it was possible to see and manipulate microorganisms in the lab, so Ehrlich needed only a variety of chemicals and considerable persistence to test his idea. In 1909, in his 606th attempt to find a drug that selectively killed bacteria, he identified Salvarsan, which could be used to treat syphilis. Salvarsan is an arsenic derivative that did poison the host but usually managed to finish off the syphilis bacteria first. Because its toxicity was not selective enough, Salvarsan was far from the ideal chemotherapeutic agent, but it was sufficient proof of the principle to motivate searches for less poisonous antimicrobials. Ehrlich proposed that, because some pathogens could be selectively stained, dyestuffs might provide a clue to specificity. He was right.

In 1935, the German pathologist Gerhard Domagk uncovered the antibacterial activity of the red azo-dye prontosil. Working in cooperation with clinicians and other scientific researchers, he soon discovered that the active principle was a colorless sulfonamide derivative. This research led to the development of an almost limitless line of "sulfa" drugs. In 1928, British bacteriologist Alexander Fleming discovered that *Penicillium* mold oozed a chemical that caused bacteria to swell and burst. The development of penicillin took longer than that of sulfa drugs, but it was accomplished once the drug could be produced and purified.[9] Penicillin was rapidly followed by other antibiotics, including tetracycline, an extremely broad-spectrum agent, and streptomycin, the first drug with activity against the bacteria that causes tuberculosis.

Bad news soon began to creep in with the good, however. Clinicians noticed resistance to sulfa drugs in the late 1930s, only decade few years after widespread use of these drugs had begun. An alarming 1939 report describing sulfapyridine-resistant pneumococci was followed by a case report of a death due to meningitis in which resistance emerged during therapy. During World War II, the armed forces' use of penicillin to prevent soldiers from developing scarlet fever was followed by the emergence of resistant flesh-eating bacteria.[10] Streptomycin could not be used alone to treat tuberculosis because resistance arose in infected patients before the bacteria could be eliminated. These and other reports demonstrated that resistance could arise easily, and that it was associated with drug use. In particular, when inadequate quantities of drugs are used, microorganisms can undergo stepwise progression toward full resistance.

It is particularly unfortunate that "magic bullets" and other chemical tools against infectious disease came into common use and abuse at the height of European colonization of Africa. Insecticides and antimicrobials were seen as cheap solutions to infection and infestation, so colonial medical systems deemed it superfluous to invest in the public health resources that had dealt with these problems in Europe and North America a century before. Within weeks of European health teams' arrival at some Nigerian villages, everyone had received penicillin in an attempt to eliminate yaws. Sulfa drugs were mass distributed in northern West Africa, across the meningitis belt, to ward off meningococcal meningitis, and the antibiotic tetracycline was widely distributed as a cholera panacea in East Africa. Chloroquine, one of the most effective antimalarials of all time, was disseminated everywhere the disease was endemic. Antimicrobials could be distributed without refrigeration and administered without special training or devices. As late as the 1960s, disease-preventing vaccines rarely made it to remote rural parts of Africa, but tetracycline and penicillin did. Medical practitioners, community health workers, and quacks dispensed antimalarials and antibiotics in clinics with equal alacrity, feeding an insatiable appetite for cheap *gbogbo-niṣe* (Yoruba for cure-all) drugs that developed at a time when the problems resulting from their overuse were not widely known.

In and outside Africa, the belief that pharmaceutical innovation was sufficiently robust to overcome the problem led to damaging delays in efforts to avoid or limit drug resistance. Not until the 1980s did scientists, clinicians, and health policymakers admit that the antimicrobial honeymoon was over: microbes were winning the war against infectious disease.[11] There were virtually no new antimicrobial drug candidates, and the pharmaceutical industry was diverting its efforts from discovering antimicrobial drugs to developing drugs for chronic disorders or lifestyle problems such as hypertension, high cholesterol, attention deficit disorder, and erectile dysfunction. These disorders require medicines that must be taken for months, years, or even decades by long-living, affluent patients in developed countries, while anti-infective drugs are only needed in short courses and more commonly taken by low-income patients in tropical countries. It takes, on average, ten to fifteen years and US$800 million to bring a candidate drug from the laboratory to the pharmacist's counter. Antimicrobials, although urgently needed in Africa and elsewhere, are far less profitable than medications for chronic conditions. A malign combination of economic factors and technical difficulties that deter antimicrobial drug development means that new antimicrobial drugs, which are critically needed, are not available.[12]

In September 2001, WHO gathered information from experts all over the world and released a global strategy for the containment of drug resistance.[13] As the report outlines, a continuous supply of new drugs is sorely needed, and resistance to existing drugs must be contained through judicious antimicrobial use and by infection control. Most countries have yet to implement most, or even any, of these recommendations. For example, very few health practitioners actually refrain from overprescribing antimicrobials.

Ideally, the etiologic microbe that infects a particular patient would be isolated and identified. Then susceptibility testing would determine which antimicrobials are effective. The prescriber would know what was causing the disease, whether antimicrobials were required, and which drug to apply. Using conventional methods, this process takes at least two days. In practice, the ideal approach is seldom used. For minor infections, it is possible to wait for susceptibility testing results, but physicians often do not routinely order susceptibility tests in these cases. Sometimes they, often erroneously, presume that tests are not cost effective. In other instances, the prescribers bend to patient pressure to offer an antimicrobial immediately, without confirming infection. Even though treatment of microbial infections is cheap, and side effects are uncommon, it is now becoming clear that testing to ensure that the patient is infected with a susceptible microbe often can be justified by the long-term, intolerably high cost of future untreatable infections.

Waiting for susceptibility test results is not an option when the patient is very sick and some therapy must be given immediately. Where possible, empiric choices will be informed by data from previous similar infections that have been collected from previous patients or from sentinel surveillance sites. Poor countries generate less susceptibility testing data, even though they collectively treat more infections. Therefore there is often little or no data to inform empiric prescribing: the most effective medicines available to "evidence-based" allopathic medicine are used without any evidence at all. Calls for antimicrobial conservation through rational drug use must address diagnosis as well as prescribing, since diagnostic shortfalls are often a primary reason for antimicrobial misuse.

Neonatal Infections

The oldest and the youngest among us are least able to fight infections without medical assistance. In Africa, infections are the most common cause of death in the first month of life, and these often preventable deaths take a huge toll. Neonatal infections are less likely to occur in affluent countries, but they almost always prompt both immediate empiric therapy and an order for culture and susceptibility testing. Western pediatricians routinely update their knowledge on local and global susceptibility patterns to make sure that they make the right choices for critically ill babies.

Much of what is known about the epidemiology of pediatric infectious disease on the west coast of Africa comes from a single medical research facility in The Gambia, a small country adjacent to the Gambia River, which is surrounded by Senegal. The Medical Research Council–Gambia has its main campus in Fagara, as well as several outposts. MRC-Gambia is an affiliate of the British MRC and is supported by the council and additional grants from research councils and philanthropies. Its well-cultivated lawns and state-of-the-art laboratories are a welcome oasis in something of a biomedical desert, providing model research infrastructure, health care, and educational facilities. Unlike other coastal West African countries, The Gambia boasts only one fledgling university and has very little homegrown research capacity and therefore this institution has a tremendous impact. MRC-Gambia, along with a few other research centers in Africa, demonstrates that diagnostic testing on the continent not only is useful but can be implemented and sustained.

Diagnostic testing is less common outside the MRC, but The Gambia has its own health care facilities. Like many central government or tertiary care institutions in The Gambia, the Royal Victoria Teaching Hospital in Banjul is reasonably well equipped. It has all the standard tools needed to diagnose most endemic infections and is well staffed by a combination of Gambians and technical employees who come predominantly from other developing countries such as Nigeria and Cuba. Upriver, away from Banjul and the coast, communities are poorer and public services less accessible. At the end of the twentieth century, childhood mortality during the rainy season could reach ninety-nine per 1,000. Many deaths were due to malaria, but almost a third of the children who died were newborns who may have had bacterial infections. The burden from these infections has been somewhat ameliorated by vaccines introduced at the end of the twentieth century whose deployment was informed by decades of pathogen surveillance at the MRC.[14]

A bumpy main road runs from the coast to the interior, paralleling the Gambia River and stretching past about a dozen villages until it passes by the splendid archway at the entrance to the Sulayman Jungkung General Hospital. Patients who come here would find it difficult to get to the MRC or the Royal Victoria Hospital, particularly during the rainy season. One dry season, I was in a group of five road-weary scientists who made a pit stop here on a Saturday and asked to see the hospital lab. Although it is open only on weekdays, we found the room refreshingly well equipped, and a technician who lived nearby was kind enough to take us around. The laboratory had six microscopes, a centrifuge for separating blood, a colorimeter for chemical tests, a few reagents, adequate refrigeration, and a record book. The walls were adorned with photocopied pictures of parasites and motivational messages. A proud technician informed us that the lab did thick films for malaria, hemoglobin levels to test for anemia, stool microscopy for intestinal parasites, and, in a separate room, sputum smears for tuberculosis bacilli. It was well stocked with HIV diagnosis kits. The technician's pride was justified: effective diagnostic work was proceeding on a very low budget, when it is almost entirely absent from many other hospitals in West Africa. Most important, this lab was equipped to diagnose the "big three"—HIV, malaria, and TB—with reasonable precision. "Unfortunately," moaned the technician, "we cannot culture bacteria nor can we do susceptibility testing." In the light of the facilities available, his complaint had previously been brushed off as reflecting an unrealistic expectation. But there was nothing to inform prescription of roughly half the drug classes dispensed to patients at the hospital, especially those prescribed for infections in the youngest, most vulnerable patients. Malaria is responsible for the greatest burden of disease in The Gambia, but bacteria are a close and often underappreciated second, particularly in children.[15] High rates of neonatal death could be drastically reduced in the resource-poor countries of Africa and South Asia by the use of preventive measures and the judicious use of effective antimicrobials.[16] Although treatment of life-threatening neonatal infections must be empiric, knowledge of local susceptibility patterns ensures that empiric therapy selected by prescribers will work.

The diagnostic hole in Sulayman Jungkung General Hospital is replicated across the continent. A 2009 review of thirty-seven health labs in the Tanga region of Tanzania revealed that although thirty-four could perform a blood smear for malaria and seventeen could test for HIV, not one was equipped to perform blood culture and sensitivity of blood. A 2004 survey of Ethiopian laboratories made similar findings.[17] Authors of a third report, this time from Muhimbili National Hospital in Dar es Salaam, Tanzania, and published in 2007, wrote, "There was no formal empirical regimen for the treatment of sepsis at the hospital, partly because of the scarcity of local studies on antimicrobial resistance of relevant bacterial isolates."[18] In that study, bacterial bloodstream infections were a leading cause of death among neonates and young children.

Bacterial infections may cause almost half the deaths among children under five years old in Africa.[19] Location-specific data on drug susceptibility is often absent, even though testing technology is simple, and the continent has the greatest need for chemotherapeutic drugs. Physicians must use treatment as a diagnostic tool where cure confirms diagnosis, reminiscent of ancient medical practice. More than three millennia after the ancient Egyptian Ypres papyrus suggested that a diagnosis of the relatively innocuous condition of night blindness could best be made after successful treatment,[20] analogous diagnostic methods are still employed for potentially lethal bacterial infections: successful antimicrobial therapy confirms presumptive diagnoses. This practice is tantamount to negligence, particularly since medical science has developed alternatives. In an impassioned plea for laboratory support, Dr. Richard C. Brown, a physician practicing in Kinshasa-Gombe, Zaire, wrote: "Clinicians in developing countries often treat infected patients on a trial and error basis, which may be costly, time consuming, and dangerous. It would be preferable if clinicians knew with reasonable certainty to which organisms specific organisms are susceptible."[21]

Even those who advocate for diagnostic development often underestimate the contribution that bacteriology laboratories could make to health care. For example, an otherwise excellent review of diagnostics for the developing world included the unfortunate statement that "[bacterial infections] can often be treated syndromically with broad-spectrum antibiotics or with combinations of antibiotics."[22] This diagnostics-free protocol has missed fatal bacterial infections and allowed the most cost-effective antibacterial drugs to be misused almost to extinction, that is until their therapeutic use has been overtaken by drug resistance. Far from being superfluous, new diagnostic tests for bacterial infections including respiratory infections and diarrhea could save over three million disability-adjusted life years annually if paired with today's treatments.[23] For the future, diagnostic testing will make it possible to use narrow-spectrum antimicrobials, which kill specific microbial species while having no effect on other microbes. These drugs are a powerful tool for limiting resistance,[24] but they cannot be used unless the infecting pathogen is identified. Another proposed strategy has an even more pointed focus. Instead of killing pathogens, a chemical agent that disables them can be used to treat the infection. This strategy requires laboratory infrastructure for pathogen identification because these drugs have extremely specific targets.

Divining without Seeds

The Yoruba oracle of Ifa is consulted in western Nigeria and is famed beyond its domicile, with adherents as far away as Brazil. A patient or applicant visits a diviner, who reads a metaphysical diagnosis from the patterns of palm kernels cast during the consultation. In Tanzania, the Kigoma region has practitioners who use the patterns of seven thrown seeds as the basis for divination; in Swaziland, the *Inyomya* make a diagnosis by reading the patterns made by thrown bones.[25] Diviners learn to recognize hundreds of patterns and to link each pattern with a specific diagnosis. An Ifa diviner masters a materia medica of 256 diagnostic poems or *Odu,* each of which translates a pattern to a diagnosis and then prescribes the specific treatment or spiritual atonement that must be performed.

The diviner's consultation approach, the process linking diagnosis to treatment, and the long and rigorous training associated with the healing profession have parallels in Western medicine. Skeptics might claim that in Western medicine the practice of diagnosis and cure is based on scientific tenets. A West African patient with bloody diarrhea, for example, could have one of many hundreds of infections, or even a noninfectious condition, but according to existing, albeit dated, documentation it is most likely that the patient is infected by *Shigella* bacteria (bacillary dysentery) or with the protozoan *Entamoeba histolytica* (amoebic dysentery). We know this because the role of these pathogens in bloody diarrhea has been evaluated in animal and clinical experiments as well as in controlled epidemiological studies. Both infections can be detected in a very basic diagnostic laboratory, provided that the facilities are available and the appropriate tests are ordered. Amoebic dysentery is typically treated with metronidazole (known as Flagyl), *Shigella* with an antibiotic; the treatments are not interchangeable.

Although these two diagnoses may be the most likely, they are not the only possibilities. Any physician who treats dysentery without the benefit of laboratory investigation probably has less than an even chance of getting it right the first time. Medical schools, particularly those in tropical countries, teach students to suspect *Shigella* or *Entamoeba histolytica* when a patient first presents with bloody diarrhea and to confirm or refute these possible diagnoses with laboratory support. In Africa, many prescribers omit the essential laboratory component and more or less randomly select one course of therapy, or administer both therapies to the patient. This practice is equivalent to a diviner proposing one or more treatments without casting seeds. An Ifa diviner would not do this because it would render his knowledge of the *Odu* irrelevant and would represent disrespect for the deity. So, too, in conventional practice prescribing drugs without prior diagnosis violates the basic principles of scientific medicine.

In the absence of a laboratory and surveillance data, two levels of diagnostic insufficiency are associated with sporadic bloody diarrhea. First, the diagnostician has no way of determining whether *Shigella, Entamoeba,* or some other cause is responsible for the illness. This uncertainty is significant since the patient might have an infection caused by enterohemorrhagic *E. coli* (such as *E. coli* O157), in which case antibiotics for *Shigella* could worsen his prognosis, or a hemorrhagic viral infection, in which case failure to isolate the patient could initiate an epidemic. Even if the physician makes *Shigella* his or her reasonable guess, he or she has no information about which antibiotic is effective against the offending *Shigella* strain. Prescribers with access to laboratory facilities can order susceptibility tests or, more likely, use previous test data from recent, local *Shigella*-infected patients to inform their guesses. Because they do not have recent and locally relevant susceptibility data for *Shigella*, most physicians in Africa cannot make rational choices. As *Shigella* strains often acquire resistance to multiple antimicrobials, particularly the affordable ones,[26] the likelihood of picking the right antimicrobial without supporting information is small. A physician could increase his or her chances of achieving a cure by selecting a newer drug, when one is available, but doing so increases the cost of treatment substantially. The drug selection problem, when coupled with the significant probability that the physician may not have made the right etiologic diagnosis in the first place, means that only a minority of patients will receive appropriate therapy on their first prescription. The others will have to depend on their immune systems to resolve the infection, return to this prescriber, or visit another practitioner; at worst, they will spread the disease while suffering adverse and, perhaps, chronic or even fatal consequences. An Ifa diviner who knows all 256 *Odus* would never select one at random from a set of eight or more, but medical doctors work with these odds every day in Africa.

The Feasibility of Susceptibility Testing

Diffusion or dilution susceptibility testing methods are the diagnostic seeds for bacterial infections. The tests are used to generate patterns of susceptibility for bacterial isolates, which dictate the antimicrobial agents that might be used to treat an infected patient. In diffusion tests, the antimicrobial is placed on a lawn of bacteria seeded onto a plate.[27] If the organism is susceptible, a clear zone of no bacterial growth is produced around the antimicrobial. The size of the inhibition zone is proportional to the effectiveness of the agent, and official standards determine "breakpoint" inhibition zones that mark the border between susceptibility and resistance.[28] Presently, most laboratories purchase standardized, commercially available discs and media and use them in accordance with guidelines from official laboratory institutes. If an organism produces a zone of inhibition diametrically smaller than the standard breakpoint, it is considered resistant. The test is based on the premise that inhibition zone sizes can be correlated with concentrations of the antimicrobial required to inhibit the organism. However, zone sizes are also influenced by other factors, such as test media composition, the solubility and diffusion coefficient of the agent under test, and the quantity and quality of organism growth. Standardization and quality control are critical to the use of disc diffusion tests, and patient isolates must be tested alongside control strains of known susceptibility.

In dilution tests, standardized cultures of test organisms are sown or "inoculated" in, or on, graded concentrations of antimicrobial agent in culture medium.[29] The lowest concentration completely preventing the growth of the test organism is referred to as the minimum inhibitory concentration, or MIC. The basis for the test is that the concentration of antimicrobial agent that reaches the site of infection must exceed the MIC for the drug to be deemed effective. The materials required for routine dilution or diffusion testing are not sophisticated or expensive. Media solidified with the gelling agent agar allows multiple organisms to be inoculated at separate positions on each antibiotic plate. Recent developments to make susceptibility tests less labor-intensive or more rapid[30] have not displaced traditional ones, which are inherently simple and are performed today essentially as they were almost seventy-five years ago, before sophisticated laboratory equipment was developed. Once the modest requirements for standardization, rigorous testing, interpretation, and safe handling can be fulfilled, testing can be performed anywhere.

Following the imposition of structural adjustment programs by the International Monetary Fund and the World Bank during the 1980s, it became increasingly hard for African countries to procure "luxury items" from abroad, including many materials that are necessary to proper medical practice. African nations had very little capacity to produce diagnostic reagents locally. Consequently, laboratory diagnostic tests are expensive in many parts of Africa. The small size of today's market exacerbates the problem. Performing tests more commonly would enable manufacturers to produce or procure these materials in larger quantities and sell them more cheaply. When testing is so expensive, blind drug prescribing appears cheaper, even when it is dangerous to the patient and deleterious for public health. In 2005, discs for susceptibility testing cost at least ten times as much as antimicrobials for oral administration in many African markets. Since less of the same chemical is in each disc than in a tablet or capsule, and the formulation of the test disc drug is usually simpler, the cost of component materials does not account for this discrepancy. It is even harder to procure organisms with known susceptibility patterns, which are essential for quality assurance, and media for sensitivity testing in some cases cost more than a technician's monthly salary. As a result, laboratories that once performed susceptibility tests no longer do so, and academic institutions are providing their students with woefully inadequate practical training.

Tertiary care hospitals typically have facilities for susceptibility testing that are used routinely—or at least most of the time. However, most primary and secondary institutions that serve the majority of the populace in Africa do not generate any susceptibility data. Belete Tegbaru, Hailu Meless, and their colleagues audited twenty-eight hospital and six regional laboratories in Ethiopia and found that only seven performed any kind of bacterial culture and susceptibility testing.[31] Many of the laboratories that perform susceptibility tests, as well as several private laboratories that partially address this need, have inadequate quality assurance. Were the simplest diagnostic support to become routine, a new and viable market for diagnostic products would be created and a diagnostic test community that could include networks to boost quality assurance could be built. Even in light of the current high cost of reagents, physicians are often unaware that susceptibility testing still yields savings in patient costs. At the Komfo Anokye Teaching Hospital in Kumasi, Ghana, where testing is available, expensive antimicrobials were routinely prescribed because doctors would not order cheaper tests that would have made it possible to use less expensive drugs for some patients.[32]

Perhaps the best evidence that susceptibility testing can be easily and routinely performed in remote hospitals are the dusty storerooms in those institutions containing corroded incubators that previously housed plates of growing bacteria and autoclaves once used for media preparation. Most secondary care and many primary care public hospitals once had susceptibility testing facilities, but have ceased to perform bacterial culture and sensitivity testing.[33] Presently, because many of the government hospitals and clinics on which Africa's poor depend do not offer testing, specimens from patients who have failed to recover after chemotherapy must be sent to private laboratories, where the cost of testing is high and quality assurance is at best suspect. In 2006, fifty of seventy-two inspected laboratories in the Nigerian cities of Abuja and Benin were shut down as part of "a crack down on illegal and substandard medical laboratories providing poor and inaccurate tests".[34] In spite of the poor state of affairs at present, capacity building for bacterial susceptibility testing is feasible at all levels of care in Africa. Advocates for diagnostic development in Africa acknowledge that assistance may be required to set up surveillance and reporting systems, to obtain consumable supplies, and to train personnel, but they argue convincingly that susceptibility tests and quality assurance can be performed at local and regional levels.[35]

During the 1980s and 1990s, a number of international research projects temporarily enhanced laboratory capacity in Africa, including susceptibility testing, but these gains were not sustained. Popular among methods used in these programs was the E-test, an easily performed hybrid diffusion-dilution method employing standardized, commercially available strips. E-tests provide an MIC and have been favored by many researchers conducting brief studies in Africa because they are easy to transport and use and their quality is relatively easily assured. E-test strips are pricey; it can cost over US$3.00 to test one isolate against one antibiotic (compared to less than US$1.00 for up to six antibiotics using conventional dilution or disc methods). Although this expensive method precludes the need for extensive monitoring and quality control and is cost effective for small labs in Europe and North America, it cannot be sustained by collaborating African laboratories. The microbiology laboratory at the University of Ghana Medical School and the laboratory for sexually transmitted bacteria at the University Teaching Hospital in Lusaka, Zambia, have both previously collaborated with foreign labs to study drug resistance using E-tests. After the projects ended, the Accra lab reverted to earlier used disc-testing protocols and had to retrain personnel in order to commence minimum inhibitory concentration estimations by dilution methods. In Lusaka, two years after completion of a high-quality international collaborative project, the Sexually Transmitted Bacteria lab was unable to provide any susceptibility testing at all. Diagnostic development should feature cheap, conventional susceptibility testing methods with a proven record of sustainability in developing countries.

Antimalarial resistance presents an additional diagnostic dilemma because plasmodia are less readily cultured and tested than bacteria. There are no effective traditional methods that could be applied in clinical settings. Instead, susceptibility is monitored at sentinel sites. Sadly, the effectiveness of this monitoring actually declined from the 1970s to the 1990s. Earlier guidelines called for parasite-based analyses but, as laboratory capacity eroded in malaria-endemic parts of Africa, these were replaced with clinical guidelines in 1996.[36] Since malaria diagnosis was also almost entirely clinical at that time, the quality and applicability of some of these data are questionable. With increasing awareness of the limitations of clinical diagnoses, parasite-based diagnoses is regaining popularity, and this time, molecular technology offers hope that it could be broadly implemented. Molecular testing by the polymerase chain reaction (PCR) to identify resistance genes is potentially the most applicable diagnosis for drug-resistant malaria, and modern technology could confirm a diagnosis of malaria and generate susceptibility results within four hours.[37] Although PCR-based testing can only detect resistance due to known mutations and novel resistance mechanisms will therefore be missed, it has proved to be valuable in diagnosing returning travelers in nonendemic areas. If available in malaria-endemic areas, PCR would enhance surveillance and even make it possible to use cheaper drugs for some patients.[38] Currently, molecular tests are out of reach in the most malarious parts of the world, where only a few research laboratories are equipped for molecular biology.

When resistance to chloroquine and sulfadoxine-pyrimethamine emerged and spread across Africa, international donors of health aid initially did not support the introduction of artemisinin-based combination therapies (ACTs) at the point of need because of their high cost. Donors continued buying and supplying ineffective drugs until WHO was publicly accused of medical malpractice,[39] and then African countries were advised to switch to ACTs. However, as some policymakers have warned, these drugs must be used appropriately to curtail resistance or "the potential benefits might be outweighed by the negative consequences."[40] ACTs are expensive, but because they are yet to be compromised by resistance, they are cost effective. Their useful life could be extended by using diagnostic tests to ensure that they are employed only when indicated.

Most people understand that a computer with no software has virtually no practical applications; today, computer hardware is commonly sold with basic software already installed. Antimicrobial drugs and diagnostic tests are similar. If antimicrobials would be more rationally employed when partnered with diagnostic tests, why are they not developed and marketed together? In the long term, diagnostic support increases the life span of drugs by reducing selective pressure and the appearance of resistant strains. However, injudicious drug use leads to higher levels of consumption and a greater income for the companies that discover and develop new anti-infective drugs. For a company marketing a patent-protected drug, potential short-term profits are more important than long-term earnings, which can be meager for antimicrobial drugs. The pharmaceutical industry has historically not supported activities that highlight diagnostic microbiology, much less the resistance problem, unless it specifically spotlights its own products.[41]

Despite the commercial disincentive to avert drug resistance, society at large benefits when infections can be cured because untreated or improperly treated infections spread. Thus cure benefits the patient and his or her society, that is, pathogen susceptibility is a common resource. Prescribers, the "gate keepers" of this resource, have to be the advocates for susceptibility testing and create the incentive for biotechnology companies to develop and market appropriate diagnostics. When use of a common resource accrues moderate benefits to individuals, the absence of incentives for a more valuable common good can lead to consequent societal catastrophe. This "tragedy of the commons" paradigm, outlined by Garrett Hardin in 1968, applies to a number of common resource problems, including antimicrobial resistance.[42] According to Hardin, the first step in resolving a "tragedy of the commons" is the "recognition of necessity." In the case of antimicrobial resistance, diagnostic testing and surveillance are essential to this recognition. Prescribers could act as self-policing gatekeepers for the antimicrobial susceptibility resource if they would agree to prescribe certain antimicrobials only when diagnostic testing supported their use. Alternatively, regulatory and professional organizations could legislate diagnostic testing, or at least require surveillance to avert a "tragedy of the commons" in the form of drug resistance.

The inadvertent and deliberate distribution of substandard antimicrobials is a recently highlighted problem that is pervasive across most parts of Africa. Diagnostic insufficiency and poor drug quality assurance are unfortunately synergistic in their contributions to poor health care delivery. Although each problem has a different origin and must therefore be addressed separately, many of the consumables and equipment used for laboratory diagnosis can also be used to determine antimicrobial drug efficacy, at least rudimentarily. Although physicochemical assays are less labor intensive, laboratories employing a suitably qualified scientist can conduct microbiological assays for drug content and quantity.[43] The additional infrastructure that will be needed for a basic drug-quality surveillance laboratory attached to a regional or reference clinical laboratory is small in comparison with the potential benefits. At the very least, a diagnostic lab can confirm the diagnosis and determine when a drug product *should* have worked.

Major African hospitals are frequently a hub around which pharmacies, private diagnostic laboratories, and their unsanctioned counterparts congregate. The area around the Lagos University Teaching Hospital and the sixteen-hundred-bed Korle Bu Hospital of the Ghana Medical School is replete with them. A proportionately smaller number of these institutions are found within easy walking distance of Lagos's smaller and less-well-endowed Ikeja General

Hospital (now Lagos State University Teaching Hospital). These "strategically positioned"[44] premises take advantage of the hospital's deficiencies in diagnosis and drug supplies. Hospitals readily send patients to these sources of medications and testing, but they exercise no responsibility or oversight, and patients pay exorbitantly. Underpaid health professionals who work full time at hospital clinics moonlight at these establishments, assuring a ready pool of part-time employees. In some cases hospital staff with up-to-date information on the needs that their institutions cannot supply actually own these premises. In spite of the obvious conflict of interest, those outlets are among the best managed.

The convoluted health marketplace in African cities is vulnerable to invasion by fraudsters. The question of pharmaceutical quality has been broached, but the quality of diagnostic reagents marketed and used in Africa has yet to be evaluated, even though counterfeit diagnostics have been documented elsewhere. A spot test for gonorrhea purchased from a sex shop in Shanghai, for example, was unable to detect a million *Neisseria gonorrhoeae* bacteria in WHO labs even though samples from patients with gonorrhea are likely to have much lower bacterial counts. Counterfeit tests for visceral leishmaniasis have also been found in the Indian subcontinent.[45] In 2006, an Indian company, Monozyme, was accused of repackaging old pregnancy test kits as tests for HIV and hepatitis B.[46] Over one hundred patients were given wrong diagnoses with fake kits, and some of these were in a position to donate blood or transmit their diseases. Calcutta police recovered ninety thousand expired diagnostic and pregnancy test kits, less than half of those estimated to have been obtained from hospitals and distributed by the criminals. Poor quality reagents compromise diagnosis, treatment, drug quality assurance, and even drug development, since many diagnostic reagents are used in research. The near absence of a market for laboratory reagents makes needed chemicals and other consumables difficult to procure, so counterfeit or substandard diagnostics are unlikely to be detected, and a deliberate search for them could well uncover a more extensive problem.

VIRAL HEMORRHAGIC FEVERS

These outbreaks illustrate the high price exacted by introducing modern medicine...without due attention to good medical practice.

— S. P. Fisher-Hoch et al. "Review of Cases of Nosocomial Lassa Fever in Nigeria" (1995)

Only the wealthiest African patrons of allopathic medicine can afford to have personal physicians. The rest visit overburdened and understaffed health institutions, usually only when they are very young, pregnant, or severely ill. Patients do not necessarily visit the same institution each time, so that whatever facets of their medical history are documented tend to be fragmented, and prescribers have very little opportunity for patient follow-up. Prescribers rarely express concerns about the difficulties inherent in charting patients' progress, however. For the most part, they simply do not have the time or resources to do so.[1] Typically, the health system processes patients visiting overburdened health institutions as if they were faceless components on an assembly line. The final step before the patient is released is taken at a dispensing counter.

Each patient eventually leaves the health institution with bottles, plastic packets, or envelopes of medicine in hand. He or she is regarded as "treated" irrespective of whether cure is assured, likely, or even possible. In response, patients often view the health care system as an impersonal institution rather than a cooperative service rendered by different professionals. Drugs are frequently unaffordable outside of government-funded or publicly subsidized hospitals, so the simple desire for palliative medicine is enough to motivate clinic visits. Private practitioners, too, earn more by marking up medicines than by charging consulting fees. Obtaining medicines has become a principal objective of seeking health care. A cure—or, better still, a positive state of health[2]—is a much more distant goal; patients are often unlikely to think that the institution is even invested in achieving it. Prescribers, for their part, cannot feel guilty about failures from whose consequences they are detached, or of which they are unaware; the inadequacy of any treatments offered is not their responsibility. For all these reasons, lack of diagnostic technology is pervasive, condoned, and almost entirely unrecognized, at least when infections are acquired outside the hospital.

Portrait of a Hospital

In 1990 Sir Mobolaji Bank-Anthony, OBE, a Nigerian philanthropist, donated a maternity wing, Ayinke House, to Ikeja General Hospital in Lagos.[3] The hospital, then owned and managed by the Lagos state government, served the urban poor but also functioned as a secondary center that accepted referrals from private institutions and community clinics. At the time Ayinke House was completed, I was one of several National Youth Service Corps members, recent graduates whom Nigerian law requires to serve the country for a year before embarking on independent careers. The National Youth Service Corps guarantees recent graduates work experience and provides the underserved in Nigeria with health workers, teachers, and administrators. Lagos state government hospitals serve the least affluent patients, in one of the world's largest cities, with very limited resources. Over two-thirds of the medical and pharmacy staff at Ikeja General were interns, residents-in-training, or Corps members. In 1990–91,[4] Ikeja General Hospital had about half a dozen physician corps members, one graduate nurse, four pharmacists, one dentist, and one physiotherapist. Conspicuously absent from our contingent were medical laboratory technicians. Most of the hundreds of biological scientists in our Youth Corps camp served as school teachers. The Youth Corps members added to a workforce of several dozen nurses, about six pharmacists and pharmacy attendants, and about sixty doctors, almost half of whom were interns. Most of the staff moonlighted at private institutions in order to make a living. The general hospital did have a lab, but it was very small and only occasionally functional.

On the day that the ribbon at the gate of Ayinke House was cut, I stood with other hospital staff along the road to the building to wave to the motorcade of dignitaries. A precious half hour of nonemergency service had been sacrificed for the biggest event that Ikeja General had seen in many years. Hospital expansions and upgrades are few and far between in Nigeria. The new building's stark whiteness was almost blinding against the dull green backdrop of the rest of the hospital. The maternity wing was only the second two-story building on the entire campus. A week later, dispensing in the shiny pharmacy for the first time, I realized that Ayinke had served up even more than we had anticipated. Water flowed from sparkling taps, a generator supplied electricity whenever the main supply failed, tiled surfaces could be wiped clean, and the medicine cupboards were latched and rodent-proof. The very idea of rodents in Ayinke was preposterous.

Just a week before, I had been working at the Old Pharmacy, where things were not as fancy, and, despite our best efforts, the occasional rat scuttled across the floor.[5] Usually I sat on a hard, high stool at an outpatient counter, which had peeling green paint, dispensing medicines through a small window. When the electricity supply was interrupted, I leaned out of the window to catch the light and kept my feet off the floor. Angry-looking patients and their guardians watched me suspiciously, sliding toward my window on what looked, from my vantage point, like endlessly long wooden benches. After my first week, I learned that they were not angry at me, just exhausted. By the time they reached the pharmacy, they had been waiting for three to eight hours, which included less than ten minutes of contact time with all the health professionals combined. With the exception of inpatients, tuberculosis patients, and pediatric patients, who had separate pharmacy facilities, every one of several hundred patients each day had their prescriptions filled, or converted to shopping lists, at this counter. At any given time, there were at most two pharmacists or pharmacy attendants on outpatient dispensing duty at the Old Pharmacy counter.

While hundreds of outpatients poured into the clinic each day, the staff also cared for critically ill patients admitted to the wards. The pharmacy unit had other staff dedicated to inpatients, but whenever we were even more understaffed than usual I had to close the window for an hour or so to take medicines to the wards. These clinical pharmacy rounds were a welcome change from the monotony and pressure of counting out tablets, mostly antimalarials, to patients on an unending line and dictating instructions in my broken Yoruba. I felt relieved to be able to stretch my legs without being plagued by guilt about leaving an endless line of tired patients. On my occasional trips through the tightly packed wards, I was accompanied by a student or intern, whose major responsibilities included running back and forth between the pharmacy and the ward to bring in intravenous fluids that could not fit on our tiny cart and ensuring that the three-and-a-half wheeled contraption did not overturn. As I walked by the patients, their relatives, who were typically camped outside the wards, said hello through the windows. Since we were constantly fighting shortages, I dispensed what few medicines were available and translated unfilled prescriptions into shopping lists for patients' guardians to procure the rest elsewhere.

Our inventory of cheap generics and vetted donations did cover the most heavily prescribed medicines, but there were still some essential drugs that were only sometimes, or never, in stock. We were perpetually short of surgical disposals, and only rarely did we have a stock of gloves for surgical procedures. In the early 1990s, everyone had heard of AIDS, but no one thought it had reached Nigeria. We were aware that other diseases lurked in the hospital and took some precautions to protect ourselves and our clients. Staff that wore lab coats procured their own. Patients were asked to procure gloves for their own procedures and were even given their doctor's size, but every now and then a doctor would work without gloves in an emergency or to save a poor patient some money. At the pharmacy, we staff members bought our own soap, disinfectant, and, on occasion, kegs of water.

No one was ever turned away from Ikeja General Hospital. For the many patients for whom the heavily subsidized hospital services were still out of reach, fees could be waived by completing "Pauper" forms. Considering the vast numbers of patients who pushed through its gates each day and the meager resources allocated to their care, Ikeja General Hospital was remarkably clean and efficiently run. Working in the conurbation of Lagos, where medical and allied practitioners are not scarce, I did not face the challenges that classmates of mine posted to more remote areas had to endure. There, a hospital might have only one doctor and no nurses, so the pharmacist was forced to give injections, stitch cuts, and even attend births if the doctor happened to be otherwise engaged. We had postgraduate medical residents, certified midwives, and a handful of consultant specialists. The hospital was chronically understaffed and overcrowded, but it offered better care than many private institutions.

Through my experience at Ikeja General Hospital, I later became acutely aware of how easily infectious pathogens might travel from one patient to another and to hospital staff during an outbreak. We had no untrained practitioners and easily avoided needle sharing and grossly unsafe surgical practices, but in most wards at Ikeja General we could not implement infection control at a standard necessary to contain highly virulent and transmissible pathogens. Reaching these standards routinely and reliably was attainable in parts of the new Ayinke wing, but the older buildings, which were more representative of urban public hospitals in Nigeria, lacked a reliable water supply, surgical disposables, or enough staff. Patient beds were too close together, and relatives walked in and out of the wards bringing essential supplies that had to be procured from outside.

Many patients admitted to hospital wards in sub-Saharan Africa come with a nonspecific fever. Most of them recover, even if they are still undiagnosed when they leave. If their illness is caused by malaria parasites or blood-borne bacteria, precautions taken in well-run institutions such as Ikeja General are sufficient to protect medical staff and other patients from becoming infected. In the uncommon event that a more easily transmitted pathogen is responsible, however, proper infection control is essential, particularly if the unexpected agent cannot be identified. Hospital-based outbreaks of viral hemorrhagic fever result from conditions in which infection control is desirable but difficult. This situation has repeatedly been highlighted in reports describing hemorrhagic fever outbreaks in Africa, in spite of the growing emphasis on infection control. Viral hemorrhagic fever outbreaks are promoted by the prevalent mode of medical practice in which etiology is only of interest when a cure fails, and not always even then. Because of the challenges associated with infection control and patient diagnosis, in typical African hemorrhagic fever epidemics the death toll is high and the spread throughout the hospital has already begun before the cause of the outbreak is known or even suspected.

Allopathic medical institutions are only one of several options available to the sick African. Indigenous practitioners and unsanctioned providers also can be consulted; they often cost less and are closer to the patient, which are significant benefits. Although hospitals are greatly revered, especially for their surgical proficiency, they are also viewed with some suspicion and fear.[6] When an unusual infectious disease appears, it is difficult to tell whether the bad turn of events is inevitable or a consequence of treatment. If an illness is acquired within a hospital, however, the finger of blame can be pointed directly at the institution. The blinders that obscure the otherwise inconspicuous deficiencies of allopathic medicine are removed when death is linked to the hospital.

During a 2005 Marburg outbreak in Uige, Angola, in which almost four hundred people were infected and about 88 percent died, a local pastor explained to personnel from Médecins Sans Frontières and WHO why people were fleeing the hospital: "They say that Marburg is in the hospital; that there is a large reservoir of blood there; and that anyone who approaches it dies."[7] Just as London's John Snow was able to link cholera to the Broad Street Pump in the nineteenth century, even though he had no idea that a bacterium caused the disease, deductive epidemiology was all the people of Uige needed to link Marburg hemorrhagic fever to their hospital. In 2007, a Ugandan primary health center was attacked by locals who blamed it for an Ebola outbreak and chased five potentially infected patients, who were at the time under quarantine, from the hospital. In the same outbreak, patients were reported to have fled from the hospital to use indigenous therapies.[8] In those uncommon but significant instances when iatrogenic illness leaps out of control, patients as well as health care workers flee hospitals. Infection control remains far from optimal in many places, but at least an understanding of its importance exists within health-professional circles. Diagnostic insufficiency has yet to achieve this basic level of appreciation.

Viral Portraits

The best known African viral hemorrhagic fevers are yellow fever, Marburg, and Ebola.[9] Yellow fever is an ancient viral disease whose etiology and mosquito vector were discovered in the early twentieth century.[10] Patients suffer from a high fever, headache, and bleeding in the skin. They often become jaundiced by the third day, resulting in the yellowness of the eyes that gives the disease its name. Yellow fever originated in tropical Africa but was transported to the Americas, where it rapidly became endemic in every locale inhabited by *Aedes aegypti* mosquitoes. It killed thousands of people, usually in the summer months. Mosquito control is one option for intervening in transmission but, as with many other mosquito-borne diseases, had limited success outside the United States.[11] Yellow fever deterred the construction of the Panama Canal. This disease, along with malaria, led to West Africa being labeled "the White man's grave." Intensive global research on yellow fever was vital to serve the goals of empire and was stimulated by its major architects. The causative virus, vector, and life cycle were worked out principally by researchers in the Americas. Successful control of yellow fever came largely through the development of an effective vaccine, 17D, an attenuated variety of a strain obtained from a Ghanaian patient, through research at early colonial laboratories in West Africa.[12] A monkey reservoir exists in rain forests of Africa and South America, and the *Aedes aegypti* mosquito continues to inhabit these parts of the world. For these reasons, yellow fever cannot be eradicated, and occasional outbreaks still occur in South America and Africa.

In contrast to yellow fever, which has been known for centuries, Ebola and Marburg hemorrhagic fevers are postcolonial or "emerging" infectious diseases. Both are caused by filoviruses, tiny, threadlike microbes capable of killing up to 90 percent of the humans they infect. Ebola and Marburg viruses look remarkably alike but have very different surface proteins. This means that infection caused by one will not protect against subsequent infection by the other, although known outbreaks have been few and none have overlapped. As yet, there is no protective vaccine for either disease. Outbreaks of Ebola and other African hemorrhagic viruses have been the subject of moving nonfiction chronicles.[13] Fear of these diseases is rooted in the knowledge that there is neither a cure nor a vaccine and that their mortality rates, which range between 50 percent and 90 percent, are among the highest for any known illness. Intense terror emanates from the painful and grisly suffering of infected patients. The disease follows a terrible course, after days or weeks of fever:

> The victim soon suffers profuse breaks in small blood vessels, causing blood to ooze from the skin, mouth and rectum. Internally, blood flows into the pleural cavity where the lungs are located, into the pericardial cavity surrounding the heart, into the abdomen, and into organs like the liver, kidney, heart and spleen, and lungs. Eventually, this uncontrolled bleeding causes prostration and death.[14]

Ironically, the efforts of relatives and health care providers to care for the sufferers of Ebola and Marburg hemorrhagic fevers are especially dangerous because these activities often foster transmission. The high rate of person-to-person transmission via infected body fluids is well documented, but the disease is not always identified until it is too late to prevent outbreaks in health care settings.

Filoviral threads often settle in the shape of a question mark, taunting scientists at the other end of the microscope by posing numerous questions. Where did Marburg and Ebola come from? How do the viruses spread? Where do they live between outbreaks? Some have supposed that Ebola virus has always been hidden in the forests of central Africa, thriving and circulating in a less susceptible or symptom-free host population. This school of thought contends that contact between the reservoir and humans or susceptible apes (gorillas and chimpanzees) is normally an unlikely event but has increased because of habitat disturbance or climate change. Another school proposes that Ebola is a new virus that did not exist anywhere before its sudden emergence the 1970s. That hypothesis is supported by the genetic similarity among viruses from outbreaks between 1976 and 2004, but this could also mean that the virus is under evolutionary pressure that does not support change.[15]

Almost as enigmatic as the origin of these filoviruses is their normal habitat. Viruses cannot exist on their own; they need a living host that can support them until they can be transmitted. Humans and primates succumb to infection too rapidly to transmit the virus to many other individuals; these diseases' rapid transmissibility and high case-fatality rates imply that we are merely incidental hosts.[16] As there is a holding period between epidemics when no one shows signs of disease, a reservoir that can transmit the virus without being killed by it must exist somewhere.[17] When a reservoir is unknown or uncertain, it is impossible to predict the advent of epidemics or to prevent and control them. It took over thirty years to identify the bat species that are the Ebola and Marburg reservoirs.

The Ugly Picture: Viruses in Hospitals

In 1995, Dustin Hoffman and Renee Russo starred in a movie called *Outbreak,* a thriller about the fictional Motaba virus that was transported from Africa to the United States via an infected monkey. In this cinematic scenario, scientists dressed in space-age suits used the latest technology to protect America against the dread disease. This somewhat absurd fictional account can be viewed as an exaggeration of an outbreak that occurred in Reston, Virginia, when an Ebola outbreak occurred in a research institute's monkey colony.[18] In contrast to outbreaks that occur in Africa, the actual and fictional United States outbreaks did not lack high-tech facilities to protect scientists and health-care workers and make sure diagnoses were accurate and treatment prompt and efficient.

All the principal Ebola outbreaks and most Marburg outbreaks have occurred on the African continent, except for a few relatively unremarkable laboratory outbreaks in Western countries.[19] Marburg was identified in 1967 during one such laboratory outbreak in Germany. There were sporadic cases of this disease in southern Africa and Kenya in the 1970s and 1980s, but the first outbreak caused by the virus was documented in 1998, in the Democratic Republic of Congo (formerly known as Zaire). In 2005, the largest known Marburg outbreak erupted in Angola.

Ebola outbreaks were first recorded in Yambuku, Zaire, and across the border in Maridi, Western Equatoria, Sudan, in 1976.[20] The first human case, called the "index" case, came from the forest to the Yambuku Catholic Mission Hospital, a facility managed by devoted but unsupervised Belgian nuns. The hospital was popular "because it maintained a good supply of medicines"[21] but the staff's limited medical training meant that they did not appreciate the importance of aseptic procedures and infection control. In an attempt to stretch scarce resources and serve more patients, they used a sparse stock of injection paraphernalia—five syringes in all. These were sterilized by boiling just once a day, so that almost every patient in the hospital had a near 100 percent risk of infection once the index case was admitted.[22] Before long, the virus was transmitted from patients to nurses. By the end of the outbreak, most of the hospital staff, including all the health-worker nuns, had died.

The concurrent Sudanese Maridi outbreak, by contrast, featured multiple cases of community-acquired hemorrhagic fever associated with a cotton factory, followed by some hospital amplification. Patients who were stricken by the mysterious disease were taken to the district-level hospital in Maridi. Early in the epidemic, a telegraph message was sent to the central medical services in Khartoum, and WHO was notified. A team headed by Dr. Ali Idris, Sudan's director general of epidemiology, and including public health specialists, epidemiologists, and laboratory scientists, as well as doctors and nurses, was immediately dispatched to Maridi.[23] A third of the health care employees at the hospital—seventy-six of 230 staff—became infected; forty-one eventually died, and most of the rest fled.

Even though the etiologic agent of the infection was unknown to science at the time, Dr. Idris was especially prescient in requiring that barrier precautions be taken very seriously by every member of this team. A strict quarantine was instituted, and all specimens were collected and handed aseptically so that the epidemic was confined to Maridi and containment was relatively rapid.[24] An important observation in the 1976 outbreaks was that, for reasons unknown, hospital-acquired infections appeared to be more lethal than community-acquired Ebola hemorrhagic fever.[25] Hemorrhagic viruses have greater reach today than at any other time in history because of very recent medical advances; Western medicine must ensure that it protects patients and practitioners from these deadly agents by detecting outbreaks early, before they spread in the hospital.

Why are tests necessary in order to ascertain that infection control must be heightened around a patient bleeding from all orifices? Because patients infected with Ebola or Marburg viruses do not begin to bleed early in the course of infection. They present with high fever and nonspecific malaise indistinguishable from malaria, typhoid, and other severe blood-borne diseases. By the time the patient shows definitive signs of hemorrhagic fever, his or her prognosis is poor. Even more important, the patient is likely to have been admitted to a hospital and to have shared accommodations, health care staff, and, far too often, infectious milieu with a roomful of other severely ill patients.

In 1995, an Ebola epidemic occurred in Kikwit, Zaire, a city of between two hundred thousand to six hundred thousand people. The deadly disease made its impromptu appearance at a resource-poor hospital, but the epidemiological investigation of the Kikwit outbreak was superior to most investigations in Africa. Communications had improved considerably since the 1976 Maridi and Yambuku outbreaks. Although several weeks went by before the outbreak was known to the world, the Kikwit Ebola epidemic offered more opportunities for epidemiologic investigations, and even for some preliminary inquiries into disease reservoirs.[26] In an exemplary case study in epidemiological sleuthing, the index case, a charcoal pit worker, was identified even though he had died months before the international investigation team arrived. Later in the outbreak, an international team was commissioned to propose and implement interventions and to perform epidemiological investigations. However, clinical care for most of the dying patients was furnished by volunteer Zairian doctors and nurses, who came in from the capital, Kinshasa, after the staff at Kikwit's hospital had either died of the disease or fled from it.

In addition to caring for the dying, local doctors conducted a high-risk clinical experiment that may well have succeeded. At the tail end of the epidemic, a nurse who had cared for infected patients became feverish. Clinical diagnosis in the context of the epidemic strongly suggested that she had contracted Ebola hemorrhagic fever. Since the death rate was then about 80 percent, her colleagues were devastated and acutely aware of their own vulnerability. Their helplessness to do anything to change the clinical course of the deadly disease in someone who had battled it alongside them sunk home and motivated them to handle her case aggressively.

The Zairian clinical team decided to transfuse the nurse with blood from a recovering patient. The idea was that the patient would have protective antibodies against Ebola virus in his or her blood that could offer some protection to the newly infected nurse. During the first Ebola outbreak, in Yambuku, a variation of this procedure was tried on two patients but very little information was available to judge the value of this therapy.[27] The principle has been used to treat other infections for which there is no cure, such as Lassa fever, but in those cases the source blood is screened for blood-borne pathogens and, as in Yambuku two decades before, the therapeutic antibodies are purified away from whole blood. The Kikwit hospital did not have the facilities for either of these safety protocols but, if the procedure were to work at all, the patient needed to receive the antibodies immediately.

The few patients who survived Ebola hemorrhagic fever were still quarantined at the hospital because the virus remains in body fluids for several weeks after recovery. The clinicians had a decent pool of convalescent patients and found a compatible donor. The blood was screened for HIV, but not for hepatitis and other blood-borne viruses. Although the hospital typically transfused malaria patients with severe anemia, it lacked the facilities necessary for more complete screening. For these and other reasons, the international scientific team strongly disapproved of transfusion. Not only was there little evidence to support this radical approach to treatment, there was real risk of doing harm. Indeed, well into one of the largest Ebola outbreaks of all time, and two decades after the virus had been discovered and characterized, there was still no way to confirm that the nurse had Ebola.[28] It was likely that she had the disease, but it was impossible to rule out malaria, typhoid, or some other infection. If the nurse had something else, transfusion with blood from a convalescent Ebola patient could infect this already ill patient with the deadly virus. The Zairian medical crew and its nurse-patient weighed the pros and cons and eventually chose to go forward with the transfusion against the advice of the international scientific team. They were probably slightly desensitized to the dangers; they had performed risky transfusions in the past, although perhaps none as risky as this.

The transfused nurse and seven of the eight patients who were treated similarly recovered. Had the team stumbled upon an effective treatment for Ebola? The entire episode deserved to be aired in the pages of a prestigious medical journal, but, as one witness observed, there was no way to know whether the therapy had worked or not. Without laboratory backup for this key experiment, which cannot be replicated because of ethical considerations, it is impossible to tell whether the patients who recovered at the tail end of the epidemic were cured by the transfusion therapy, had a different type of Ebola infection, or never had Ebola at all.

Contracting the Ebola virus might not be the worst thing that could happen to a person during an outbreak. Anyone who came down with a curable infection, whether with malaria, bacteremia, or enteric fever, was likely to be housed with Ebola patients with similar signs and symptoms and could then be infected with an incurable disease. These ill patients would probably be hypersusceptible to Ebola infection. In the most likely scenario, neither these patients nor their caregivers would ever know that the disease was acquired after, and not before, admission to hospital.

Compared to malaria, typhoid, and many other fever-causing diseases, Ebola hemorrhagic fever is uncommon, so some may argue that routine diagnosis for the disease is not cost effective. The lack of a cure also could be put forward as an argument against investing in Ebola-specific diagnostics. However, experts insist that early diagnosis allows for tailored supportive care that reduces mortality, and the evidence from treated cases supports this position. When an epidemic is occurring, rapid and precise diagnostics are essential to contain it.[29] At the inception of an epidemic, routine use of diagnostic protocols that are rigorous enough to rule out common infections would hasten the identification of a new outbreak. Certain populations should be targeted for more rapid and rigorous routine diagnostic protocols. For example, many of the people who have been sickened by Ebola and Marburg viruses are health workers on the front line in battles against the unknown. Health workers in Africa are too few to serve their populations and very expensive to train. From a purely economic standpoint, it makes sense to ensure that these skilled professionals are protected from on-the-job infection and that they receive the most effective care when they fall ill, particularly when hospital transmission is suspected. Even though health workers are not more "valuable" than other people in the community, their exposure to infectious microorganisms is greater because they are in contact with so many ill patients, and their illness could serve as red flags for hemorrhagic virus outbreaks. Health workers are also in a position to spread any diseases that they carry, so diagnosing them rapidly and precisely is an important way to contain hospital outbreaks.

The need for a simple but reliable test that can be used during an Ebola epidemic, or to screen high-risk subpopulations, has long been appreciated in scientific circles. Toward the end of the 1976 Yambuku Ebola outbreak, WHO commissioned a scientific team to conduct fieldwork and define the syndrome caused by the deadly new virus. The scientists were obliged to use hastily assembled and improvised equipment, but still prioritized the development of a diagnostic test to differentiate people infected with the new virus from those with fever of other etiology. Within two weeks of their arrival at Kinshasa, the team devised an immunofluorescence-based field test. The test was used to estimate the scale of the epidemic, as well as to identify people who had previously been exposed to the virus who could provide antisera to treat the newly infected. Unfortunately, the hastily developed test was insufficiently sensitive; its use had to be discontinued, and no replacement test was developed. Twenty years later, diagnostic testing was unavailable in the Kikwit epidemic, even to validate or at least safeguard experimental therapy.[30]

The gold standard for identifying any causative microbe in an infection is amplification of live organisms to detectable levels in a test tube, a technique known as culture. Routine detection of the Ebola virus by culture is out of the question; it is simply too dangerous to amplify the virus to necessary levels outside a Biosafety Level 4 containment facility. Level 4 represents the highest biosafety level and is used to protect scientists and technicians working with deadly pathogens, including Ebola virus. Level 4 labs are hermetically sealed off from the outside environment. Like the actors in *Outbreak,* technicians wear impervious space suits and work with samples in chambers that suck out potentially infected air. In the absence of these and other safety features present in a Biosafety Level 4 lab, surrogate methods that do not require viral amplification must be used for diagnosis.

The best available technology for routine filovirus diagnosis is probably a reverse transcriptase-PCR (RT-PCR) test, which measures viral load, in which portions of viral genetic material are amplified for detection.[31] Amplifying sections of viral genetic material in this way is safe and reliable and can be conducted in ordinary clinical laboratories. The absence of alternatives before the RT-PCR technique became routine is one explanation for the lack of progress in this essential area. In 2004, an RT-PCR test for Ebola was described in a paper authored by Ebola specialists, who are aware of the poor results from the earlier immunofluorescence assay.[32]

RT-PCR is a promising approach, particularly as viral load determinations for HIV, using the same method, are increasingly sought in Africa. Facilities and resources that are being developed for this purpose could be adapted for use with filoviruses. Presently, the dearth of molecular facilities in African hospitals presents a major roadblock to routine use of RT-PCR tests: most HIV-positive patients cannot yet access viral load testing. In the absence of suitable facilities to detect the virus itself (or viral nucleic acid) in blood specimens, surrogate serological or immunological diagnostic tests for filoviruses are theoretically possible but are rarely applied because of challenges associated with making them sensitive enough. Many patients do not develop antibody levels sufficient to be reliably detected until they are close to death or recovery. Patients who have previously been infected by the same or a similar organism have high antibody levels, resulting in false positives.

Gulu Learned Little from Kikwit

It is not enough merely to develop diagnostic tests; they must be deployed at the point of need. The Kikwit outbreak, during which 245 of 317 documented infected patients died,[33] was highly publicized and has featured prominently in the scientific literature. One epidemiologist, reviewing recent advances in laboratory testing, commented that the power and speed of modern diagnostics "is spectacularly demonstrated by the rapid response" to this outbreak: "glycoprotein sequences from the Kikwit strains were obtained within 48 hours of the virus arriving at the CDC in Atlanta."[34] A key point that this epidemiologist appears to overlook is that the epidemic's index case died four months before the CDC's evaluation and one month after about one hundred health workers were felled by the disease. Although the technology required for the rapid confirmation of Ebola existed outside Africa, the "ability to isolate and identify quickly new pathogens" was not called in until the epidemic was approaching its fifth month (table 1).[35]

Uganda documented its first Ebola hemorrhagic fever epidemic in 2000. By that time, Ebola virus had been known for a quarter of a century, longer than HIV. Following the extensively televised 1995 Kikwit outbreak, the virus was routinely featured in U.S. undergraduate microbiology classes, and the U.S. Public Broadcasting Service (PBS) had prepared curricular resources about Ebola epidemics for high schools.[36] In spite of extensive human experience with the virus, at least 425 people ultimately contracted the disease in and around Gulu, Uganda, and roughly half of them died. As with the previous human Ebola epidemics in Africa, the identification of the disease was delayed by misdiagnosis of early cases. Although Ebola was no longer an unknown virus, the delay from the appearance of the first patient until a diagnosis of Ebola hemorrhagic fever was made was an astonishing *six weeks.*[37]

Table 1.   Kikwit Ebola outbreak of 1995

KEY EVENT	APPROXIMATE NUMBER OF NEW CASES SINCE PREVIOUS EVENT
January 13: Death of index case	4 in 12 days
April 10–14: Identification of first cases among health personnel	33 in 90 days
April 27–29: Emergency message sent to health authorities; lab technician dispatched	89 in 14 days
May 1–3: Preliminary lab findings and clinical signs establish a diagnosis of viral hemorrhagic fever	141 in 3 days
May 4–5: First blood specimens sent to CDC; first antiepidemic measures taken	38 in 7 days
May 9: Specimens arrive at CDC	
May 10: Results of serological and RT-PCR tests confirming Ebola hemorrhagic fever conveyed to Kikwit	
June 30: No more new cases reported	100 in 50 days

Until a definitive Ebola diagnosis was pronounced, patients with hemorrhagic fever were variously diagnosed and treated as if they had malaria or typhoid fever by indigenous as well as allopathic health providers. Patients and their contacts were not isolated or quarantined, and the disease spread with ease. The situation was not helped by the fact that this was Uganda's first Ebola outbreak. That outbreaks of Ebola and other viral hemorrhagic diseases frequently occur in nearby Congo and Sudan, and that circulating Ebola antibodies had previously been found in eastern Ugandan residents, was not sufficient warning for the nation's health system.[38] During the 1976 Sudanese outbreak, patients at Maridi hospital were treated for malaria during their first week of illness and for typhoid fever during their second. By the third week, when patients began to hemorrhage and die, it became clear that this infection was caused by an unusual, as yet unidentified pathogen.[39] Twenty-four years later, by which time the Medline database of biomedical literature had indexed almost five hundred scientific and medical publications on Ebola, infected Ugandans met a similar fate.

The World Health Organization and the U.S. Centers for Disease Control (CDC), the principal international agencies that respond to outbreaks, recommend that viral hemorrhagic fever isolation protocols begin only *after* patients do not respond to therapy for malaria and typhoid.[40] In a typical African health care setting, following this course can result in a delay of over two weeks. In situations where drug quality is not assured and resistance has been documented, the delay could be longer, as physicians sequentially experiment with different therapies. If Ebola, by then a well-characterized virus, could not be identified in Uganda in 2000 because of its local novelty, the failure to rapidly rule out malaria and bacterial infections, which could have been done by the simple laboratory tests that are needed to manage those conditions, extended the period of ignorance and the opportunity for the infection to spread. Ebola virus was eventually confirmed through laboratory tests performed in South Africa. An internationally assisted field lab, surveillance, and containment strategies were established within a week of this confirmation, and the epidemic waned shortly thereafter.[41] The rapid demise of both the Gulu and the Kikwit outbreaks following diagnosis demonstrates that, in spite of its transmissibility and high mortality rate, Ebola is controllable once detected. In contrast to viral hemorrhagic fevers elsewhere, the repeated failure to identify and quarantine patients infected with Ebola and other African hemorrhagic viruses precipitates alarming, oversized outbreaks that perpetuate the stereotype of Africa as the infectious continent.

In 2000, it took only six days to confirm Ebola in Uganda once viral hemorrhagic fever was suspected. This time span was acceptable, allowing for unfamiliarity of Ebola in the locality and the need to ship samples to a specialist laboratory in another country. The lag time that was responsible for massive amplification of the epidemic elapsed before Ebola was suspected and might have been shortened if an early warning system had been available:

> By and large, once an outbreak has been recognised by the public health authorities there are well-tried processes and procedures that come into play that serve to contain further spread of the infection and limit additional cases of the disease. This was shown spectacularly in the case of the SARS outbreak, in which not only was the disease controlled but the novel causative agent was identified, both within a few months. But as Lamunu and colleagues [in their 2000 chronicle of the Uganda Ebola outbreak] make clear, the most difficult aspect of the outbreak control is the initial recognition of the disease: diagnosis depends on the astute health-care worker who notices an unusual clinical picture, or more usually, an unexpected cluster of cases.[42]

Severe acute respiratory syndrome (SARS) was rapidly identified as a new disease in 2003 because other respiratory infections were ruled out with considerable help from laboratory and radiological diagnostics in Asia and North America.[43] The same conclusions might have been reached had testing been delayed, but the effect of such a delay would almost certainly have been catastrophic. The vision of an "astute" African health care worker who is responsible for recognizing a potential Ebola outbreak is bound to be clouded by numerous cases of malaria, typhoid, and other infectious diseases that continue to flow in whether or not an epidemic of viral hemorrhagic disease is under way. Jerome Groopman, who has studied physicians' decision-making behavior, notes that "availability heuristics" are among the most common causes of medical error[44]: simply put, a diagnostician is less likely to come to the correct diagnosis when he or she sees a test case in the midst of many "detractor" cases that present with similar symptoms but have other causes.

Kikyo health center in Bundibugyo district was at the epicenter of Uganda's most recent Ebola outbreak, which raged from August 2007 until early January 2008. Kikyo health center has no doctors, and its nurses treat about 850 malaria cases a month, in addition to patients with dysentery and meningitis. Between August and November 2007, patients sickened by what was later discovered to be a new subtype of Ebola did not bleed as Ebola patients typically do. Concerned by the high mortality rate, but oblivious to the fact that the outbreak was caused by a deadly virus, health workers without adequate protective clothing tended the patients and collected infectious specimens for shipment to the CDC. One experienced clinical diagnostician was convinced that the outbreak was typhoid fever. His guess was wrong: he contracted Ebola, and five more health workers—including almost all of the staff in this small health center—were sickened by the disease before a diagnosis was made. This outbreak was caused by a new strain of Ebola, a fact that has been blamed for diagnostic delay. However, it has been observed that the disease may have been circulating before the first diagnosed case, and, although the CDC was unable to identify the causative agent within twenty-four hours, as in other recent outbreaks, Ebola was identified within three days of receipt of specimens. Testing began earlier than in the 1995 Kikwit and 2000 Gulu outbreaks, but it did not begin early enough to prevent 149 infections and thirty-seven deaths.[45]

A patient infected with even the better known strains of Ebola or Marburg initially presents with a fever, general malaise, and perhaps some diarrhea. That the patient does not have malaria, typhoid, or some other fever might only become apparent when internal organs begin to dissolve and blood starts to trickle from bodily orifices, by which time it is too late to intervene in a way that might change the course of this infection or protect others from exposure. The high prevalence of pathogens that produce similar early symptoms means that even the best clinical surveillance will detect that something is amiss only when the number of deaths spikes, by which time the outbreak will be well under way. It was the high mortality among clusters of patients that led doctors to suspect that both the 2000 and 2007 Uganda epidemics were caused by filoviruses. Clinicians working without laboratory support noticed that something was amiss before Ebola was confirmed, but not early enough to block its rapid dissemination.

Surveillance for viral diseases with epidemic potential is today of global interest, with increasing focus on influenza viruses with pandemic potential, including those that can infect birds as well as humans, the avian influenza strains. In a sense, the existing "warning system" for much more lethal viral hemorrhagic fevers in Africa is analogous to that for avian influenza, with the notable exception that a human, rather than a bird, die-off indicates an epidemic. Even if the health system did not routinely test for Ebola, a spike in the number of patients with febrile illnesses that could not be attributed to malaria or other endemic diseases could form the basis of a more effective and acceptable early warning system. Early warning systems are valuable for rare yet deadly infectious diseases, as well as for newly emergent diseases. We know enough to predict that the next emergent pathogen will most likely be an RNA virus with a broad range of hosts and will probably appear in a part of the world where human beings are being pushed to interact with unfamiliar animal species because of ecological and/or demographic change.[46] These risk factors are very likely to converge in Africa, where a new Ebola subtype emerged in 2007.[47] Preparedness for new diseases and new forms of known diseases requires, at the very least, strong surveillance systems for existing endemic infections.

Without proactive containment of a hemorrhagic virus, the hospital, which should be central to managing a disease outbreak, becomes the focus of an epidemic and is disengaged from the community as potential cases avoid treatment and quarantine. Patients with severe malaria or bacterial bloodstream infections do not need to be placed in isolation (and the cost of doing so would be prohibitive for most African hospitals), but it is imperative that patients with hemorrhagic fevers be identified early and isolated. Health workers also need to use strict protective protocols when collecting and handling body fluids, including those required for testing. Where tests are routinely performed, these precautions are normal protocol. In cases where blood, stool, and urine are almost never collected, a directive to collect laboratory specimens in a suspected outbreak could have lethal consequences.[48]

In Western countries, the risk of hospital transmission is low. When one patient who exported Lassa fever to the United States died before a diagnosis was made, no hospital staff members were infected because routine infection control procedures were sufficient to prevent nosocomial spread of most highly virulent and transmissible agents, and health workers were familiar with protocols for specimen collection and handling. A similar course of events unfolded more recently in Europe and South Africa.[49] There are considerable, ongoing efforts to improve infection control around the world, but prevailing conditions in most African hospitals are not sufficient to prevent the initial spread of a virulent pathogen. However, African hospitals can step up infection control to stem an epidemic when one is identified. Of the approximately one hundred cases of Ebola reported among health workers at one Kikwit hospital, only one infection occurred after the etiologic agent had been named and barrier precautions had been taken by health workers. Burial practices in the community can also be temporarily modified in the event of an outbreak.[50] Unless these measures are put in place in the very early stages of an Ebola epidemic, rapid spread and high mortality will almost inevitably ensue.

Some have proposed that Western notions of contagion and the need for isolation cannot always be applied in the context of many African cultures.[51] Through patient care, sharing household utensils, and ritual instruments, but most importantly during the intricate preparations employed by some peoples prior to the burial of the dead, Ebola and similar pathogens can be rapidly disseminated through a community. Although these risk factors have been associated with the epidemic spread of hemorrhagic viruses, it has been repeatedly demonstrated that, with reasonable justification, African societies will modify customs to preserve life and health. "Ignorance" is often blamed for public health failures where the word is taken to mean the lack of public health education. In truth, ignorance arises from the failure to convey the necessary information or justifications to promote behavioral change. Too often, the outcome of an epidemic itself is the only source of information that people have. Investigators of the 1976 Yambuku Ebola outbreak were pleased to find that villagers were voluntarily enacting an effective quarantine and burying corpses away from communities.[52] In Kikwit, almost twenty years later, appropriately protected workers were permitted to perform potentially risky burial rites. Refusal to comply with potentially lifesaving public health orders can often be traced to mistrust of the Western health care delivery system.[53] Providing clear messages following precise diagnoses is one way to build trust.

After the 2000 Gulu Ebola epidemic, viral hemorrhagic diseases were added to Uganda's list of notifiable diseases,[54] and local health workers attended a one-day course on Ebola prevention and containment. Although both responses were essential and commendable,[55] it is not clear how primary health care workers can be expected to delineate future viral hemorrhagic fevers from malaria and other endemic diseases. In spite of the obvious benefits that could result from stronger laboratory support, modifications to the Gulu hospital after the outbreak focused on the development of isolation facilities: "A new purpose-built 28-bedded room and one single room isolation unit was put up. The medical ward was extended to allow more space per patient. Although there was no significant change in the laboratory aspects, the originally suspended laboratory activities during the Ebola outbreak returned to normal a few months after containment."[56]

The filovirus knowledge base has yet to generate a vaccine or cure, but we know what is needed to contain an Ebola epidemic: "barrier-nursing techniques, health education efforts, and rapid identification of cases."[57] Gulu has everything in place to isolate future Ebola cases, but no practical way to identify them. A late-arriving field lab staffed by the CDC offered on-site diagnostic testing, the first time that these facilities were available in an Ebola outbreak.[58] But there, as in Kikwit five years earlier, the internationally supported field lab was dismantled after the epidemic. Just as the 1995 Kikwit experience did little to inform events at Gulu in 2000, very few lessons learned from the 2000 epidemic were applied to the Ebola outbreak in rural Bundibugyo in 2007, where all that was received was a few years' worth of disposable protective supplies.[59]

Doctors at the Mercy of Lassa Virus

A Nigerian physician contracted a deadly infection while working in the village of Jalingo in Taraba state, northern Nigeria. On February 6, 2007, the doctor was admitted to a national hospital in the country's capital, Abuja, with a fever.[60] In a manner that is atypical for Nigeria, malaria and viral hepatitis were ruled out by testing, so a bacterial infection was the most likely diagnosis. By February 15, it became clear that the antibiotics he was receiving were not addressing his illness. He suffered renal failure and received kidney dialysis. Four days later, he was flown to South Africa, where Lassa fever, a viral hemorrhagic disease that is less well known but just as ghastly as Ebola, was diagnosed by RT-PCR and serology. He was immediately isolated and given appropriate supportive therapy. This physician was lucky on several counts. He managed to evade the almost routine prodrome of antimalarial therapy, which could have delayed his diagnosis. He was flown to a medical center that could diagnose, manage, and contain his infection. Many other West African doctors have not been so fortunate. The deaths of at least five physicians and seven nurses infected by undiagnosed patients in Nigeria and Sierra Leone have been chronicled in the medical literature;[61] many more deaths may be undocumented.

The genetic information in the core of Lassa virus, like that in Ebola and Marburg, is carried by single-stranded RNA, rather than the double-stranded DNA that carries the code in humans and other higher organisms. But the resemblance ends there. Lassa virus is an arenavirus having a granular, more compact appearance than the threadlike filoviruses.[62] The outer proteins of filoviruses and arenaviruses are completely different, so cross-immunity cannot occur. Lassa fever was first described by Jeanette Troup and her co-workers in 1970.[63] Troup, a missionary doctor in the Jos highlands of Nigeria, tended patients with what was then an unknown disease marked by fever and terminal bleeding. She investigated and documented the outbreak, but became infected and eventually died. The index case in that epidemic is believed to have come from the village of Lassa, which lies between Jos and Nigeria's border with Cameroon. Through contact with this patient, a missionary nurse became ill and eventually died in a Jos hospital. Health and laboratory workers associated with early definition of the virus and the disease in Africa and the United States contracted the deadly condition, and very few of them survived.[64] Lassa fever developed a lasting reputation for its "proclivity for killing doctors and nurses."[65]

Since the Nigerian outbreaks of 1969, most Lassa fever outbreaks have occurred in West Africa. Lassa fever is more prevalent than either Ebola or Marburg disease: a tentative estimate suggests that over three hundred thousand cases and five thousand deaths can be attributed to this disease across West Africa each year.[66] Like many "emerging" infectious diseases, Lassa fever existed long before humans noticed and named it. Lassa fever viruses from Sierra Leone and Nigeria are considerably divergent, supporting the idea that Lassa is an ancient disease. Eight unconnected Lassa fever cases or outbreaks were reported in the five years that followed its initial description. Sporadic cases and even outbreaks of the disease probably occurred before 1969 but were missed or misdiagnosed.[67]

Epidemiologic data collected in the two decades following the discovery of Lassa fever virus, including European studies showing antibodies to Lassa virus in the blood of returned expatriates, demonstrates that the pathogen is endemic in Nigeria, Sierra Leone, Guinea, and Liberia. (The use of returned travelers to estimate disease endemicity in Africa and other parts of the world has been likened to estimating the girth of a hippopotamus from its eyes as they peer above the water.[68]) The primary Lassa virus reservoir, the brown mastomys rat (*Mastomys natalensis*), is known, so human contacts with it can be controlled. It proved easier to identify the reservoir of Lassa than of Ebola because circumstantial evidence associating *Mastomys* with humans and the disease made the rodent a likely candidate for testing. This success, however, owes much to research conducted on the ground in endemic areas by African as well as visiting scientists. Many of these scientists were based at a viral research center of excellence, at Nigeria's University of Ibadan, where laboratory capacity has declined since the 1970s.

The first documented Lassa fever outbreak was amplified in a hospital; staff became infected while conducting autopsies, rather than through poor infection control. As with Ebola, hospital outbreaks of Lassa fever continue to occur, although available evidence suggests that they are typically less extensive and less likely to be overtly caused by medical procedures.[69] In a particularly ghastly instance, injections were identified as a risk factor for infection in two 1989 nosocomial outbreaks in eastern Nigeria, suggesting that needles were being reused. The poor quality of facilities, sterilizing equipment, record keeping, and auxiliary staff supports this inference. Retrospective analysis revealed that patients from one hospital who received the same injected drug from the same nurse on the same day were more likely to die of Lassa fever. Until every one of the medical staff and patients had either been infected by Lassa fever virus or fled the premises, Lassa fever was not diagnosed. The physicians never thought to refer their intractable patients to specialists, but treated them with antibacterial and antimalarial drugs, as well as fever reducers, for up to two weeks, largely administering the drugs through shared needles. When the doctors themselves fell ill, they were referred to the University of Nigeria Teaching Hospital. Lassa fever was suspected, but only confirmed posthumously in all three cases. A team of experts that investigated the outbreak months later concluded that it "mirrored the 1995 outbreak of Ebola hemorrhagic fever in Zaire, where introduction of the virus into a poorly run hospital led to several generations of infections."[70] Patients in such atrociously run institutions fare particularly badly when their diagnoses are unknown.

Lassa fever is clinically indistinguishable from Ebola or Marburg disease. However, the arenavirus Lassa appears to be restricted to West Africa, while filoviruses are more common in central and southern Africa. The real diagnostic challenge is that, particularly in the early stages, all three diseases share signs and symptoms with almost thirty other serious infectious conditions.[71] Outside a confirmed outbreak, a Lassa fever diagnosis is most commonly made in a patient with prolonged fever that does not respond to antimicrobial therapy. Drug resistance is becoming more commonplace among bacteria and malaria parasites, so using the patient as a diagnostic test tube in this manner becomes more and more unreliable over time. Lassa fever can kill within ten to fourteen days after symptoms start, so two courses of serial chemotherapy are sufficient to bring an undiagnosed patient precariously close to the grave.

Today, despite advances in treatment, 15 percent or more of Lassa fever patients that visit a health institution are likely to die, and mortality rates in facilities that lack diagnostic technology can exceed 50 percent. In southern Nigeria, a populous endemic epicenter for Lassa fever, investigation of epidemics in 2009 revealed that only two facilities were equipped to diagnose the disease.[72] Ribavirin, an antiviral drug, or convalescent sera from previously infected patients increase a patient's chance of survival by 90 percent if administered within six days of the onset of the disease. A Sierra Leone study found that "delays between onset and admission resulted in most patients not receiving ribavirin within the critical first six days," and a similar problem was noted at the Irrua Specialist Teaching Hospital, a Lassa fever treatment center in Nigeria.[73] West African hospitals cannot afford to administer ribavirin just in case: it has nasty side effects, including severe anemia, is complicated to administer, and an unsubsidized course cost about US$1,000 in 2007, twenty times the per capita expenditure on health care.[74] Diagnostic delay reduces the odds of a patient's survival and increases the possibility that the disease will be spread before it is identified.

Kenema Government Hospital, in Sierra Leone's third-largest city, is the world's center for Lassa fever treatment and has served as a site for clinical research on the disease for over thirty years. Diagnostic support and quality of care have fluctuated considerably during this period. In its early days, investigators from the CDC used the hospital as an outpost to study the epidemiology and ecology of Lassa fever virus, providing the baseline information that frames much of what is known about the disease. At that time, Lassa and other African hemorrhagic viruses may have been of interest not only because of scientific curiosity directed at a new and deadly disease but because of their potential as biological weapons.[75] Interest in Lassa fever research in both United States and Soviet scientific circles declined after the end of the cold war, diminishing the research and diagnostic capabilities at Kenema Government Hospital.[76] Retrospective laboratory confirmation of clinical diagnoses remained available until services at Kenema were severely disrupted by armed conflict in Sierra Leone.

Retrospective laboratory data has been important for understanding the epidemiology of and in highlighting a recent decline in the accuracy of clinical diagnosis of the disease. In the 1980s, clinical diagnosis of Lassa fever in highly endemic areas was estimated to have a high predictive value.[77] Prior to 1998, between six and seven of every ten presumptive Lassa fever cases were subsequently confirmed by laboratory tests. By 2000, the figure had dropped to about five in ten, suggesting that "apparent changes in infection patterns must be interpreted with caution." As Lassa fever can account for up to 15 percent of hospitalizations among adult patients in endemic areas,[78] diagnostic errors are not trivial. Unfortunately, laboratory diagnosis, which would resolve the uncertainties, is rarely used to enhance individual patient care in West Africa. A precise diagnosis is more likely to be obtained in South Africa, Europe, or North America than in places where the disease is endemic.

Compared to many other diseases endemic to West Africa, Lassa fever is still relatively uncommon, and few health workers are trained to diagnose, treat, and contain the disease. Until recently, Dr. Aniru S. Conteh was a principal occupant of that vital niche. The Sierra Leone–born, Nigeria-trained Lassa fever specialist was a well-placed authority in the Lassa fever field for a quarter of a century. On April, 4, 2004, the sixty-one-year-old physician died after a brief illness with fever, diarrhea, renal failure, and bleeding. Conteh had contracted an infection from a patient following a needle-stick injury. Presumptive Lassa fever was diagnosed, but the antiviral drugs and supportive care he received did not save him.

Dr. Conteh had spent most of his career battling to save the lives of hundreds who had the misfortune to be infected by the Lassa fever virus.[79] His clinical research and treatment advances contributed greatly to an 80 percent reduction in mortality from the disease by 2000. Indeed, this devoted physician's work was so profoundly admired and widely respected by the communities he served that his hospital was deliberately spared during multiple attacks on the city by antigovernment forces. It is shocking to learn that in order to confirm the presence of Lassa fever virus in the blood of Dr. Conteh, and the patient who infected him, specimens had to be sent from Sierra Leone to the National Institute for Communicable Diseases in South Africa, from the undisputed center of Lassa fever to a country where this infection never occurs naturally. Three years later, a Nigerian doctor was flown to South Africa to have his Lassa fever diagnosed and treated, placing numerous people involved in his evacuation and care at risk.[80]

Why is it that Lassa fever and its reservoir, first documented in Nigeria, where the disease remains endemic, cannot be identified at the national hospital in that country nearly forty years later? Why was the Nigerian hospital unable to detect an endemic virus, even though the same hospital was equipped to successfully implement the complicated procedure of kidney dialysis? Why is it that even though Nigeria probably has the most cases of Lassa fever in the world each year, in 2009 almost all cases defied diagnosis because only two laboratories had the necessary capacity? Why was the laboratory capacity to diagnose the disease not an integral part of Dr. Conteh's 2004 Lassa fever ward at Kenema Government Hospital in Sierra Leone? Conteh and his collaborators at the CDC had coauthored a study published in the *Journal of Clinical Microbiology* that focused specifically on the development of a diagnostic test for Lassa fever.[81] Why were effective diagnostic facilities unavailable at the station where they were most needed four years later?

Dr. Conteh is remembered for his dedication and resilience in fighting this deadly disease in the face of violent conflict, funding challenges, the changing priorities of international collaborators and donors, and limited facilities. His death engendered many concerns for the future. Obituaries published in leading medical journals lamented the loss of this key base for treating Lassa fever patients and the near impossibility of replacing a scientist-physician who pursued research and clinical care conjointly—and did so on African soil.[82] Patients voted with their feet and paid with their lives. The number of patients admitted to Kenema's Lassa fever ward declined from 321 in 2004 to nineteen in the first half of 2007. The same period saw a rise in the proportion of fatal cases from 25 percent in 2004 to 58 percent in 2007.

Finally, three Lassa fever–endemic countries, in a consortium that included virologists from Tulane University, the U.S. Army Medical Research Institute of Infectious Diseases, and the WHO, established the Mano River Union Lassa Fever Network, with a primary objective of increasing laboratory capacity in the "Mano River Countries" of Guinea, Liberia, and Sierra Leone. The first priority has been to replace the essentially derelict Lassa fever treatment and research facilities, which shut down when Conteh died. It took a couple of years to build the requisite Biosafety Level 3 Kenema lab and longer to equip it, but by the end of 2007 the consortium was able to announce that the lab was functioning and that comparable facilities were planned for Guinea and Liberia.[83] This development offers much promise, even though some of its impetus comes from biosecurity, rather than public health concerns.

Many physicians in Africa are highly skilled diagnosticians whose clinical guesses are often, but not always, right. They cure many patients but could address the illnesses of very many more if they were not handicapped in ways that could be resolved by simple tests. These tests are often described as impractical but, in fact, are both essential and feasible. Patients in endemic areas bear the brunt of this handicap and, in some cases, know it. A survey of "knowledge, attitudes and practice" conducted by the British charity Merlin, a principal supporter of Dr. Conteh's Lassa fever work at Kenema Government Hospital, reveals that laypeople in Sierra Leone are well informed about the risks posed by the disease and the need for more rigorous diagnosis. Patients, sufficiently aware of diagnostic imprecision, used the term "guessing" to describe the prevalent mode of diagnosis.[84] One patient group pleaded for a lab: "We are begging for a Lab, so we can go there for a proper check up...so we can be serious and fast to know which is the sickness, instead of giving blind treatment to people."[85]

Even people without medical training are aware that the most pivotal roles that a hospital could play are early and precise laboratory diagnosis and the administration of antiviral or supportive care in a safe environment. These services are never available outside of allopathic medicine and should be available within any scientific medical care system worthy of the name. Although emphasis is frequently on therapeutics, two complementary areas of deficiency loom large: diagnostics and infection control. Instead of meeting the charge to diagnose, contain, and manage disease, African hospitals have too often served to amplify epidemics, unwittingly mediating person-to-person transfer via diagnostic imprecision and suboptimal infection control. Infections acquired in this manner are more likely to be fatal than those acquired in the wild, and their impact detracts from the many more patients that hospitals bring to health.

Bringing the Diagnosis Home

In the last three months of 1984, a hospital in the small Brazilian town of Promissão admitted about two dozen children with conjunctivitis, high fevers, intestinal disturbances, and purple skin from bleeding capillaries. Many of the children died within twenty-four hours of reaching the hospital. Promissão hospital, and then the state of São Paulo, ruled out meningococcal meningitis and a number of other known diseases that have similar clinical presentation. By the time the U.S. CDC was called in to assist in investigating the strange epidemic of "Brazilian Purpuric Fever," it was clear that this was a new disease and that it was very likely caused by an unfamiliar strain of bacteria: *Haemophilus influenzae* biogroup aegyptius, which was isolated and identified from some patients. Presumptive identification of this bacterium prompted use of antibacterials to treat the strange syndrome, ultimately saving some patients' lives. Continuing research in Brazil and at the CDC confirmed this bacterium as the cause of the new disease, and, within three years, a rapid diagnostic test for the disease was deployed. The test was used to chart the epidemiology of the new pathogen inside and outside Brazil over the next twelve years.[86]

In contrast to Brazilian purpuric fever, diagnostic expertise for African hemorrhagic viral fevers has until very recently been based almost exclusively at locations that are far away from the places where they are endemic. Rather than augmenting local efforts and providing specialized technologies for confirming unusual or new diagnoses, Western centers of excellence are providing primary and secondary level care support for African patients. The prevailing model has been one in which outbreaks of hemorrhagic fever are identified after a considerable delay, and then experts in space suits are flown to the scene, where they work from laboratories housed in tents. Although these personnel provide valuable expertise and selfless service, their arrival is often accompanied by demoralization of local health workers, who have been struggling for weeks or months to contain an unidentified epidemic at great personal risk. Sometimes international experts even work independently, neglecting to communicate with local personnel, even though the two groups have the same goals.[87] Time and time again, field laboratories are set up to manage outbreaks and to procure specimens for distant laboratories, only to be dismantled when the epidemic wanes. Ebola and Marburg are localized in central and southern Africa, and Lassa fever is endemic to West Africa, so diagnostic and research facilities should be centered in these regions. Having laboratory capacity on the spot is the only way to mount continuous surveillance and recognize outbreaks early. Moreover, functional laboratories in endemic areas are better placed to provide testing with appropriate quality assurance, which is difficult to ensure in emergency outbreak labs or for small numbers of hurriedly shipped specimens.

A more useful and responsive diagnostic strategy would have frontline medical and laboratory personnel in local laboratories appropriately trained to recognize African viral hemorrhagic disease, respond to sporadic infections, and contain outbreaks quickly. The need to ship dangerous strains and specimens, as well as infected patients, would be reduced. The safety of local health workers, and their confidence in the health systems that employ them, would be better assured. Transmission patterns and reservoirs would be much more rapidly and effectively studied. Despite these obvious advantages, it was not until 2001 that an epidemiologic surveillance system for hemorrhagic fevers was set up to cover Congo and Gabon.[88] The network's mandate was to identify potential human and primate Ebola cases, relying on local hunters to report carcasses of suspected infected animals. Between the inception of this surveillance network and 2003, five human outbreaks of Ebola were reported, and in all but one of these index cases had likely contact with infected primates. The initial network has successfully predicted high-risk periods for human outbreaks from the occurrence and density of primate infections. The centers were also bases for recent research pointing to bats as reservoirs for Ebola and Marburg.[89] The surveillance enterprise has placed much-needed diagnostic and protective infrastructure on the ground, ensuring that it is available where and when outbreaks occur.

A 2004 Ebola outbreak in southern Sudan had a considerably better trajectory than earlier outbreaks because preliminary identification at a Kenyan lab hastened the confirmation of the epidemic. Community-based social mobilization and education began immediately, and no more than seventeen cases, seven deaths, and four generations of transmission were documented by the end of the outbreak. Diagnostics were unfortunately not available in the field, but the regional lab was still able to reduce the time from initial case presentation to diagnosis to less than a month, even in a remote area.[90] The laboratory development initiatives of the Mano River Union Lassa Fever Network may offer similar promise for Lassa fever diagnosis in Guinea, Liberia, and Sierra Leone. These projects need to be nurtured and used as a template for clinical laboratory development elsewhere on the continent. For example, the urgent need for diagnostic support to manage and control Lassa fever and other hemorrhagic infections is yet to be addressed in other endemic countries, including Nigeria, where the most virulent strains of the virus are believed to exist.[91] Similarly, not every country at risk of Ebola or Marburg outbreaks can identify hemorrhagic fevers caused by those viruses.

Africans are moving deeper into forests, and improved travel networks mean that an individual can move from the heart of the forest to a city with international connections in just a few hours. Contact with wildlife and the risk of contracting and spreading Lassa, Ebola, Marburg, and as yet unknown zoonotic infections will continue to rise. Repeated nosocomial outbreaks demonstrate that modern hospitals are sites where critically ill patients and their caregivers may face heightened risks of infection by blood-borne viruses when housed with infected but undiagnosed patients. At the time when yellow fever was a major scourge in Africa, three of the seven major yellow fever labs were located on the continent.[92] Even though the science of virology was only emerging at the time and a number of research roadblocks had to be surmounted, the vector was identified, and a vaccine was produced. Repeated flying in of space-suited superheroes equipped with mobile temporary laboratories is not a rational way to manage or learn from epidemics caused by emergent viruses. Floundering health workers and hospital amplification engender a justifiable lack of confidence in local health systems and are detrimental to containing the damage caused by these epidemics. The services of international expert teams are likely to be required in future large epidemics, irrespective of any diagnostic development, but sole dependence on this slap-dash protocol is not wise. In addition to time delays, considerable risk is associated with intercontinental transport of infected specimens harboring as-yet unidentified and possibly lethal viruses. Although the best scientific research is a global achievement, it is essential to focus diagnostic support and research in countries where the diseases occur in nature.

DETECTING COVERT INFECTION AHEAD OF THE FINAL DIAGNOSIS

> Now the bulk of the deaths were boringly similar. They were the
> deaths of lies. We heard there was the feared AIDS pandemic
> stalking the homesteads. Yet no one died of it. Or anything related
> to it.... At the funerals I mourned; the dreaded four letters were
> never mentioned, only TB and pneumonia and diarrhea. People died
> of silence. Of shame. Of denial. And this conspiracy resulted in a
> stigma that stuck like pubic lice on both the living and the dead.
>
> —Zakes Mda, 2007

One of the pathologist 'Ṣẹgun Ojo's lifelong gripes has been the steady decline of medical laboratory science in Nigeria. Aware of the pressing need to train a generation of competent laboratory diagnosticians and researchers, he committed himself to building the expertise necessary to remedy diagnostic insufficiency. I initially encountered Dr. Ojo in graduate school, when he was a lecturer, researcher, and consultant pathologist at western Nigeria's Obafemi Awolowo Teaching Hospitals complex. Formally and informally, he mentored residents and students working in subdisciplines as diverse as clinical chemistry, biochemistry, microbiology, and pathology, and encouraged many young practitioners to pursue careers in laboratory medicine. Ojo was subsequently appointed to head the department of Morbid Anatomy and Forensic Medicine at Obafemi Awolowo University, and named professor of anatomical pathology. Several years later, I spotted an article in the Nigerian *Guardian* newspaper reporting on his inaugural address, delivered a few years after he was elevated to the chair. Ojo's lecture, "The Pathologist, the Misery, the Mystery and the Final Diagnosis—An Interminable Quest for Excellence," outlined his work on the diagnosis and epidemiology of hepatitis B.[1]

Viral hepatitis is an inflammation of the liver caused by any of six or more viruses, hepatitis A, B, C, D, E, or F. Acute viral hepatitis, which many doctors can diagnose clinically, manifests as a rapidly debilitating illness with yellowed eyes, dark urine, and severe tiredness. The more common chronic form of the disease is less dramatic, so unseen infection persists until it manifests as liver cancer. Chronic hepatitis can only be diagnosed in the precancerous stage by measuring liver enzyme concentrations in the blood (as enzymes spill from damaged liver cells) or by detecting the viruses. Ojo, with other liver experts, determined that in Nigeria the disease is commonly caused by hepatitis B virus. Preventing infection is key, and a vaccine is advocated for use by health workers and any other at-risk populations. Diagnostic resources for blood screening also reduce the threat from the disease by preventing transfusions with infected blood. According to data collected by Ojo and others, as many as 15 percent to 20 percent of Nigerians may be chronically infected with hepatitis B virus, and most of them are unaware of their infection status. The virus is responsible for 50 percent to 80 percent of all liver cancers in Nigeria, and liver cancer is one of the most common cancers in that country.[2]

Across Africa, hepatitis B is among the most important causes of death in middle age. This disease is controllable, even technically eradicable, and it can be treated—but only at a cost that most Nigerians cannot afford. As decades can pass between the time of infection and the point of diagnosis and death from liver cancer, prevention and early diagnosis are key. In his inaugural lecture, Professor Ojo enunciated the great need for control of the hepatitis B virus and explained the central role that the laboratory must play in its control, prescreening all transfusion blood and testing and vaccinating health workers and other populations at risk. He emphasized the importance of creating at least one national liver care center with up-to-date diagnostic and therapeutic equipment.

The diagnostic dilemma posed by hepatitis B is also seen in many sexually transmitted diseases, for which symptoms in at least some infected people are few or none but long-term infection can be devastating or irreversible. Bacteria that cause sexually transmitted diseases are difficult to culture or manipulate genetically, making vaccine development a real challenge. Quick identification of infected people and prompt treatment, which in most cases is cheap, effective, and easy to administer, is an important way to diminish spread. Social stigma prevents many patients from seeking care overtly and frequently. Patients that are correctly diagnosed and treated in a single health-center visit are least likely to be lost to follow-up, a persistent problem with sexually transmitted infections.

Diagnosis is the lynchpin for disease control. Women infected with *Treponema pallidum,* the corkscrew-shaped bacterium that causes syphilis, can remain oblivious to their status until they bear a child that acquires the disease during delivery. A woman with syphilis can be easily treated with a single, inexpensive dose of penicillin, even while she is pregnant, so no child should have to begin life battling congenital syphilis. Testing and penicillin are cheap and assure the health of the mother and child; therefore, testing every pregnant woman is worthwhile, even where syphilis is rare. For gonorrhea and chlamydial infections, infected women, again usually asymptomatic, can become sterile or end up with dangerous ectopic pregnancies if their fallopian tubes become blocked by the disease. Babies born to women with these infections can catch them and in some cases are rendered blind. Again, usually irreversible damage can be prevented by timely diagnosis and treatment with effective medicine but most Africans with a sexually transmitted disease cannot access testing.

Underutilization of diagnostics for sexually transmitted diseases exacerbates gender disparities in health. Men with sexually transmitted diseases are more likely to have symptoms, and therefore symptom-based diagnosis can be effective. Women rarely show symptoms, and are more likely to suffer irreversible damage if not diagnosed with an appropriate test. Many existing tests do not serve women well. Urethral discharge from a man with gonorrhea can be fixed to a slide, stained directly and examined microscopically to reveal red pairs of spherical *Neisseria gonorrheae* bacteria. Results are available in minutes and all that is required for the test are the stains, slides, and a microscope. Swabs and discharge from women, however, even from symptomatic women, rarely detect *Neisseria* when they are present. Tests that will detect these bacteria in vaginal swabs are expensive and often too sophisticated or too unreliable to be used at regional health facilities in Africa.

Collecting samples and sending them to a reference lab means that some will be damaged during shipment, and that patients, who often have no symptoms and therefore little motivation, must return later for test results. When they do not return, the costs incurred in specimen transport and testing are wasted, and patients can continue to spread the disease. Therefore, rapid, point-of-care tests for syphilis, gonorrhea, and chlamydial disease are sorely needed. The impact that these tests could have goes beyond controlling these diseases and the irreversible damage they can cause. Lesions produced by these devastating but nonlethal sexually transmitted pathogens create portals for the AIDS virus.[3]

Surveillance and Denial of HIV/AIDS

The human immunodeficiency virus (HIV), the etiologic agent of AIDS, has come to emblematize present-day discourse on disease in Africa. In some circles, the mere mention of Africa conjures up images of emaciated people in their last ebb of life. Some foreigners have a vision of an entire continent's adult population passing away, leaving only helpless and neglected orphans, many of whom carry the virus themselves. Visitors with this vision of the continent who arrive in an African city and find citizens going about their daily lives with alacrity and ease are astounded. Depending on the country and the city, a visit to the local hospital could also contradict this highly publicized portrait of a dying continent. The disparity between the situation on the ground and the picture that has been so commonly projected is a baffling reality for many Africans as well. How could a wasting and ultimately fatal disease be endemic, yet so few persons be visibly ill? This disparity has led to skepticism about the nature, etiology, and epidemiology of AIDS. The skeptics, such as South Africa's former president Thabo Mbeki and his health minister, Dr. Manto Tshabalala-Msimang, appear almost ridiculous to the medical mainstream, and those directly affected by the disease find their skepticism incomprehensible and their inaction outrageous.[4] In other circles, particularly those with close ties to certain parts of West Africa, skeptics are heroes.

For far too long, and in too many critical instances, Africa has been considered as a continuous whole, with each African a unitized part of that whole. Because thousands upon thousands of people were dying of AIDS in parts of East Africa and southern Africa, many outsiders assumed that the disease was taking the same toll in towns and villages in Mali, Ghana, Nigeria, and Sudan. Data derived from relatively small and biased studies in the places where HIV infection was prevalent and AIDS appeared first were extrapolated to apply to those countries and then to the whole continent. Many of the figures and images suggested that every African must have a loved one who had perished from the disease, even if he or she was not ill or infected. In fact, in 2002 much of the population of Africa had not yet seen a case of full-blown AIDS. Whereas many people in Uganda and Botswana found the reports of HIV overtaking their continent perfectly consistent with the rising number of sick people, burials, and orphaned children, many West Africans who listened to the figures regarded them as what Benjamin Disraeli might have catalogued as "lies, damned lies, and statistics."[5]

Unfortunately for the credibility of Western medicine on the continent, the historical record is replete with instances in which European colonial officials falsely alleged that epidemics of sexually transmitted infections were occurring in Africa. Anxieties about sexually transmitted diseases were part of a colonialist mentality that regarded Africans as members of a "primitive race" who were unable to exercise rational, moral control over their bodily sexual impulses.[6] In 1897, for example, the supposed rapid and widespread dissemination of syphilis in colonial Africa caught the attention of British medical practitioners. Megan Vaughan has drawn attention to a series of papers published in London about a syphilis outbreak that allegedly was ravaging the Baganda, a people of the Buganda region in present-day Uganda. The population in question was presumed to have had no previous exposure to the disease; the epidemic was said to be occurring on "virgin soil," so it spread especially rapidly. According to the initial report by army medic Colonel Lambkin, 80 percent of adults were infected, and the entire clan was perilously close to being wiped out. Lambkin's article was followed by a series of papers ascribing the epidemic to causes including the decline of traditional gender norms, resulting in an uncontrolled expression of women's "strong passions," and the failure of the people of Buganda to embrace Christian morality.[7]

This racist and sexist discourse continued in Britain's foremost medical journals for months, with contributions from clergymen as well as medics. The vast majority of the "syphilitic" Baganda presented with skin lesions, and the cure rates following administration of mercury injections were much better than has previously been documented for sexually transmitted syphilis, or the congenital form of the disease. Unfortunately, these observations, although carefully noted, did not suggest to the medics engaged in "saving" the Baganda that they were dealing with an entirely different disease. It is now clear that the Baganda rarely, if ever, had sexually transmitted syphilis; rather, they had some other form of treponemal disease, perhaps yaws, or more likely a less severe version of syphilis produced by a tradition of deliberately inoculating children with *Treponema* to produce a mild disease that would protect them from more virulent infections later in life.[8] What was never clarified to the avid readers of the *Lancet* and the *British Medical Journal* is that the basis for this stigmatizing epidemiology was clinical presentation and a positive Wassermann reaction, a serological laboratory test that cannot distinguish true venereal syphilis from treponemal diseases that are not sexually transmitted.[9]

The unfounded assumptions and unwarranted inferences that underlie the discussion of the supposed syphilis epidemic in Uganda at the turn of the twentieth century are evident in the initial reports about AIDS in Africa as well, and Africans' well-founded concerns about the invidious intent and systematic errors of colonialist medicine have shaped their responses to reports about the epidemic.

Recalling numerous instances similar to the supposed Buganda syphilis epidemic, many Africans concluded that the AIDS epidemic was a new stereotypical and subjugating Western fiction. It did not help that other subpopulations commonly associated with the disease—gay men and injection drug users— were marginalized in Western culture. Many members of Africa's intelligentsia, including physicians, familiar with earlier case studies labeling Africa "the infectious continent," stubbornly refused to accept the "myth" of AIDS. In too many cases, the very people who might have spearheaded HIV intervention programs derided them. Persons living outside regions where HIV-related deaths are commonplace have on occasion refused to be tested or to protect themselves from the virus, believing that condoms and abstinence messages are being used to curb Africa's population growth. In the 1980s, AIDS, called SIDA in French, was variously described as the "American Idea of Discouraging Sex" or "Syndrome

Imaginaire pour Déscourager les Amoureux," the Imaginary Syndrome to Discourage Lovers.[10] Health care workers have even been reported as taking inadequate precautions to protect themselves and other patients from infection.[11]

Initial HIV antibody tests occasionally drew false positives. This is a common problem with antibody tests in general—the Widal test for typhoid fever, for example, is even more nonspecific than the earliest HIV tests. During development, diagnostic tests are typically developed and validated using samples from non-African patients so that even tests that perform well elsewhere can perform less well in Africa. The difficulty in deciphering the cause of AIDS when the disease first appeared, coupled with the urgent need for a test to diagnose the infected and screen transfusion products, meant that AIDS diagnosis was particularly prone to insufficiently specific first-generation tests. Today's tests are much more reliable than their predecessors, and at least two tests, one of which is not an antibody test, are needed to confirm each HIV infection.[12] There were unavoidable but marked social implications of using nonspecific tests for HIV in Africa, where similarly nonspecific Wasserman tests had led to overestimation of syphilis prevalence rates several decades before. Among them was the muddling of the problem of test limitations, which were rapidly resolved, with denialist hypotheses that discounted the existence of the virus altogether.

Most recent epidemiological studies adequately address the problems with HIV tests and, whether the results are required for patient care or research, it is standard practice to use more than one test to confirm the results. Therefore, people documented as HIV positive from the 1990s are indeed infected with the virus. However, the final figures presented in some reports have inflated HIV prevalence continent-wide because of sampling bias. It makes sense to start by seeking cases in a high-risk catchment group and conduct small point-prevalence studies in order to establish or disprove the presence of a disease. However, after the presence of HIV had been established, samples were still far too often drawn from antenatal clinics in urban centers, where HIV research and health delivery services were justifiably located. Research focused on HIV prevalence in young, pregnant, urban women—one of the most sexually active subpopulations, and the least able to protect themselves from sexually transmitted diseases. In malaria-endemic areas, this subpopulation is also among those most likely to receive blood transfusions, so this group is exposed to multiple risk factors for HIV.

Other overestimations arose from HIV tests performed only on patients with symptoms that suggested they might have opportunistic infections, again the product of convenience sampling. One study in Nigeria recorded a 25 percent prevalence of HIV in this subpopulation.[13] This figure appears low given the test population, but if viewed outside its original context it can be misinterpreted to mean that HIV prevalence is extraordinarily high. At the regional level, more data comes from countries with high HIV prevalence than from those with fewer patients with full-blown AIDS. Researchers did not always assume that data based on antenatal testing or other skewed samples accurately reflected prevalence rates in the general population, but, in the absence of sentinel surveillance or the kinds of generalized testing programs that were established in Europe and North America, these were the only data available when public officials made projections and reporters needed a sound bite.[14] When testing is uncommon, data used to inform health policy or by the media is more likely to be inaccurate.

Obtaining unbiased data is extremely difficult in the case of a pathogen as biologically and socially complex as HIV. Drawing data from people who volunteer to be tested could show higher prevalence rates than the general population because people with risk factors or symptoms may be more likely to request a test. In places where AIDS is heavily stigmatized, volunteer testing could underestimate prevalence. Nonetheless, even this type of data, which can be procured from health systems in countries where appropriate laboratory tests routinely accompany diagnosis, is a preferable substitute when population-based data is unavailable.

Making unwarranted generalizations from data collected in high-prevalence parts of Africa may have done as much harm as good. A more region-specific and precise mode of data collection might have provided information that locals could reconcile with their own environments, giving them a realistic view of their actual risk. In Senegal, where testing at four sentinel sites began in 1989 and was coupled with aggressive AIDS education and intervention programs, HIV prevalence rates may have been held down.[15] The failure to rapidly provide adequate and accurate support for the then hypothesis that HIV was present and spreading in some parts of Africa helped alternate hypotheses gain dangerous ground. Among the most popular are denialists who claim that AIDS is not caused by HIV and therefore cannot be managed with antiretroviral drugs or contained by limiting viral transmission. (Any reader still swayed by denialist claims that HIV does not cause AIDS or that antiretrovirals do not prolong the lives of AIDS patients should read the article by Pride Chigwedere and Myron Essex, which systematically and directly addresses these and other denialist arguments[16]).

Although we must acknowledge holes in surveillance, the present state of HIV diagnosis is perhaps the best example of diagnostic development on the continent. In contrast to other common infectious diseases of which less than 5 percent of the infected are diagnosed with a test, laboratory diagnosis now occurs in the majority of patients who are told they are HIV positive. Nonetheless, the diagnostic resources for HIV in most parts of Africa are insufficient to catalog the demographic and socioeconomic effects of the disease, or even to ensure that apparently healthy people can easily be made aware of their infection status. Diagnostic support for treating HIV-positive people is grossly inadequate, and HIV surveillance remains suboptimal. Some commentators have argued that gathering precise figures would be a merely academic exercise. They contend that if the line is too long to be reasonably attended to, it really does not matter how long it is. However, a recent theoretical model suggests otherwise: universal testing and access to antiretrovirals would lower transmission rates.[17] Moreover, exaggerations of the state of the HIV epidemic in both directions—underestimates and overestimates—have been extreme, and they remain dangerous because they undermine intervention programs, which today are necessarily largely focused on changing behaviors. Inadequate surveillance data are fostered by continuing diagnostic insufficiency and adversely affect prevention and treatment of the disease, irrespective of how widespread it is at different localities.

Death Emerges from Its Pouch

The presence of HIV-infected persons throughout Africa is indisputable, although the extent to which the documented prevalence of AIDS reflects actual epidemiology is open to debate. Awareness of risk has come quite belatedly, an unfortunate result of the skepticism that attended early reports. As recently as 1996, health workers in Nigerian primary, secondary, and even tertiary care institutions were not taking sufficient precautions to protect themselves from HIV and other blood-borne diseases. Although some information suggested that local people were becoming infected with the virus, most West Africans did not encounter anyone with the disease until 2002 or even beyond. The average Nigerian remained ignorant of the threat from HIV/AIDS; too many were denialists. The images of emaciated patients projected from several countries in East Africa and southern Africa were attributed to greater tourism in those areas, as AIDS was seen as a Western import associated with the "foreign" cultures of homosexuality and intravenous drug use. Just as the United States received its belated kick in the pants from actor Rock Hudson's HIV infection, Nigeria's first AIDS reality check came not from the health ministry but from popular music. Most Lagosians can recall exactly where they were on August 3, 1997, when the world was told that Fela Anikulapo-Kuti was dead.

In the 1970s, in spite of their English teachers' best intentions, Nigerian elementary school children acquired their first words in creole or pidgin English, a fashionable lingua franca of unschooled and urban professionals alike, by singing Fela's smash hit "Suffering and Smiling." In the face of back-to-back repressive military regimes, many of these children later gained political awareness by interpreting its lyrics. Fela's life and work were shaped by a striking mix of talent, energy, obstinacy, and scandalous behavior that in some eyes branded him a scoundrel. Devising his own genre of music, Afrobeat, he rapidly achieved international fame. Fela set up a music studio within his self-proclaimed "independent" Kalakuta republic, which was destroyed by Nigerian soldiers in 1977. He was repeatedly harassed by successive Nigerian military governments, and once convicted, but he would not be silenced. Fela's best music was political satire, and Nigeria's tumultuous postindependence regimes gave him much to make music about. Even more entertaining than his many recordings were the works he performed live at his Lagos Shrine, as well as on tour with his Africa 70 and then Egypt 80 bands. The Afrobeat king is also famed for his numerous concubines and wives; he married twenty-seven of them in a single day to commemorate Kalakuta's destruction.

Fela was born into the illustrious and multitalented Ransome-Kuti family in 1938. His father, Reverend Ransome-Kuti, was a minister and high school principal in Abeokuta. His mother, 'Funmi Ransome-Kuti, was the first Nigerian woman to secure a driver's license and one of her country's earliest and best known feminist activists. His two brothers, Beko and Olikoye, were internationally renowned physicians.[18] Beko remained a popular left-wing political critic until his death in 2006. Olikoye, a public health specialist, pioneered primary care initiatives in Nigeria and remained, until his death, one of the few incorruptible Nigerian public officials.

Claiming that the first part of his hyphenated surname had slave origins, Fela changed it from Ransome to Anikulapo, that is, one who carries death sealed in a pouch. It was a huge shock to all who knew of him when, in 1997, before his fiftieth birthday, the seemingly invincible Fela died. In a clear departure from the typical obituary following death at an early age, Fela's demise was not attributed to an unnamed "brief illness." His brother Olikoye publicly announced that Fela Anikulapo-Kuti, the world-renowned musician and sociopolitical critic, had died of complications from AIDS. In a cultural climate in which AIDS was considered foreign and heavily stigmatized, the family's statement was uncharacteristically open. Nigerians received the news with profound shock. Fela himself, like most Nigerians of that time, was a well-known denialist,[19] but his death from AIDS made it increasingly difficult not to believe that HIV might lurk in Lagos. Lest anyone remain of the opinion that the HIV virus was completely absent from Nigeria or that the medical community had the epidemic under control, a decade later Adewunmi Eniola was projected from obscurity when he became the much-publicized, not-so-proud father of an HIV positive baby. The case garnered more publicity than most because Eniola claimed that he and his wife were HIV negative and that the baby must have been infected at the Lagos University Teaching Hospital.[20]

By the end of 2004, although the reported prevalence rate had started to level off (a drop from 5.8% to 5.0% had been reported), the statistics were grim and the Nigerian media had begun a campaign to encourage people to believe them. This report from the Nigerian United Nation's Development Program office was published in *This Day,* a Lagos newspaper:

> According to official statistics, 3.5 million Nigerians already live with HIV and AIDS, which is more than the entire population of some countries. About 300,000 Nigerians die annually of AIDS-related diseases and 1.5 million Nigerian children have been made orphans as a result of these deaths. The fact that Nigeria's prevalence rate is in single digit [*sic*] can be misleading and can give a false sense of security. In real fact, Nigeria has the second highest number of infection [*sic*] in Africa, going by the actual figures, not the percentages. Also, the 3.5 million Nigerians living with HIV and AIDS account for about 10% of the 40 million people infected worldwide and 20% of those affected in Africa, the world's most affected continent.[21]

Other estimates place HIV prevalence in Nigeria at between 3 percent and 4 percent.[22] Nonetheless, all but a dwindling number of denialists concur that a large number of people are at risk in Africa's most populous country. Regardless of how low prevalence rates might be, in the face of continued diagnostic insufficiency they translate into large numbers of incognizant infected people who could spread the disease and have limited access to preventive interventions and treatment.

Diagnosis, "Cure," and Treatment of HIV/AIDS

It is not clear why the AIDS epidemic in Nigeria—just as in some neighboring West African countries—appears, by all measures, to be less extensive and/or more recent than the epidemics in such countries as Botswana, Uganda, or Zambia. A recently identified protective effect of male circumcision is likely to have contributed to some degree. Other credible hypotheses about contributing causes include religious and cultural differences, less contact with tourists, less effective health systems for documenting disease, and lower rates of contact with nonhuman primates. Still other explanations that have been proffered for the higher rates elsewhere include infection due to indigenous or allopathic surgery, blood transfusion, or sharing injection needles in health centers. What is clear from the diversity of theories is that the burden of disease attributable to AIDS varies across the continent.[23] The magnitude, causes, and implications of this variation are not well understood, mostly because they have not been studied systematically.

Because antiretroviral drugs were largely unavailable at the time AIDS emerged from partial seclusion in West Africa, the demand for anything that could help AIDS patients was insistent and unsatisfied. In response, providers stepped rapidly into the vacancy. The disease was new and frightening, patients were desperate, the ineffectiveness of many spurious treatments was not proven, and regulatory oversight was weak. Anyone courageous and foolhardy enough to claim they had a cure for AIDS was able to make such assertions with relative impunity. All over the continent, spiritual, herbal, and other cures were advertised and paid for. Although Nigeria had barely acknowledged the presence of the disease, many local "experts" claimed to know exactly how to cure it.[24]

A group of concerned researchers investigated awareness, diagnoses, and treatment modalities among indigenous medical practitioners. Their study was performed in Ile-Ife, the "cradle of the Yoruba race," the origin of Yoruba traditional religion and of the Ifa priesthood, as well as the home of one of Nigeria's most prestigious universities and its teaching hospital. Professor of pharmacy Anthony Elujoba and his colleagues interviewed fifty-one indigenous healers, most of whom claimed to have acquired their training in the management of sexually transmitted diseases and HIV/AIDS from their ancestors or during their apprenticeship—even though the disease emerged after they became healers. Twenty-two practitioners, almost half of those interviewed, stated that they had treated at least one AIDS patient.[25] Fifteen said that they typically relied on an allopathic practitioner to determine the HIV serostatus of their patients, but clinical signs and symptoms played a large part in the diagnosis of AIDS by indigenous practitioners. Five admitted that their diagnoses were based on patients' "confessions," and fourteen, including some of those who received "confessions" from some patients, had "guessed" that their patients had AIDS. Interestingly, all the practitioners claimed that their patients were cured, but verification was in most cases based on clinical observation alone, on the patient's testimony, and/ or on a supernatural source. Only eight claimed to have requested that a hospital verify that the patient was cured.

Although all the practitioners interviewed claimed to have cured AIDS, most had not notified anyone about cures in specific cases. Five practitioners told other traditional practitioners, but four admitted to being unsure that their treatment was efficacious. Two-thirds (fourteen) stated simply that there was no need to advertise the feat, and two practitioners said that no one would believe them. The researchers concluded that "it is rather difficult to accept or reject traditional practitioners' claims of caring for people with HIV/AIDS as some of the diagnostic symptoms used can neither be confirmed nor rejected as being valid in the absence of confirmation of positive HIV serostatus of clients."[26]

This dilemma exists across Africa. Kenyan Arthur Obel claimed that his Pearl Omega drug could cure AIDS; the Gambian head of state has offered a spiritual cure for AIDS; and a Ghanaian herbalist was reportedly slain in connection with intellectual property disputes surrounding his therapy. Before antiretrovirals were sanctioned by its government, the most popular AIDS treatment in South Africa was a pair of herbal mixtures called uBhejane.[27] The mixtures were not evaluated in clinical trials, but the first was reputed to increase $CD4^+$ counts and the second to lower viral load. Low counts of the $CD4^+$ cells that are depleted by HIV, and increased viral loads, are laboratory indicators that are used to determine the point at which HIV-infected individuals progress to AIDS. Even though the value of many cure claims is stated in units defined by Western laboratory medicine, in far too many cases diagnostic shortfalls have made it impossible to validate or disprove them.

Another widely publicized claim, perhaps second only to uBhejane, has come from a practitioner of "orthodox" allopathic medicine. In 1999, Nigerian physician Jeremiah Abalaka contended that he had devised a vaccine-based protection and cure for AIDS. Like the indigenous practitioners interviewed by Elujoba and his colleagues, he refused to disclose the nature of his medicine. Public health officials and the Nigerian media emphasized the need to validate Abalaka's claims by studying his "curative vaccine." No effort has been devoted to pre- and posttherapy testing of his bevy of patients, which would have been one way to validate or dispute his claim without his cooperation. Abalaka's case, which could easily have been verified or disputed by biomedicine was instead mediated by the courts.[28]

Abalaka has published his "Attempts to Cure and Prevent HIV/AIDS in Central Nigeria between 1997 and 2002: Opening a Way to a Vaccine-Based Solution to the Problem?"[29] In this unusual scientific paper, Dr. Abalaka was careful to state that his findings did not represent a systematic clinical trial but rather a report of his practice over five years. He noted that $CD4^+$ cell assays, which validate HIV infection and serve as a measure for the progression of AIDS and as an indicator of patients' general health, as well as all other laboratory tests, had been procured off-site, at patients' expense. Abalaka observes that "in Nigeria, there is no free laboratory investigation or medication for any person including those with HIV infection."[30] Although his critics, myself included, debate the rest of the report, the lack of access to laboratory diagnosis and appropriate treatment is undeniable. Essentially, Abalaka, his cure, and cases like this thrive because of deficits in laboratory medicine.

Diagnostic insufficiency in relation to HIV has other risks. Estimates of how many people acquire the disease following transfusion of tainted blood range from eighty thousand to 160,000 worldwide. In many parts of Africa, the need

for transfusions is high because of endemic *falciparum* malaria, but 2007 estimates of banked blood tainted with HIV range from under 1 percent in South
Africa, Rwanda, and Namibia to 2.5 percent in Nigeria and 7 percent in Mozambique.[31] Other blood-borne viruses, including hepatitis B, are even more likely
to be transmitted. The capacity to store donated blood is often limited, so donations are often made at the point of need by family members or paid donors.
A test that can verify the safety of blood within minutes is vital.

Western medicine still offers no generally applicable cure for AIDS, but HIV
infection is no longer an automatic death sentence. Today, in most of Europe
and North America, HIV-infected people can live relatively normally, and they
survive much longer than their counterparts did two decades ago. A huge debate
ensued over whether life-saving antiretrovirals should be supplied to the poor in
countries that could not procure them at the high prices charged by the pharmaceutical companies that initially developed them. The lack of infrastructure
and personnel for laboratory monitoring was frequently cited as a reason for
withholding antiretrovirals from Africans, a claim that is becoming as irksome as
the earlier insinuation that Africans could not tell time well enough to take their
medications on schedule. Although it is true that laboratory services are needed
to use antiretrovirals properly, they are also needed to use antimicrobials that
have been available in Africa for decades. In those cases, as well as in the case of
HIV, WHO director general Jim Yong Kim's criticisms of those who compare
price with patients' economic means, weigh human lives against money, and
enounce the prevention versus treatment "false dichotomy" all apply.[32]

The argument against providing antiretrovirals because of the absence of appropriate laboratory support for their administration became the most popular reason to deny AIDS patients in poor countries life-saving medicines. This
argument could be supported by evidence, and was less unpopular because it
criticized systems rather than people. The fact that this point gained so much
ground in the debate illustrates that there are health policymakers who believe
that the infeasibility of diagnostic development justifies the deaths of thousands.
This argument has been tacitly accepted for many other infections for decades,
but the antiretroviral lobby—one of the most effective in developing-country
health—has been able to overcome it for HIV. It is now generally acknowledged
that even though testing facilities are still scarce, they can and have been set up in
the most resource-poor parts of the world, and should be expanded.

At Makerere University in Kampala, Uganda, the infrastructure had not been
updated in thirty-five years until a new AIDS center was commissioned in April
2004. The center was provided with state-of-the-art diagnostic and patient management facilities through generous donations from industry and many nongov-
ernmental organizations. The opening of the center in August 2004 was extremely
timely, for it provided the facilities necessary for the conduct of clinical trials of

antiretroviral drugs and AIDS vaccines. Thus, the donation of US$15 million from Pfizer, a major developer of anti-AIDS treatments, is as much a simple act of charity as a matter of self-interest. Notwithstanding, this center and others like it have greatly boosted biomedical science in Africa. Importantly, the center demonstrates that sophisticated diagnostic and treatment facilities are not out of place or unnecessary in Africa, and its success shows that it is not the white elephant that such facilities were often predicted to be.

Optimal Laboratory Testing Promotes Control

People who know their HIV infection status can be empowered to assist in containing the spread of the virus. Unfortunately, not every African who needs antiretrovirals has access to them today, and not every African who is taking anti-retrovirals has access to supportive diagnostic resources. Each patient should have a positive HIV test (determined by at least two methods), a CD4$^+$ count, and, if possible, a viral load estimation before commencing antiretroviral therapy. The last two parameters need to be periodically monitored during treatment. Many patients in Africa are started on antiretrovirals based on clinical criteria alone. The lack of laboratory verification has clinical consequences because patients who are not correctly "staged" before they start antiretroviral therapy may fare worse than patients who receive a proper laboratory workup. CD4$^+$ T-cells are the immune-system cells invaded, and destroyed, by the AIDS virus. In order to determine which patients are precariously close to immune deficiency, the CD4$^+$ cells in a blood sample from the patient are labeled—to distinguish them from other white blood cells—and counted by a laser in a machine called a flow cytometer. Flow cytometry is expensive but offering this service for HIV patients is cost effective because antiretroviral drugs are essential but expensive. If patients' CD4$^+$ levels can be precisely monitored, costs associated with starting therapy too early or too late can be avoided. Laboratory monitoring is also essential to determine when the treatments of patients who are on antiretrovirals need to be updated.[33]

Globally, diagnostic requirements for HIV-infected patients have moved beyond ascertaining infection and estimating CD4$^+$ counts and viral loads. Because drug-resistant viruses have become widespread, clinicians of newly diagnosed or unresponsive patients in the West order genetic testing on viruses infecting their patients. From the DNA sequence of viral target genes, clinicians can predict which antiretrovirals a patient's virus will be susceptible to and therefore which drugs to prescribe. This type of personalized medicine, often touted as the medicine of the future, is available in Western HIV clinics today. HIV replicates rapidly and mutates quickly, but patients must receive drugs for life. Therefore, drug resistance is an inevitable consequence of antiretroviral therapy, and only by sequence typing of viruses can we be sure that every patient receives effective treatment, and that resistant viruses do not become more commonplace than susceptible ones. With so many HIV-infected people and the most difficulties in ensuring antiretroviral access, many countries in Africa are at greatest risk of being overwhelmed by resistance if diagnostic infrastructure and requirements are not strengthened.

In 1988, before the diagnostic development forced by the antiretroviral access debate, the WHO recommended that, in the absence of the necessary diagnostic testing resources, a set of standard clinical indicators be used as a surrogate for diagnosing AIDS. The clinical case definition (CCD) for AIDS includes tuberculosis, Kaposi sarcoma, and other opportunistic infections. Supra-infections in AIDS patients vary with location, so considerable local modification is essential to implement this model.[34] Even when region-specific definitions are incorporated, the effectiveness of CCD has always been questionable, but it continues to be used in some parts of Africa today. In a Tanzanian study, the CCD protocol was shown to have a very high positive predictive value and specificity (both over 90%), but an extremely low sensitivity (36.6%)—that is, almost all patients with late-stage, full-blown AIDS were readily identified, but two-thirds of those with less obvious symptoms of HIV infection were missed. Patients who fit the clinical profile recommended for diagnosing AIDS were close to death. Those whose infection might be treated and who might be enabled to avoid transmitting HIV to others were not identified. Nor were individuals coming to the end of the asymptomatic stage, whom Brandy Rapatski, Frederick Suppe, and James Yorke[35] have proposed are principal drivers of the HIV pandemic, because they have a high viral load but no symptoms.

HIV infection and the imminence of AIDS can be diagnosed with virtually 100 percent precision by detecting the virus and by measuring CD4$^+$ levels. There are very basic tests for HIV, and many can be used in resource-poor laboratories or even at the point of care. Late-stage clinical diagnosis of AIDS on the other hand places clinicians on par with laypeople, including quacks, all of whom can clinically diagnose a case of AIDS at the time of death with precision.[36] But responsive health systems need to be able to spot HIV infection before it is too late to intervene. Presently, as with hepatitis B–induced liver cancers and congenital syphilis, too many patients discover that they are HIV positive only when they develop AIDS. Diagnostic development and the distribution of antiretroviral drugs have begun, but they must be closely coordinated as well as accelerated in order to stem HIV epidemics in Africa.

DIAGNOSTIC CERTAINTY AND DISEASE CONTROL

Before attempting the heroic cure of disease, we seek first to ascertain its true nature.

—Ronald Ross, 1905

Despite media images that portray Africa as a disease-plagued continent and the concerns expressed, even by medical and public health experts, that in Africa health targets are often set but rarely achieved,[1] some well-planned and properly implemented programs have met with success. Smallpox was eradicated, guinea worm and polio have almost disappeared, and campaigns to control other vector-borne or vaccine-preventable diseases, notably measles and river blindness, are making impressive progress.[2] Many effective strategies for disease control are disarmingly simple: clean water, adequate nutrition, and depletion of the vectors, such as mosquitoes, that transmit infection. These interventions, which have been primarily responsible for infectious disease control in the West, can break the chain of transmission for many communicable diseases at once. Vaccines, insecticides, and medicines that target specific diseases augment these measures.[3] Laboratory science often plays an important behind-the-scenes role in disease control, particularly when it involves biomedical tools that are necessary components of today's ambitious disease eradication programs.

Globally, we have attempted to eradicate only a handful of human diseases and have not yet succeeded in eliminating most of them.[4] The social and economic benefits of eradication are so great, however, that the single success—smallpox—and the few near successes more than justify all failures. Eradication offers the supremely attractive prospect of never having to deal with a disease, or its causative organism, ever again. Premature deaths and disabling illnesses are prevented, and resources that would have been expended on preventing or treating the disease can be diverted to other causes. Eradication campaigns must be built on a practical foundation. As experience has repeatedly demonstrated, the worst scourges are not always the easiest to eradicate.

Eradication Successes

Smallpox, which killed or disabled and disfigured countless people throughout most of recorded history, probably emerged around 10,000 BCE, when human societies shifted from the dispersion and seasonal migration required by hunting and gathering to more permanent and compact agricultural settlements. Because the virus infects each person only once and cannot survive for long outside the human body, it can maintain its existence only in settled and interconnected communities. According to the best estimates, a population of roughly two hundred thousand humans connected by not more than fourteen days of travel was needed to sustain smallpox. The dumbbell-shaped virus, which perhaps evolved from a rodent pathogen, seems to have been spread from Africa to India by Egyptian merchants in the last millennium BCE. Muslim clergy inadvertently carried smallpox across other parts of Africa and to Europe during the Middle Ages, and in 1519 Spaniards took the virus to the Americas. In Mexico City, then known as Tenochtitlan, a disastrous epidemic that both the immune *conquistadores* and the vulnerable Aztecs found shocking led to the fall of the fortified capital. Indeed, smallpox was the principal weapon that enabled the Spanish to subjugate the indigenous peoples. Within a single generation, it had wiped out a third of Mexico's native population. International trade in spices and other exotic items and the growing traffic in enslaved Africans ensured that by the eighteenth and nineteenth centuries smallpox had spread around the world. This single scourge accounted for one-tenth of all deaths and took a higher toll during epidemics. In the mid-twentieth century, just before the global smallpox eradication program began, the disease killed two or three million people and disfigured or disabled another ten to fifteen million every year.[5]

Interest in smallpox eradication emerged in the early nineteenth century, but it was not until 1967 that the WHO made its formal, landmark commitment to that goal. The program began just as an expensive malaria eradication effort was clearly failing, which raised doubts about the very idea of eradication. However, the proposal to eliminate smallpox was supported by substantial evidence of success: by the 1960s, smallpox had been eliminated from Europe, North America, East Asia, and North Africa. The elimination of the disease from the Soviet Union convinced the World Health Assembly to revisit the idea of eradicating smallpox from the thirty-three countries in Asia, South America, and sub-Saharan Africa that were its "last frontier."[6]

The major innovation that made smallpox eradicable was an effective vaccine. The first vaccinations, which were actually variolations, used material derived from smallpox and entailed significant risks. Those seeking to attain lifelong immunity inhaled dried powdered scabs or, more commonly, had their skin scarified and inoculated with fluid from active pustules. Variolation usually produced mild disease, but it could also cause full-blown and potentially fatal smallpox. The Vedas, the sacred Sanskrit texts of ancient India, contain the following passage: "put the fluid from the pustule onto the point of a needle, and introduce it into the arm, mixing the fluid with the blood; a fever will be produced but this illness will be very mild."[7] Although more is known about variolation in Asia and western Europe than in Africa, several African ethnic groups had developed vaccination protocols before extensive European contact, and the practice probably reached the Americas through the slave trade. Indeed, the feared Yoruba Ṣọpọnọ cult, banned by special ordinance in 1907, could deliberately spread the disease without becoming infected themselves, suggesting that variolation may have been part of initiation rites.[8]

In 1798, Edward Jenner, observing that people who got cowpox never seemed to catch smallpox,[9] developed a remarkably successful cowpox-based vaccine, which was the precursor of the vaccine used for smallpox eradication. Even in the unusual cases when protection was incomplete, only 3 percent of those vaccinated with Jenner's vaccine were likely to die of the disease when they became infected, as opposed to 30 percent of the unvaccinated. Vaccination is much safer than variolation; it does not leave pockmark scars and vaccinees do not need to be quarantined. Jenner's procedure was so safe and effective that, despite initial fears that it might be as risky as variolation, it had been widely accepted by 1840. Variolation was soon considered criminal, and political leaders were predicting that the vaccine could be used to eliminate the disease.[10]

Vaccination, unlike variolation, was invented at one site (or possibly a very few sites) and distributed widely. It was difficult to maintain vaccine efficacy during long-distance transport because the live vaccine virus can only survive in living cells. As humans are the only host for smallpox, variola vaccines had to be maintained in people. In 1806, King Charles IV supported the transportation of variola vaccine from Spain to Latin America by the sequential inoculation of twenty-two orphans, who were brought on board ship specifically for this purpose. Jenner's cowpox vaccine could be transported as impregnated threads or in live cows, so it could be disseminated before other preservation methods were developed. Ultimately the eradication program was greatly served by the development of a heat-stable, freeze-dried portable vaccine. Additionally, the invention of the bifurcated needle produced an inexpensive inoculation device that could be used by relatively unskilled personnel to scratch the vaccine into the skin. The result of these developments was a safe smallpox vaccine that conferred lifelong immunity and could be transported to any part of the world in a stable and deliverable form.

In addition to the technical advantages conferred by the vaccine and its delivery system, smallpox eradication was enabled by the convergence of pathogen, host, and political conditions that, in retrospect, offered a narrow window of opportunity. Whereas a proposal to eradicate smallpox had failed to garner unanimous support in 1953, every country committed itself to the eradication campaign at or immediately after the World Health Assembly of 1965.[11] Biologically, humans are the only hosts of the smallpox virus; it has no subclinical form and no hiding place in the environment. Transmission can be interrupted by vaccination, and both vaccination and infection provide lifelong immunity. An often overlooked but important fact is that people infected with the smallpox virus can easily be identified, even by laypeople, by the characteristic pustules, and individuals are infectious only when their condition is visibly identifiable. Smallpox was a disease of virtually complete diagnostic certainty, and the ease of diagnosis was a key factor that enabled its eradication.

The original strategy for smallpox eradication was to vaccinate the entire human population, or at least very close to it. This strategy was effective in eliminating the disease from Europe and North America, but it is unlikely that this plan would have achieved global eradication because too many at-risk people lived in remote areas. Because smallpox is transmitted only through close personal contact, it became obvious during the campaign that aggressively finding active cases and immunizing the people around them would suffice. A revised "identification, confinement and local immunization" strategy eventually achieved complete eradication.[12] Case-finding was easy: showing laypeople photographs of smallpox patients was sufficient to train them to find cases. The new "search and destroy" strategy was enormously effective in low-income regions: seventeen of the twenty-one West African countries eliminated smallpox in just two years.

In October 1975, three-year-old Rahima Banu of Bangladesh recovered from the last infection of the more severe form of smallpox, variola major. By 1977, the war-torn Horn of Africa was the last remaining focus of the disease. Early that year, the success of a concerted program to vaccinate Somali Muslims ahead of the Hajj (the annual pilgrimage to Mecca) ensured that the last natural viruses were contained within a limited geographic area. Aggressive case-finding turned up the penultimate case of naturally acquired smallpox. In October 1977, a Somali child with smallpox infected health worker Ali Maow Maalin. Maalin achieved international fame as the last case of smallpox on earth.[13] Thirty months later, WHO boldly declared smallpox gone for good.

Smallpox was vanquished just in time: within the next decade, the spread of HIV produced an immunocompromised subpopulation that cannot be vaccinated. In economic terms, eradication was highly cost effective. Countries that had been plagued by the disease as recently as the 1970s gained from the productive lives that were saved. Where the disease had been eliminated, countries could save money by ending their vaccination programs. The value of smallpox eradication to people alive today is inestimable. Monetarily, almost US$1.4 billion is saved each year, fourteen times as much as was spent on the eleven-year campaign.[14]

One important lesson to be learned from the smallpox eradication campaign is that mass methods do not necessarily guarantee effective results.[15] Megan Vaughan (1991) has observed that during the colonial period Africans were unitized for the purpose of administration and health care delivery. Unitization is directly opposed to individualization, since it presumes that all individuals are identical for the purpose of the intervention. In the places where medicine and public health are most efficiently administered, arguably in Scandinavia, individualization of health care delivery is the norm. It is likely that the individualization that diagnostic development requires would improve the delivery of public health interventions. The shift from the campaign's original goal of immunizing everybody on earth to a strategy of case-finding and contact immunization changed the smallpox eradication campaign from a unitized to an individualized program: people were vaccinated only if they might have been exposed to the virus. In some places, less than 10 percent of the population needed to be vaccinated.

Among the many lessons from the smallpox eradication campaign that inform disease control today, the lesson most relevant to the problems facing Africa is the central role that diagnosis plays in public health and disease control. Smallpox, with its easily identifiable pustules that appear early in the infection and its lack of an infectious subclinical stage, is the diagnostician's ideal.

Dracunculiasis, or guinea worm, is another disease that can be diagnosed by the untrained eye. When the one-to-three-foot-long adult female worm is ready to lay her eggs, she bores her way out of the skin of the limbs of infected people, causing disabling inflammation and superinfection and announcing the diagnosis to the patient and anyone else who can bear to look. Guinea worm is not a killer, but the crippling "disease of the empty granary"[16] keeps workers away from their farms and children out of school. There is no vaccine or preventive treatment, but it is possible to interrupt the parasite's life cycle. People become infected by the worm when they drink water contaminated with cyclops, a type of plankton, which are infected with Guinea worm larvae. The larvae make their way from the intestine to the connective tissues of the infected person, usually in the legs, and mature there. If people in endemic areas do not drink water contaminated with larvae, if infected people do not shed eggs into public water supplies, and if freshwater cyclops that carry larvae are destroyed, the worm can be eliminated.

The U.S. Centers for Diseases Control began a guinea worm eradication program in 1980. The Carter Center soon became the program's chief advocate and made a formal commitment to see eradication through in 1986. In the same year, the World Health Assembly put forward a resolution to eliminate the disease, upgrading the objective to eradication in 1991.[17] Thus the parasitic infestation guinea worm became the fifth disease that public health authorities and governments worldwide committed to eradicate, after yellow fever, yaws, malaria, and smallpox. With guinea worm, as with smallpox, diagnosis was no problem. In Cameroon, 19 percent of cases were detected within twenty-four hours in 1991. When cash prizes were offered to people who reported cases, 70 percent of cases were reported within one day.[18]

Once identified, guinea worm is eliminated by treating people with infestations and keeping their limbs away from communal water supplies, by providing safe water, or by supplying filtration devices that remove cyclops from the water. The eradication program is behind schedule but steadily advancing toward the goal of eradication. The tally was less than nine thousand cases in 2007, down from just over 150,000 in sixteen African countries in 1996 and almost one million in 1989. In 2008, only four countries—Ghana, Nigeria, Sudan, and Mali—reported cases of guinea worm. By 2009, there were only 513 cases worldwide and Nigeria, acknowledged as one of the most challenging countries at the last frontier, did not report a single case.[19] Problems have arisen with funding and in reaching affected populations, particularly those cordoned off by violent conflicts. But while the guinea worm eradication campaign does face challenges, the ease of diagnosis is a key reason for the program's success so far.

Eradication Challenges

In 1988, two years into the guinea worm eradication campaign, a bold step was made to begin the eradication of poliomyelitis, with a target completion date of 2000. In the first half of the twentieth century, amid a marked decline in the incidence of other infectious diseases in North America, thousands of middle-class children and a few adults were killed or crippled by the paralyzing disease—most notably, future president Franklin Delano Roosevelt. This epidemic spurred fund-raising for a concerted research effort to develop a vaccine, with American scientific heroes Albert Sabin, Jonas Salk, and Hilary Koprowski at the front lines.[20] These well-supported and largely political efforts resulted in several effective vaccines and the elimination of the disease in the United States by 1979. In 2001, 575 million polio immunizations were administered in ninety-four countries as part of the worldwide eradication effort.

Unlike smallpox and guinea worm disease, patients who can transmit polio can be reliably identified only by laboratory tests. Although a high prevalence of lameness in a population points to endemic poliomyelitis, less than half of seriously ill polio patients are paralyzed, so paralysis is not a sensitive enough diagnostic sign.[21] The virus is transmissible during the early stages of the illness, when symptoms often resemble those of other common conditions such as influenza. Recognizing this problem early in the campaign, WHO issued a statement explaining why it was essential to integrate laboratory and clinical approaches. High-burden countries, including many in Africa, would not necessarily need laboratory support to verify each infection, although local isolates should be preserved in order to track infections during the final mopping-up phase. Toward the end of the campaign, when most countries would be polio-free and some would have a few cases, laboratory support would be fundamental. In this strategy, polio eradication could begin even with diagnostic insufficiency in many endemic areas, but diagnostic development in the most troublesome spots would be essential to complete the campaign. A global laboratory network was an integral part of this plan.[22] As an editorial observed, "Progress achieved by the network has demonstrated that high-quality virology in support of public health activities can be made accessible to all areas of the world, including war-torn countries and countries without organized government or health infrastructure."[23] With sufficient support and motivation, laboratory diagnostics can be used anywhere, even for a viral disease such as polio. Polio surveillance has increased laboratory capacity for diagnosis and surveillance of other infections in many parts of Africa.

Polio eradication is now at a challenging last stage. Insufficient access and political will are the preeminent roadblocks, but there are biological challenges as well. The poor immune response of Indian children means that their vaccines must be carefully crafted and more frequently administered. The return of an eradicated polio subtype warrants reintroducing a discontinued vaccine in Nigeria. Viruses are periodically exported from the last four endemic nations (India, Nigeria, Afghanistan, and Pakistan) to other countries that have eliminated the disease.[24] All of these problems were identified, and are being addressed, using the results of laboratory tests that confirm infections, vaccine-derived immunity, and fingerprint poliovirus subtypes. Only with this real-time monitoring at the laboratory bench will we eradicate polio.

Measles, a virulent viral infection that is often fatal in very young children, is also high on the list of eradicable diseases. A population of two hundred thousand or more is needed to sustain the measles virus because it has no nonhuman reservoir. An effective vaccine was developed by researchers at Harvard University in the 1950s, and infection or vaccination can produce lifelong immunity. Measles is highly contagious; it is caused by an airborne virus that infects up to 90 percent of exposed nonimmune people. Infected infants have a significant risk of dying from measles, and there is a severe risk to the unborn children of infected pregnant women. Individuals infected as adults often suffer long-term effects, including testicular damage in men and blindness. Not only is the disease itself debilitating, it precipitates a temporary immune deficiency during infection that makes patients susceptible to activation of latent infections such as tuberculosis or infections by other organisms. The historical impact from measles has been high and includes the depletion of isolated immune-naïve populations in Greenland and the Fiji islands.[25]

Until recently, the association of measles with a characteristic rash was thought to be sufficient for diagnosis, but the accuracy of clinical diagnosis can vary substantially enough to make laboratory verification valuable. Laboratory support is also needed for other facets of a measles eradication program, such as calibrating the optimal timing of vaccination. Most babies are born with antibodies acquired from their mothers during gestation, which protect them against the measles virus until the antibody concentration declines, at about nine months of age. If measles vaccine is administered before this decline, the infant's maternal antibodies will inactivate the vaccine before the child can develop a protective immune response. Administer the vaccine too late, and a child could be left unprotected. For most children, vaccination at nine months works well, but infants born of HIV-positive mothers may be vulnerable before they reach their ninth month because they did not acquire sufficient passive antibody protection in utero. For this reason, WHO has advocated vaccinating these children at six months. However, laboratory tests performed in Zambia demonstrate that measles antibody concentrations in the children of HIV-positive mothers may be much less predictable. HIV infection status must be determined before vaccination, but often cannot be verified by six months. Vaccination of this growing subpopulation poses multiple diagnostic dilemmas that are becoming increasingly important as mother-to-child infection rates drop and survival of HIV-positive people improves.[26]

Determining the best way to deploy measles vaccines for underprotected babies is one of the most challenging problems that must be solved in order to eradicate the disease. Other more pedestrian challenges can, and will, be overcome. In 1999, 61 percent of the 871,000 measles deaths documented worldwide occurred in Africa. The WHO African region aimed to improve vaccination, case management, and surveillance, with the goal of halving deaths due to measles by 2005. Most countries that immediately began supplementary immunizations increased vaccine coverage from between 30 percent and 50 percent to over 60 percent within five years, and improved surveillance allowed lab verification in up to 80 percent or 90 percent of cases.[27] The end result was an impressive reduction in the number of clinical measles cases in thirty-two African countries by 2005.[28] Overall, deaths from measles worldwide fell by 68 percent, with the greatest declines in Africa. The reduction was partly due to closing the disparity between suspected cases identified clinically and cases confirmed in the lab. Being able to differentiate measles from other maladies is a first and essential step toward implementing control and monitoring progress toward the 2020 eradication target.

Yaws is a contagious bacterial disease caused by a close relative of the etiologic agent of syphilis. An early attempt to eradicate yaws was unsuccessful because, although the disease itself produces clearly discernable lesions, symptomless or subclinical infections also occur, resulting in a hidden reservoir for the spiral bacteria that cause the disease. The energetic yaws eradication campaign lacked the targeted case-finding that enabled successful completion of the final, mopping up phase of smallpox eradication. The experts who planned that campaign were aware of the problem posed by subclinical infections, and the strategy applied in most areas where yaws was endemic included treating the contacts of infected people. Since there is no vaccine, the tool for eradication was procaine penicillin, an antibiotic that kills the Treponemal bacteria that cause the disease.[29] This plan was efficacious in areas of high endemicity, where everyone was presumed to be a contact, but as laboratory tests were not used, contacts had to come forward voluntarily. Unfortunately, in addition to failing to reach all those who were spreading the disease, it is likely that the campaign was instrumental in producing selective pressure for the development of penicillin-resistant bacteria in many parts of the world, as well as a preference for injectable medicines.

A control program that is implemented without precise diagnostic support can reduce disease prevalence only when a large proportion of the population is infected. In the final phase of an eradication campaign, when previously uncommon illnesses with similar symptoms become more prominent than the target disease, accurate diagnosis with laboratory support becomes essential. If the laboratory does not participate in case-finding at this crucial stage, the disease could rebound and the campaign could face a huge loss of financial investment and morale. Yaws was never eradicated. Although containment varies from place to place, it is largely a forgotten scourge that remains a threat to poor countries, including some that had almost completely eliminated it. For example, yaws was resurgent in Ghana in the 1980s, and over 1.6 million people had to be injected with procaine penicillin between 1981 and 1983 to contain the disease.[30]

Controlling the Ineradicable

The fortuitous diagnostic certainty of smallpox and guinea worm was a key factor in eradication campaigns for those diseases. One of the hard lessons from less successful eradication programs is that diagnostic precision is a prerequisite for eradication. Not every case of poliomyelitis or measles can be diagnosed clinically with certainty, so the campaigns against these diseases are developing diagnostic capability. Which diseases should we tackle next, and how? In theory, any infectious disease can be eradicated as long as human infection can be interrupted and there are effective and practical means to diagnose it. Some diseases are not presently eradicable but may become so when effective tools to interrupt transmission are developed. We cannot eradicate pathogens that have a nonhuman host from which the organism cannot be simultaneously eradicated, or if people can carry the organism undetected. Diseases that are transmitted too efficiently to permit a practicable intervention may also be ineradicable. Although public health advocates often refrain from mentioning matters of finance up front, cost-effectiveness is as paramount to sustaining eradication and elimination campaigns as are political and societal will.[31]

Infectious diseases that cannot presently be eradicated can often be eliminated within a restricted geographic area. This distinction is important: eradication is the "permanent reduction to zero of the worldwide incidence of infection caused by a specific agent as a result of deliberate efforts";[32] elimination refers to similar clearance in a specified geographical area. Control refers to reduction, but not to zero. Unlike eradication, continuing interventions are needed to maintain elimination or control.

Even when case-specific diagnosis is of limited benefit, population-level surveillance may be critical for disease control. This has been exemplarily illustrated following surveillance of bacteria that cause respiratory infections, which are among the most important causes of death among African babies. One way to reduce antimicrobial use and get around the mounting problem of resistance is to develop and apply effective vaccines against life-threatening bacterial infections. Among the most dangerous pathogens are *Streptococcus pneumoniae* and *Haemophilus influenzae* type B (Hib), which can cause bloodstream infections, meningitis, and pneumonia, as well as more innocuous ear infections, which are the most common manifestation in the West. Both bacterial species can be carried asymptomatically by some individuals, who unwittingly transmit the bacteria to susceptible children, but there are effective vaccines for both.

Having used laboratory-based surveillance to demonstrate that Hib was a major cause of childhood deaths in The Gambia, the Medical Research Council research center in Fagara was able to show that, within seven years of deploying an Hib vaccine, the disease all but disappeared. Two years later, researchers found that a new hypervirulent strain of Hib had appeared.[33] This surveillance brought to light the need for long-term assurance of vaccine programs, and perhaps for booster doses of the vaccine. Without surveillance, elimination would be ultimately unsuccessful and the investment in vaccines wasted. In Mali, Hib surveillance found that, between 2002 and 2005, 12 percent of hospital admissions and 19.3 percent of deaths could be attributed to the bacteria. This alarming data was taken from the lab to the clinic and, ultimately, to the country's presidential suite and prompted the introduction of Hib vaccination, so that by 2007 there was a 68 percent reduction in the disease.[34] African countries that had some surveillance data introduced life-saving Hib vaccines first, with impressive results. Overall, vaccines were introduced last in countries that were furthest from those nations that had data before 1995.[35] Costly but life-saving interventions are harder to justify and implement without local surveillance data, which can only be collected with laboratories.

S. pneumoniae, otherwise known as pneumococcus, presents a much more complicated problem. There are several different serotypes of pneumococcus. Each serotype is enveloped in a different sugary capsule, its cloaklike disguise from the immune system. Immune systems can be educated to recognize specific capsule types by preexposure through infection or vaccination but immunization against one serotype does not protect against others. Fortunately, less than a dozen serotypes are responsible for most pneumococcal disease, and these also include the types that are more likely to be resistant to antibiotics. When a multivalent vaccine protecting against seven types was deployed in the United States, S. pneumoniae infections declined substantially and, when infections did occur, they were less likely to be drug resistant.[36] Both the reduction in resistance and the "herd effect" were unanticipated. A herd effect is seen when individuals who have not been vaccinated, but who live in the vicinity of vaccinated individuals, are protected from the disease. With pneumococcal vaccines, this phenomenon is best illustrated by the protection of unvaccinated children attending day care centers where a large number of children have been vaccinated. When pneumococcal bacteria lost their niche in those centers, even unvaccinated children were protected.

In Africa, where pneumococcal infection often manifests as life-threatening respiratory or bloodstream infections and where complete vaccine coverage is often hard to achieve, the herd effect would be valuable. There is one major caveat: there are several dozen types of S. pneumoniae, each of which has a different, slippery, carbohydrate capsule. Each vaccine protects only against a limited number of capsular types, which must be carefully selected. Pneumococcal vaccines have been most successful when extensive surveillance precedes their deployment to ensure that the vaccine targets locally relevant types. Such studies have been done in some parts of Africa, but most are not extensive enough to adequately inform vaccine deployment.[37] Moreover, prevaccination surveillance alone is insufficient. Today's most virulent and antimicrobial-resistant types are the focus of current vaccines. When these vaccines are used intensively, new types will replace the old. This process is already beginning in the United States.[38] We must monitor disease-causing serotypes constantly in order to keep the vaccines up to date.

Tuberculosis is a disease of contemporary as well as historical significance. Contrary to nineteenth-century myths that the hectic fevers and heightened awareness of mortality that accompanied "consumption" spurred creative genius, the disease cut short the lives of many novelists, poets, and composers.[39] The 1943 discovery of the antibiotic streptomycin by Selman Waksman's graduate student Albert Schatz was the first step in turning the "white plague" into a condition that could be managed and even cured.[40] The problem of recrudescence because of resistance that emerges during treatment was conquered by the introduction of combination therapy, which followed the development of other antituberculosis drugs such as isoniazid, para-amino salicylic acid, and rifampicin. Many thought that over time TB would become less common and eventually cease to be a significant health threat. Experts in global health were startled by the emergence of multidrug-resistant tuberculosis (MDR-TB), which was entirely predictable but had been overlooked.

A third of the world's population today is latently infected with *Mycobacterium tuberculosis*. The immune systems of most of these people keep active infection at bay. The immunocompromised are not so fortunate; they will likely experience TB activation or acquire active disease after exposure. The combined emergence of drug-resistant bacteria and HIV in the last quarter of the twentieth century has made TB one of the greatest threats to public health. Adherence to prescribed TB therapy is important because even a short course of treatment takes at least six months and drug-resistant bacteria can be selected in the patient during this time. WHO declared a global emergency in 1993 and, to stop the spread of the disease and the emergence of resistant strains, proposed directly observed short course therapy (DOTS) for all TB patients. As the name of the strategy implies, patients on DOTS are observed by another person each time they take their medicine so that they do not forget doses or willfully decide to stop therapy prematurely. A regular and sufficient drug supply is essential for the DOTS program to succeed, as is the capacity to diagnose new cases and verify cures. All this requires considerable investment in support, evaluation, and reporting, as well as a national-level political commitment.[41]

Society must assume the responsibility of ensuring that TB patients recover because their highly transmissible and deadly illness poses a threat to public health. DOTS programs are therefore national endeavors that are monitored internationally. In 1992, twenty countries were implementing DOTS. By 2002, it was so obvious that DOTS was successful and cost effective that the number had jumped to 180. Although 2002 targets—to detect 85 percent of cases and successfully treat 70 percent of them—were not met in many developing countries, one Indian study showed that two hundred thousand lives and $400 million were saved when DOTS was properly implemented. The sum of lives saved from premature death and illness-related disabilities averted, called a disability-adjusted life year (DALY), is used by the World Bank as a currency for health in order to evaluate the cost-effectiveness of specific health interventions. The DALY is a unit invented by Christopher J. Murray and Alan D. Lopez (1997), who recognized that monetary estimates failed to reasonably catalog the losses from illness at the population level. Simply put, DALYs for a disease are computed by adding years of life lost and years lived with disability. By this measure, the value of DOTS was amply demonstrated by the TB control program in Beijing where the cost of saving a DALY could be reduced by 90 percent simply by applying DOTS.[42] A much understated component of DOTS is diagnosis and cure verification by sputum smear microscopy. DOTS made these successes because drugs are provided with a delivery system that includes diagnostics.

It is difficult and time consuming to grow *M. tuberculosis* in the laboratory, and therefore culturing every clinical specimen is impractical. On the other hand, because of their waxy cell coat, Mycobacteria can be distinguished by their resistance to acid decolorization after staining. Virtually all other bacteria are decolorized by acid, so the presence of acid-fast, rod-shaped bacteria in sputum is indicative of active pulmonary tuberculosis. A lab technician can smear sputum on a slide, fix it, stain it, attempt to decolorize it with acid, and then observe bacteria under the microscope. Other than a short list of inexpensive materials, the other requirements are that the setup is suitable to avoid infection of lab workers and that the slides are properly read and reported. Test sensitivity is not high, but because patients with active infection cough up high numbers of bacteria, this simple, cheap, and practicable diagnostic test will pick up most cases of the disease. Sputum smear microscopy also aids in verifying cure. By the WHO definition, only patients who are smear-negative close to and at the end of the short course of treatment are said to be cured. Those for whom this verification was negative or impossible are said to have "completed treatment."[43]

The successes of DOTS are inextricably linked to ease of laboratory-based diagnosis for TB. The effectiveness and simplicity of sputum smear staining for *M. tuberculosis* has made it possible to mount lifesaving interventions in the most unlikely places, including remote villages and refugee camps. However, in some parts of the world, including locations in Africa, access to DOTS remains difficult.

According to a 2005 report, it took more than a month to place 91 percent of tuberculosis patients from the Amhara region of Ethiopia in treatment.[44] Patients who had the foresight to go straight to the general hospital, which implemented a DOTS program including sputum smear microscopy (and lived close enough to do so), managed to avoid delay. Patients who visited local health clinics or private doctors waited from weeks to months for a diagnosis, just like the patients who visited indigenous practitioners or unsanctioned providers. In Ethiopia, the lack of diagnostic facilities at the primary health care level delays treatment for patients and facilitates the spread of disease. Similar reports have come from Ghana, The Gambia, Zambia, and Botswana.[45] The further afield testing moves from the patient, the longer the delay in diagnosis and the greater the chance that other individuals with similar difficulties in accessing DOTS programs will be infected. TB is a deadly disease, but undiagnosed or underdiagnosed TB is a public health disaster, which is amplified by each delay.

In areas where DOTS is inadequately implemented, multidrug-resistant tuberculosis (MDR-TB) emerges and spreads, with potentially devastating consequences. Patients with MDR-TB are commonly discovered only when first-line treatment does not cure them, by which time the disease has often inflicted permanent damage and has spread to other individuals. Second-line TB drugs needed to deal with resistant infections are more expensive, more toxic, more difficult to administer, and less effective. Crucially, although sputum smear microscopy is an effective diagnostic test for TB, it cannot distinguish MDR-TB from more easily treatable forms of the disease. Therefore, when MDR-TB emerges, even institutions that have good DOTS programs can lose diagnostic sufficiency.

According to British researcher Ruth McNerney, there was no routine testing for MDR-TB when drug-resistant *M. tuberculosis* emerged in Uganda. The consequent crisis is aptly described by project coordinator Edward Jones, who observed that individuals infected with MDR-TB were transmitting it in their communities and to health workers.[46] Recently, "exceedingly drug-resistant" strains, called XDR-TB, have emerged. XDR-TB strains are resistant to the first-line drugs rifampicin and isoniazid, a second-line fluoroquinolone, and at least one of the three commonly used second-line injectable drugs: capreomycin, kanamycin, and amikacin. The infections they cause are, in essence, untreatable. One of the most publicized examples of the devastation this deadly form of TB can cause was an outbreak in rural Kwazulu Natal, South Africa, where XDR-TB resulted in the rapid demise of fifty-three individuals, including six health workers who caught the infection from their patients.[47] Mathematical models have identified the slow time to diagnosis as the principal factor that precipitated that epidemic.[48]

A clear picture of the difficulties of dealing with resistant tuberculosis has been generated in many of the nation-states of the former Soviet Union, where misuse of antituberculosis drugs, with other factors, has resulted in widespread resistance. When there are no facilities for susceptibility testing, resistant infections are treated with the same drug cocktail as susceptible ones, fostering the resistance problem.[49] In an Uzbekistani study,[50] patients infected with multidrug-resistant strains were less likely to recover after completing a DOTS course, and if they survived, they were likely to experience a recurrence of TB within twenty-two months of completing treatment. Overall, infection with multidrug-resistant TB was the factor most associated with death in treated TB patients.

Currently, many laboratories that are capable of sputum smear microscopy find it difficult to extend their services to include drug susceptibility testing. The unfortunate paradox is that even though DOTS is based on a cheap and robust diagnostic protocol, a poorly managed DOTS program leads to resistance and makes it necessary to augment affordable laboratory technologies with more expensive ones. MDR-TB and XDR-TB require considerably more sophisticated diagnostics for detection and management because the susceptibility of the tubercule bacteria to different drugs must be determined when a diagnosis is made and monitored throughout treatment. Conventionally, this protocol requires expensive and time-consuming culture and sensitivity testing. Unlike fast-growing bacteria such as *Salmonella* and *Streptococcus*, which produce colonies after overnight culture, plate culture of *M. tuberculosis* on special complex media takes forty-two days to grow and requires sophisticated and expensive safety measures. When traditional methods are used, return of susceptibility testing results can take four to eight weeks.

Multidrug-resistant TB is presently uncommon in Africa. Unfortunately, commitment to the standard DOTS protocol is not common enough, and HIV prevalence is high so that resistant strains have begun to emerge and spread. Recent drug-resistant epidemics in South Africa and Botswana demonstrate that when resistant strains become commonplace, sputum smear microscopy is inadequate to support TB care.[51] It is only because these epidemics occurred in areas with some access to diagnostic facilities that they were identified at all. DOTS aims to treat 85 percent of diagnosed cases successfully; if many infections are resistant, there must be means to detect them and send them right to second-tier therapy.

Like bacterial culture and susceptibility testing methods, as well as the tests used to diagnose malaria before the advent of rapid diagnostic tests, the cardinal test for tuberculosis—sputum smear microscopy—is about a century old. Age old tests do not require expensive or labile materials; however, they are often tedious, require some specialist training, and do not always identify exceptional cases of the disease that are commonplace today but were rare when the test was developed. For example, sputum smear microscopy, a simple and informative technique, is incapable of identifying drug-resistant strains of TB. It is also in-adequate today for another important reason: it fails to diagnose tuberculosis in many HIV-positive patients, who in modern times are among those most likely to have active TB. HIV-infected TB patients deteriorate quickly and are often in-patients. Therefore, if not treated rapidly and successfully, they place health workers at risk of infection. These factors, as much as multidrug resistance, con-tributed to the much-publicized deadly outbreak of XDR-TB in Tugela Ferry, KwaZulu Natal, South Africa. Diagnostics that are more sensitive than sputum smear microscopy, more rapid than culture, and less expensive than PCR are urgently needed to contain tuberculosis in parts of Africa where HIV infection is common.[52]

Eventually drug sensitivity testing, as well as diagnosis, will be required at the point of care in most places. Simply monitoring trends from sentinel sites will be inadequate, and the international health community will have to face the prospect of making *M. tuberculosis* culture and drug susceptibility testing available throughout Africa. BACTEC instrumentation, an automated speci-men culture system devised and marketed by U.S. diagnostics manufacturer Becton Dickinson, has made TB culture faster and safer and is already in use in some African laboratories. Molecular testing also offers some promise and this capacity may need to be built in places where molecular diagnostics are not commonly used today.[53] The most promise comes from newer line-probe assays—molecular assays that don't use cumbersome and finicky equipment—and point-of-care tests that are in development.[54] Like malaria diagnostics, their quality and performance in resource-poor laboratories needs to be assured, but this cannot be done too quickly. The evolutionary innovation by *Mycobacterium tuberculosis* has far outpaced our ability to diagnose and treat the infection these bacteria cause.

Can TB, in particular MDR-TB, be rapidly and effectively detected in African laboratories using today's technology? A two-year capacity building project in Lesotho illustrates that it can.[55] Before the effort began, only seventeen clinics performed sputum smear microscopy and patients in Lesotho with MDR-TB were typically diagnosed, when they were at all, in South Africa and the United States. In 2006, new culture facilities and line-probe assays were installed in the national reference laboratory, staff members were trained, and quality control mechanisms were put in place. By 2008 the laboratory was reliably processing al-most eight thousand specimens a year. It was also providing quality assurance for sputum smear microscopy performed in district health centers, and training lab-oratory technicians from other African countries. The entire capacity-building project cost about half a million U.S. dollars, much less than the projected ex-penses for out-of-control MDR-TB epidemics.

The Ultimate Challenge of Malaria

All successful or nearly successful control and eradication campaigns have been associated with diagnostic certainty. The failure of the worldwide 1955–69 malaria eradication campaign placed malaria squarely in the category of ineradicable diseases. Transmission rates in parts of sub-Saharan Africa were so high that the interventions barely dented its incidence. This campaign relied entirely on chemical agents for which resistance rapidly emerged and spread.[56] Within five years of its commencement, mosquitoes resistant to the insecticide DDT were widespread, and *Plasmodium* parasites resistant to the drug of choice, chloroquine, had become a menace.[57] The failure to reevaluate the program's strategy, coupled with the insistence that it not extend beyond the original date for completion, left many countries to battle resurgent malaria alone. Sadly, some of these places had long suffered from endemic disease but had made real progress toward control, if not elimination.

When the program collapsed at the end of the 1960s, neither the parasite nor its mosquito vectors had been vanquished. What was closest to eradication was the community of public health officials and biomedical scientists with malaria expertise. Malaria imposed an increasing disease burden on Africa between the 1980s and 2000, but overcoming the discouraging legacy of the failed campaign and rebuilding a community of experts to address the mounting crisis took time. In the 1990s, researchers and private funders expressed renewed interest in malaria, which had become synonymous with poverty and suffering. The new impetus to attack the disease was evident at the 56th annual meeting of the American Society of Tropical Medicine and Hygiene, held in Philadelphia in November 2007. In contrast to the previous campaign's kickoff gathering three decades before, malaria researchers were in the majority and malaria was the unofficial theme of the meeting. Conference attendees included researchers from malaria-endemic countries, including Africa, who were able to participate as a result of recent improvements in research funding. The meeting rooms buzzed with reports of new developments in understanding the malaria parasite, the mosquito vector, and the course of the disease, as well as new directions for therapies, vaccines, and diagnostics.

I had browsed the schedule of the meeting ahead of time and looked forward to a veritable feast of new scientific information about tropical infections in general and malaria in particular. However, like many in the audience, I was unprepared for what we heard at the keynote lecture. Keynote lectures at large biomedical science meetings are typically well presented, even flamboyant—or, at least, as colorful as research scientists can make them. A ballroom is converted into an auditorium, and the speaker's image and Powerpoint presentation are projected on a large screen. Keynote lectures are often comprehensive and synthetic and sometimes insightful, but they rarely impart new information to insiders in the field. Many scientists attend the keynote lecture because they know everyone else will be there; it is the perfect place to catch up with old friends and former collaborators. For students, new researchers, or guests, a keynote lecture usually serves as a succinct introduction to the field.

In 2007, the society invited Tadataka Yamada, the president of the Bill and Melinda Gates Foundation's Global Health Program, to give the address. The Gates Foundation had been instrumental in the revival of malaria research as well as in delivering effective interventions, such as insecticide-impregnated bed nets and potent artemisinin combination therapies. Although conference-goers often chat quietly during a keynote lecture, Yamada's quiet but insistent voice, and his evident pain at the ravages of malaria, compelled silence. After recounting the dire statistics associated with the global burden of malaria, Yamada made a startling announcement: in spite of the failure of the 1955–69 campaign, the Gates Foundation was making a commitment to support the eradication of malaria.

Yamada's announcement followed an invitation to a select group of malariologists, who had been forewarned six weeks before in Seattle. There, the Gateses, in back-to-back presentations, challenged malariologists to eradicate malaria within their lifetimes.[58] In response, WHO's director general, Margaret Chan, announced that this global organization would share in this commitment. Considering the gravity of the announcement, which stunned some into silence, the attendees' response was either subdued or skeptical. Some gave this rich and famous couple indulgent smiles and acknowledged that their wealth and philanthropy entitled them to have pie-in-the-sky dreams. Even Chan was later quoted as saying, "It is elimination-slash-eradication, depending on the availability of tools."[59] Given the broken promises that litter the history of malaria control, scientists have been wary of making any real commitments without hard evidence of effective measures for eradication. At best, some malariologists have suggested, an eradication plan might help bolster control. But there are no models for malaria control. In Europe and North America, the disease was eliminated. In the parts of the world where malaria still plagues people, it remains uncontrolled. Perhaps, as Stephen Hoffman presciently observed, "Common use of the word [control]…represents our recognition of our inability to eradicate malaria."[60] Dr. Hoffman has complained that malaria control is a visionless goal with origins in the failed eradication effort of the 1960s.

As Dr. Yamada reiterated the Gates Foundation's determination to see eradication through and outlined a scientific framework for doing so, it was impossible not to take this proposition seriously. Yamada was able to justify the need for a new program in less than ten minutes of his hour-long presentation. The human and financial cost of the disease was great, as was the moral imperative. Quietly but firmly, he asked: "Can we sit in a world in which the vast majority of us never worry about this problem while there are people who worry about losing their children, especially as we can contemplate eradication?"

Most scientists and heath policy advocates had not contemplated eradicating malaria for forty years. At its peak, the earlier campaign had eliminated the disease from two-thirds of the globe. The recent surge in malaria research, the new disease control tools that had come to the fore, and the impressive progress from African countries such as Zambia suggested that it was time to reconsider eradication.

The technical literature describes malaria as a disease that is ineradicable for biological reasons.[61] In making a commitment to see an eradication program through before its feasibility had been certified, the Gates Foundation banked its faith on technological development. Essentially, the commitment is built on the assumption that scientific research can and will overcome all existing biological roadblocks to malaria eradication. The initial challenge will be identifying precisely what these roadblocks are. Key reasons for the failure of the older campaign include pathogen and vector resistance, secondary vectors, and a terminal loss of will and financial support. A less commonly discussed factor that must be addressed in any future malaria eradication campaign is the difficulty of diagnosing people and mosquitoes carrying malaria parasites. The difficulty of diagnosis directed the failed campaign at all individuals instead of only those who have the parasite. The smallpox campaign, by contrast, succeeded by targeting infected people and their contacts.

For malaria, mass treatment with today's tools could spell failure because intensive use of any biocide creates needless selective pressure for the development of resistance to drugs and insecticides. Biocidal agents are much more effective against specific targets. It is possible that had the application of chloroquine and DDT been more focused, their effective life spans could have been extended. Whether careful targeting would have altered the course of the malaria eradication campaign remains an open question. At a minimum, diagnostic precision would have made it clear right away that the strategy was not working in Africa and perhaps prompted a shift in approach before donor fatigue set in. Developing and deploying the tools required to monitor progress is essential to any control or eradication effort. In describing the ultimate goal for malaria, eradication, Yamada suggested an analogy between disease control and playing tennis: "If you don't keep score, you are just practicing." The score, he insisted, must be lives saved. Only with diagnostic precision can we keep score.

ORIGINS AND OUTLOOK OF DIAGNOSTIC INSUFFICIENCY IN AFRICA

My dangerous idea is that we have in hand most of the information we need to facilitate a new golden age of medicine. And what we don't have in hand we can get fairly readily by wise investment and targeted research and intervention.

—Paul W. Ewald, 2007

The chief nursing officer at Ikeja General Hospital, who was always addressed as "Chief Matron," spoke for ten minutes at a staff orientation in 1990. During her talk, she pleaded that new doctors enter at least a presumptive diagnosis into patient case notes after examination, along with their initial prescription: "A diagnosis is valuable when nursing staff have to manage emergencies," she explained. As a new pharmacist attending that orientation, I could not understand why Chief Matron devoted half of her allotted time to something so obvious. Fresh out of Nigeria's premier pharmacy school and an internship at a university health center, I found it inconceivable that a physician would commence treatment without recording even a presumptive diagnosis. None of my medical professors or textbooks suggested that could happen. Instead, they warned not to do anything to a patient "without understanding the why and wherefore."[1]

During the year I worked at Ikeja General, I came to understand this startling omission, along with many other initially incomprehensible things about routine practice in an African hospital that serves so many poor patients on a constrained budget. Patient records, which we called case notes, are written rapidly but regarded as sacred. Every entry is signed. The records are passed from one practitioner to the next; consultants use them to pick up on a referred case, or even to evaluate subordinate doctors' work. Should the need arise, case notes are admissible in a court of law. A physician would never consider writing a statement for which he or she has no evidence—including an unsupported diagnosis—in a patient's record. My medical colleagues' records were commendably thorough, even though they each typically saw up to a hundred patients each day. Signs, symptoms, histories, and prescriptions were accurately recorded, but, as Chief Matron lamented, diagnoses were often omitted.

Later I learned that omitting diagnoses from case notes was not specific to Ikeja General, or even to Nigeria. Understanding what went wrong in the period leading up to the first Ebola outbreak at the Yambuku hospital in Zaire was made difficult because diagnoses were rarely recorded. Similar omissions hobbled an epidemiological study of hospitalized pneumonia patients in the Bondo district of Kenya between 2001 and 2003: "As discharge diagnoses were rarely found in the medical records, it was difficult to assess how often the admitting diagnosis changed after review of the hospital course."[2] The question of what to do when a previous patient re-presents himself or herself looms large. After all, a patient who has never had diagnoses has no medical history. In discussing the problem of infectious diseases in Africa, science writer Laurie Garrett observed that "even sophisticated physicians often found it impossible to assign specific causes of death to their patients."[3] The difficulty arises in part from the fact that patients in high-burden areas commonly succumb to multiple infections. However, doctors' inability to determine the cause of death is closely connected with the handicaps associated with diagnosing the living, which have persisted from the inception of Western medicine in Africa until the present day.[4]

Modern allopathic medicines are powerful drugs designed to address specific indications. They act at precise targets located within or between invading microscopic cells. The antibiotic chloramphenicol, for example, inhibits bacterial growth and was the mainstay for typhoid treatment for several decades, until resistance became commonplace. It has been removed from WHO's essential drugs lists but it is still used to manage some severe infections in Africa, partly because it is inexpensive and partly because it is useful in the battle against resistant bacteria.[5] The drug works by blocking the synthesis of proteins by bacteria. Chloramphenicol molecules bind to a specific site on bacterial ribosomes, the cell structures responsible for protein synthesis. Bacteria with disabled ribosomes cannot make the proteins they need for cell structures and enzymes and eventually die. Chloramphenicol does not block protein synthesis in parasites—for example, those that cause malaria—because it cannot bind to the ribosomes in those organisms, which have a different structure similar to similarly unaffected human ribosomes. Chloramphenicol also does not kill viruses, which do not synthesize their own proteins and have no ribosomes. A patient who does not have typhoid, or an infection caused by a pathogen with bacterial ribosomes, cannot be cured with this drug. Indeed, administration of it creates a risk that bacteria resistant to the drug will be needlessly selected. Even more critically, because a small number of people treated with chloramphenicol get blood cancer through a different mechanism, overuse of this drug increases the risk of a deadly side effect. Clearly, no one should be given chloramphenicol unless it is certain that they have a life-threatening infection that can be cleared by this drug. Unfortunately, most patients with presumed bacterial infection are diagnosed based on symptoms alone, and the diagnoses are often not recorded. In the 1980s and 1990s, when chloramphenicol was highly effective, between 10 percent and 20 percent of Nigerian patients with a fever received the drug, often in conjunction with an antimalarial. There and elsewhere this potent but potentially toxic drug is often prescribed without a validated indication.[6]

In many indigenous African medical systems, the primary purpose of medical consultation is diagnosis. Indeed, defining the nature of the patient's problem is the foundation of the healer's authority. The practitioner uses clinical signs, patient history, and sometimes spiritual consultation to determine the root cause of the ailment, which may or may not be deemed physical. In their introduction to *The Social Basis of Health and Healing in Africa*, Steven Feierman and John Janzen remarked: "Whoever controls the diagnosis of illness...shapes cultural ideas on misfortune and evil. The power to name an illness is the power to say which elements in life lead to suffering."[7] An indigenous practitioner explains his or her diagnosis to the patient, and often to the family, before stating whether the problem can be treated and what is needed to resolve it. A cure might consist of herbal preparations, incantations, rituals, or some combination of medicine and spiritual therapy. The patient need not know what the components of these treatments are, and in some cases they are secret, but he or she must understand why treatment is necessary in order to be convinced of its efficacy. The diagnostic lapses in allopathic medicine, as it is practiced in Africa, do not stem from indigenous medical practice, which is built on diagnostic precision. A more likely source of allopathic medicine's tendency to utilize potent Western medicines without the necessary diagnosis is the very source of those medicines.

Portable Medicine, a Colonial Legacy

Western medical practitioners were unable to deal with tropical infectious diseases until the etiologies of these diseases were uncovered and antimicrobial drugs were developed. How could the pioneers of tropical medicine, whose work relied on microbiological science, have made such a fundamental error as to relegate diagnostic microbiology to the background? In addressing this question, we must first acknowledge that microbiology was not always tightly linked to medical practice. This illogical separation was standard until the end of the nineteenth century, when Robert Koch unequivocally linked specific bacteria to anthrax and tuberculosis. Secondly, Western medicine did not have the original objective of providing cost-effective care for Africans. Although the objectives of practice have since changed, the methods and paradigms have not.

Before the nineteenth century, people who became seriously ill in Africa recovered on their own accord, were treated with herbal mixtures, or died. Africans relied on their indigenous healers, but European colonialists did not consult African medical practitioners, whom they condemned as "witch doctors." In the early nineteenth century, as many as half of the Europeans who visited West Africa died there.[8] Increasingly, European patients who became seriously ill but did not die immediately were transported home, particularly when there were relatively few of them. Being declared medically unfit for duty and sent home for medical treatment and a long recuperation was known as "invaliding." Between 1876 and 1890, over half of the British soldiers stationed in West Africa were invalided; in 1881, a particularly bad year, fourteen of the fifteen soldiers stationed there were sent back because of illness.[9] Invaliding was uncommon for yellow fever, in part because it did not increase survival, but also because this disease could be diagnosed clinically. Patients with nonspecific fevers, including malaria, were commonly invalided.

Progress in tropical microbiology and disease control transformed West Africa and central Africa from "the White man's grave" to an environment that colonial officials and businessmen could inhabit and exploit. The first advancements that led to visible increases in the survival of Europeans in West Africa were the use of quinine for malaria treatment and prophylaxis and the emphasis on clean water. Quinine became available in large quantities after 1820, when a protocol for extracting the alkaloid from cinchona bark was devised by French chemists. A second dramatic rise in survival rates, between 1895 and 1914, coincided with the emergence of microbial science and its application in the understanding and diagnosis of infectious disease. This decrease in mortality was less pronounced than the earlier one and, interestingly, less marked than comparable declines in other parts of the world, which suggests that the potential gains from microbial science were less often applied to medical practice in West Africa.[10] Noticeably, deaths from diarrheal diseases, typhoid fever, and dysentery declined worldwide at this time, but did not decline in Africa.

To further the goals of empire, colonial health posts were frequently established at labor centers, ignoring the more pressing need for rural health centers and for maternal and pediatric health care.[11] As far as Africans were concerned, the principal goal of colonial medicine was to weed out the unhealthy in the labor force in order to protect European workers and investments. This objective was accomplished by using rapid, nonspecific, and short-term curative measures and by segregating Europeans, rather than dealing with endemic disease. Public health and medical services for Europeans advanced so rapidly and efficiently in

West Africa that, following dramatic reductions in the mid-nineteenth century, the European mortality rate fell from 206 per 1,000 in 1895 to 4 per 1,000 in 1930.[12] If success is defined in light of the specific imperial and economic goals of colonial medicine, these health policies and interventions were exceptionally successful. Tertiary care for expatriates could be obtained in their home countries, and their African workers could be replaced when they sickened and died.

Early European visitors to Africa wore a cartridge belt containing essential supplies and medicines. During the initial phase of imperialism, when Europeans imagined themselves as "explorers" in "darkest Africa," the colonial medical infrastructure consisted of a pack of portable supplies brought into Africa by Europeans principally for their personal use. By the mid-twentieth century, when more Europeans visited and resided in Africa, the scope of medical practice expanded proportionally but remained essentially portable. Medicines are eminently portable, diagnostic tools less so. Modern medications became generally available, but even rudimentary laboratory facilities were rare.

In the construction of colonial health institutions, essential health personnel were considered to be those required to provide primary empiric care without ancillary facilities: doctors, nurses, and, where they were unavailable, their less trained surrogates. Laboratory technicians and other health scientists, other than sanitary inspectors, were deemed inessential. Even when deployed, they were often considered—and considered themselves—research staff, rather than health care professionals. A research and diagnostic laboratory was established in Accra, Ghana, at the beginning of the twentieth century but was never properly staffed. In its early days, the laboratory was managed by clinicians who worked there voluntarily. Doctors and nurses can perform many essential laboratory tests, but there were not enough clinicians to fulfill consulting needs, much less staff the lab. Staff shortages in the clinic were overcome by training local African medical assistants, but when the only laboratory technician died in 1916, not a single African had been trained to work in the laboratory.[13] Training African laboratory technicians did not begin in earnest until the 1940s. When health professionals became scarce during the depression of the 1930s and the Second World War, laboratory diagnostic services in Ghana (then Gold Coast) all but shut down.[14] In 1952, the Maude Commission of enquiry into the health needs of the Gold Coast recommended a 1:9,000 ratio of physicians to the population and a 1:1,000 ratio of nursing staff, but only a 1:30,000–45,000 ratio for laboratory technicians.[15] As the category "laboratory technician" includes bacteriologists, parasitologists, virologists, histopathologists, hematologists, and clinical chemists, this ratio would preclude laboratory testing for most patients.

Shortchanging laboratory medicine extended beyond neglecting staffing needs. In most African countries, virtually no diagnostic reagents or consumables were produced locally, even after vaccines and pharmaceuticals were manufactured on the continent. Meanwhile, the costly importation of heat-labile materials declined over time. Despite the high burden of infectious disease that the colonialists encountered in Africa and the exacerbation that their presence caused,[16] the health care set up by Europeans contributed very little to the control of infectious disease and even less to evidence-based management with laboratory support.

It is fair to say that, unlike colonial governments, missionary health care posts did prioritize health care delivery to Africans. Missionaries wanted to preach, teach, and heal according to Jesus Christ's model, as well as to combat the influence of indigenous healers, whom they viewed as evil.[17] Some missionary hospitals maintained reasonably good laboratory support. For example, Our Lady of Lourdes Catholic mission hospital in rural Ipetu Modu, Nigeria, has a laboratory that performs routine blood and parasitology tests. The priority of missionaries, however, was the redemption of souls, not bodies. Therefore, they were more likely to leave models for religious practice than for health care delivery.

Dispensaries were built in remote areas by missionaries and colonial governments alike. Their name aptly describes their principal function: distributing medicine to patients, rather than providing more comprehensive health care. Dispensaries were conceived as a low-budget medical option and were more widely available than any other type of health care center; almost every African had seen one by the 1950s. As a result, Western medical practice was essentially defined by the dispensing of pharmaceuticals. Dispensing drugs and clinical practice are tightly linked in other cultures as well. In Europe and North America, the handing over of a prescription is the perceived end of a medical consultation. This drug-oriented culture has spurred misuse. In the West, however, the prescription exchange is seen as the end of a process, rather than its entire purpose. The provision of health care from dispensaries has a more deleterious influence.[18] "Dispensers," whose training was quite limited, rather than qualified pharmacists, staffed these dubious institutions. According to the Nigerian health care historian Ralph Schram,

> [Dispensaries] were never a success. It could be argued that they took the place of the town pharmacist, but they displayed, often in poorly built, ill-lit and dirty premises, a handful of mixtures outdated by several decades and usually kept in unlabelled, disused beer bottles. The dispensary assistants in charge had often had the benefit of a very poor training, amounting to watching and assisting the dispenser at a government city hospital for a year or two.[19]

Dispensaries were originally set up as hospital outposts. One account lists wounds and scabies as the sort of ailments they were designed to treat, with everything else being referred to clinics and hospitals. Since fevers and child-hood infections are the most common illnesses and hospitals were few and far between, dispensaries inevitably began to address these too. These often dubi-ous institutions are the precursors of today's popular, proliferate, and often un-sanctioned drug sellers. The major eastern Nigerian town of Calabar in the late 1940s had one hospital, six clinics, and seven affiliated dispensaries, which were regularly visited by a physician. By the early 1990s, Igba-Ora, a small agricultural town in western Nigeria, had acquired a government hospital, four maternity clinics, and four private clinics, all of which dispensed medicines in-house, as well as over fifty independent patent medicine vendors.[20] Even though only a small proportion of the town's sixty thousand inhabitants could possibly be ill at any one time and health workers were chronically short, there was at least one dispensing counter for every thousand persons.

Colonial medicine laid the foundation for diagnostic insufficiency, but to blame imperialists alone for this problem in contemporary Africa would be overly simplistic. Even the most brazen critics of the idea that Europe is respon-sible for Africa's underdevelopment admit that the British colonial office was "tight-fisted when it came to education and healthcare":[21] the health of Africans was simply not a primary objective. The real problem with the colonial model is that, although Africans were aware that colonial medical practice was not in their best interests, they allowed it to become the template for future health sys-tems. That this model remains pervasive today is exemplified by Nigeria, where, fifty years after independence, during which time over twenty medical schools and affiliated teaching hospitals have been established, the governing elite con-tinues to seek health care abroad, "invaliding" themselves for minor as well as complicated ailments, particularly when nonclinical diagnostic information is necessary. Prominent medical historians have observed that change has come more slowly in medicine than any other dimension of African postcolonial thought.[22]

After the Second World War, India's independence freed up the personnel and funds to improve Africa's British colonial infrastructure.[23] In the flurry of activ-ity that followed, programs to train medical and health care professionals were established for the first time all over Africa. New "University College" medical schools in Uganda (Makerere University College) and Nigeria (University Col-lege Ibadan) began to train doctors, nurses, and even lab technicians locally. These flagship institutions were modeled after European medical schools, such as University College London, and were equipped with labs. Established before the 1980s, they still house the few reliable laboratory services in their countries today. A few institutions were set up specifically for training laboratory techni-cians, such as the Yaba School in Lagos, which preceded Nigeria's first medical school. However, the training offered in these schools of medicine and laboratory technology did not correspond to the reality of clinical practice outside them, and the initial momentum in medical laboratory science was not sustained. Today, teaching hospital laboratories are often conceived as model space for research and teaching; in other institutions, laboratories are considered secondary to the central mission of patient care.

The timing of health care investment for Africans was especially unfortunate. In the 1940s and 1950s, dozens of antimicrobial drugs had just entered clinical use, and the rigorous etiological definition of infections that had characterized medical practice in previous decades was on the decline. This trend was dangerous everywhere, but it had less severe consequences in Europe, where public health improvements had already drastically reduced the prevalence of infectious diseases. By the 1960s, unsupported antimicrobial use was in its prime globally. Although drug resistance was known, most experts supposed that there were enough new antimicrobials in the pipeline to ensure that resistance would not become a clinically important issue. "Wonder drugs" were being prescribed for sniffles and mild stomach upsets without any laboratory diagnoses or indications for treating them as bacterial infections. The substitution of prescriptions for diagnoses had fatal consequences for diagnostic laboratories in much of Africa, where infections were rife and budgets tight. Maintaining existing laboratories and establishing new ones was not a priority; dispensing "miracle drugs" indiscriminately was mistaken for a low-budget solution to an overwhelming problem.

As African countries approached independence, the colonial basis for the design of incomplete health systems, if even acknowledged, was forgotten as altruistic attempts to expand health care resulted in more clinics being built on a faulty template. At the start of the WHO yaws eradication program in eastern Nigeria, the planners regarded the dispensary as the core of the ideal health center:

> The capital expenditure for building an appreciable network of local health centres...[has] come from the Nsùkka local authorities....These local health centres consist of a good standard dispensary, a standard 4-bed maternity home with adequate facilities for antenatal and child welfare clinics, a health office, and model quarters for their staff. A small building is also incorporated in or near the health centre for the treatment of leprosy out-patients.[24]

In the 1956 description of seven health centers that were built on this model, laboratories and diagnostic technicians are never mentioned. In contrast, when the city of Hickory, North Carolina, urgently needed a polio hospital during a

June 1944 epidemic, and a wooden hospital had to be constructed in just two and a half days, the building contained "an admissions center, a kitchen, a laundry; *a laboratory* and an operating room; isolation wards, dormitories and a therapy wing."[25]

Health clinics devoid of laboratories became the standard model in many parts of Africa. After independence, colonial dispensaries and health institutions became "government hospitals." With increasing pressure to train more health workers, many of these later morphed into teaching hospitals without an appropriate design to meet the needs of their extended functions. When they were not converted into storerooms for disused equipment, laboratories failed to expand in proportion to heath worker populations and patient load.

In existing laboratories, staff morale is often low. For example, for most of the last decade laboratory staffs in Nigerian tertiary care hospitals have been preoccupied with a turf war, as medical laboratory technologists battle consultants in pathology and laboratory medicine. The bench technologists are seeking complete and exclusive laboratory responsibility, while the consultant pathologists with laboratory specialization argue that their oversight and participation is critical to patient care. The battle has moved from hospital boardrooms to the courts,[26] even though laboratory organizational structure is something that has been worked out in most parts of the world. The turf war arises, for the most part, from the absence of a sustained model for the practice of laboratory medicine in a country that has managed infectious diseases in allopathic medicine for over a hundred years.

Accepting and Expecting Diagnostic Insufficiency

Almost two decades after Ghana became independent, medical sociologist P. A. Twumasi examined the practice of medicine in his country. Like many scholars of his generation Twumasi appropriately criticizes the prioritization of curative medicine and the neglect of preventive medicine in emerging African health systems.[27] However, his discussion of curative medicine sheds light on the all-too-common acceptance of the lack of adequate diagnostic support that accompanies Western medical practice in Africa, in spite of the obvious benefits laboratory medicine could provide. Twumasi writes that laboratory investigation is associated only with highly specialized tertiary care centers. If and when a laboratory test is ordered, it is viewed as a referral to a specialist and as a sign of the helplessness of the referring physician. Because tertiary care is generally inaccessible, the laboratory test is an obstacle to care, on the same order as an impossibly expensive trip to a distant medical center. Indigenous practitioners, according to Twumasi, were viewed as more accessible and competent because they were less likely to refer and did not order inconvenient and seemingly extraneous tests.

Indigenous practitioners do use diagnostic tools, but they themselves control these tools, so their patients seldom have to seek components of care elsewhere. All but four of the twenty photographic plates in Twumasi's book depict aspects of traditional medicine, including diagnosis by virtue of "fetish dances," spirit "possession," meditation, and even a traditional medical conference. The last picture shows a patient being examined by a "scientific medical practitioner" using a stethoscope. The caption reads: "A Doctor taking close examination of a patient; no drumming, no invocation, no mystery, as in the case of the traditional healer."[28] Twumasi interprets diagnostic protocols from which the patient is excluded as associated with Western medicine alone. However, diagnosis is a significant dimension of the culture of indigenous healing. For example, patients may sometimes observe, but they are not admitted to spiritual aspects of their diagnosis. The nature of traditional medical practice in many parts of Africa might have primed patients to accept laboratory diagnostics as an integral part of Western medicine. Indeed, laboratory diagnostics could have filled a niche vacated by the invocations, divinations, and "mystery" of indigenous medicine in a manner that would have been acceptable to patients and therefore easily implemented by practitioners.

The importance of applying diagnostic tests at the point of primary care is seldom appreciated, and laboratory facilities are available only at the most sophisticated hospitals. Twumasi describes the hierarchy of hospital facilities in Ghana: "The regional hospital has the capacity for dealing with complex laboratory examinations such as hematological, parasitic, biochemical, and bacteriological problems.... District hospitals may have only a simple X-ray for chest and extremities."[29] In this model, laboratory tests are esoteric specialist tools, while X-ray equipment, which is more expensive to install and operate, is considered appropriate for secondary care centers. Conditions that Twumasi claims are diagnosed through "complex laboratory examinations," including parasitic and bacterial infections, are in fact the most common causes of ill health in Ghana and neighboring countries. Health institutions that cannot cure patients with these conditions are largely ineffectual.

Below the category of district hospitals, Twumasi describes the primary health care center: "Its main functions are to promote healthy living conditions; to emphasize prevention through immunization, teaching better child feeding practices and early diagnoses of disease; and to be curative by treating minor ailments, which would otherwise have to be referred to hospitals."[30] Most primary care centers in Ghana aim to perform all these functions—but they cannot provide reliable early diagnoses.

Even though African health systems are criticized for their overemphasis on curative medicine,[31] this emphasis has not been translated into appropriate primary care. Referrals from primary care clinics often occur after the failure of one or more chemotherapeutic courses, by which time the patient has been severely ill for over a week. Since the primary care centers are closest to the patients, hospitals frequently have to deal with late-stage disease and its attendant complications. Because primary care centers cannot always successfully deal with common, life-threatening, but curable infections, patients juggle their attendance at these institutions with indigenous practices and faith healers. This undermines the ability of primary care centers to effectively deliver valuable preventive therapies such as vaccines, supplements, and antenatal care.

In the West, there was a relatively brief transitional period as scientific methods were introduced into routine health care. At the turn of the twentieth century, young physicians trained at medical schools that introduced the germ theory of disease practiced alongside doctors who had apprenticed to older practitioners. The public quickly realized the value of scientifically trained practitioners, and these physicians rapidly recognized the social as well as the diagnostic value of their scientific skills. As Dr. Daniel W. Cather put it: "Working with the microscope and making analyses of the urine, sputum, blood, and other fluids as an aid to diagnosis, will not only bring fees and lead to valuable information regarding the patient's condition, but will also give you reputation and patient respect, by investing in you, in the eyes of the public, with the benefits of being a very scientific man."[32]

Today, African physicians compete in a pluralistic market for health services. The care they provide must be more precise, more rigorous, and more effective than that offered by their competitors, who range from authentic indigenous practitioners to spiritual healers and quacks. If physicians fully applied the tenets of biomedicine to treat infectious diseases, they would fully enjoy the status and patronage that it confers. As long as they do not, they remain hobbled by the crippling legacies of colonial neglect and of misplaced enthusiasm for "wonder drugs" whose miracles turn into nightmares unless they are properly applied. Indeed, in the glaring light of diagnostic insufficiency, their medical practice resembles that of the nonallopathic healers and untrained drug dispensers who they deride. Prescribing medications without first diagnosing the disease violates the basic tenets of scientific medicine and vitiates the effectiveness of health care practice.

Facing Forward

It is helpful to locate the origins of diagnostic insufficiency in colonial and mid-twentieth-century medicine, but contemporary Africa should not merely look back at the baneful influences of the past. Africa needs to take a fresh look at science today and chart a new path that suits her needs. Many recent biomedical advances are well suited for diagnostic development and should be exploited to optimize health care delivery. As former Ghanaian president, statesman, and pan-Africanist Kwame Nkrumah put it in 1963:

> There is no need for us to go through all the long and complicated stages of the development of science which other countries have gone through in the past. We are, as it were, jumping the centuries, using knowledge and experience already available to us. What others have taken hundreds of years to do, we must achieve in a generation.[33]

Emerging technologies, in particular molecular biology, genomics, and nanotechnology, offer much promise to the area of diagnostics. However, recent African history, which has seen few gains from the molecular biology revolution that began in the 1950s, suggests that unless Nkrumah's words are deliberately acted upon, the want of thoughtful application could further increase health disparities between most of Africa's population and patients in the West in years to come.

When molecular technology became available, some foresaw a diagnostic revolution in the developing world. Molecular diagnostics represent the most rapidly growing segment of the diagnostic test market, and the technology exists to design molecular tests by the second decade of the twenty-first century for every organism known to infect humans or animals.[34] Indeed, a few early developers of molecular diagnostics focused specifically on improving infectious disease diagnosis in developing countries.[35] Robert H. Barker, Dyann Wirth, and collaborating specialists in tropical public health who developed a molecular probe for malaria explain that molecular methods are much less labor intensive than conventional ones: "One microscopist can read 60 samples per day; for the probe technology, we estimate that one technician can process 1000 samples per day." Still, the authors had to defend developing testing methods for resource poor laboratories as a legitimate focus of research when other scientists suggested that it did not constitute genuine innovation.[36]

Some of the potential that molecular science holds for diagnosis in Africa can be seen today, and not merely be projected into an imagined future. A 2005 visit to the University Teaching Hospital in Lusaka, Zambia, which is in many ways a model institution, demonstrates the substantial contribution that can be made by laboratory capacity and expertise. The lab itself occupies a large part of the hospital, and the department of microbiology and pathology appropriately employs more people than any other department.[37] Through a recent Japanese aid program, the tuberculosis and HIV diagnostic labs have state-of-the-art facilities for microbial and molecular analysis. The HIV unit has first-rate equipment for determining viral load and flow cytometry machines for sorting blood cells to assess immune status. Also humming in the background are two thermocyclers, electrophoresis equipment, and a sequencer so that drug-resistant viruses can be identified and subtyped. In the next room, busy technicians work with serology kits for determining HIV serostatus, and HIV screening is admirably quality-assured. Despite long lines for testing, the hospital is able to optimize patient care as well as conduct research on the evolution and spread of HIV. The tuberculosis laboratory does routine analysis and assesses the quality of smear analysis done in primary care institutions. A notice board displays recent research publications. The equipment is used routinely, consumable supplies are procured, and technical and maintenance support is obtained locally or from nearby South Africa.

These facilities demonstrate that appropriate diagnostic technology can enhance patient care in an African hospital. However, the laboratory improvements for HIV and tuberculosis did not extend to other high-burden diseases, pointing to programs that are driven by donor priorities rather than local needs. At the nearby parasitology lab, only one staff member was on duty and the diagnostic tools were limited to light microscopes. The only other pieces of electrical equipment were a decrepit weighing balance, an oven, and a radio. When we visited at midmorning on a busy weekday in 2005, only one staff member was on duty. Two record books lay on the desk, one for blood specimens for malaria blood smear screening and the other for stool microscopy, but—in stark contrast to the bustling HIV and tuberculosis diagnostic laboratories—no slides were being processed.

Overall, the priorities of donors are influenced by a myriad of factors, many of which are aimed at improving the donor's reputation in the eyes of people in rich countries who might contribute toward the donor's purse or, in the worst-case scenario, purchase for-profit materials that the donor might produce. The objective of highlighting one disease at the expense of another might even be altruistic. For example, in explaining his career focus on tuberculosis, and later AIDS, the WHO HIV/AIDS director Jim Yong Kim said:

> It made sense to focus on multidrug-resistant tuberculosis because it frightens people, even in rich countries. There is a real—although remote—possibility that you might be sitting on a plane next to someone with multidrug-resistant tuberculosis, contract it, and die or infect others. We pushed hard on the issue, not because we cared more about tuberculosis as a health problem than, for example, children dying from

diarrhea and dehydration. We were just as concerned with that problem and working on it as well, but multidrug-resistant tuberculosis allowed us to make a much larger point.[38]

The "point" as spelled out in many of Yong Kim's essays is that the developing-country infectious disease burden must be addressed, and addressed effectively. An unintended consequence of the scare-mongering approach, however, is that interventions for childhood diarrhea, the very example highlighted by Kim, are grossly underpublicized, underfunded, and underimplemented.[39]

Zambia's tropical infection research center in the Copper Belt has better di-agnostic facilities for malaria, but the absence of suitable facilities at University Teaching Hospital (UTH), the tertiary care center that serves the country's most populous city, represented a gaping hole in the country's ambitious malaria con-trol program as recently as 2005. At UTH, up-to-date technologies were applied to emerging health threats such as HIV, but diagnostic infrastructure for age-old, high-burden scourges was sadly lacking. Intestinal parasite infection rates were rising due to the AIDS epidemic, but the procedures for diagnosis had not changed even though they are insufficiently sensitive for parasites such as *Enta-moeba histolytica*.[40] Despite the great promise of biomedical advances, the histo-rian Megan Vaughn concluded in 1991, they overwhelmingly have not translated into technologies that improve health care delivery in resource-limited clinics.[41] Science is a global enterprise and diagnostic test innovation can and should occur in laboratories across the globe. However, Africans need to be at the center of deciding how testing is deployed and used in their countries, and in ensuring that appropriate technology reaches the clinic.

One Model for Diagnostic Development

Helen Lee, one of a few scientists who grasp the diagnostic challenges facing developing countries, is using modern technology to devise practical solutions to diagnostic insufficiency. Lee's laboratory at the University of Cambridge aims to develop rapid, cheap, and simple tests that can be used to diagnose infec-tious diseases in resource-limited settings. It is unusual for a research group to make diagnostic development its primary objective; most scientists who address this problem do so on their way to doing something else. It is difficult to obtain financial support for research on diagnostics itself. Nonetheless, Lee has received multiple research grants and awards from such prestigious institutions as the National Institutes of Health in the United States and the U.K.-based Wellcome Trust to support her current work on simple, rapid tests for blood-borne dis-eases, such as HIV and hepatitis B and C. Many technical challenges remain to be overcome, but her work is already showing great promise, and her interests extend beyond diseases that have received international promise to little-known "neglected" diseases that afflict some of the poorest people in the world.

Success has not come easily. It took Lee's group about five years to lay the groundwork for universally applicable diagnostic tests, and, in her words, she had to be "broad shouldered" to sustain the project over that period. Academic research institutions rarely tolerate product-directed work that takes so long to yield tangible outcomes and does not result in notable papers in premier scientific journals. Lee's laboratory focused instead on adapting science to technology that is appropriate for resource-poor areas, which is not a flashy or well-rewarded field of research.

Lee's laboratory focuses on all aspects of the diagnostic process. Noninvasive and rapid tests that can be used at the point of care are the goal. The diagnostics the laboratory develops are stable at 45°C for more than a year, making it unnecessary to refrigerate reagents or transport them through a cold supply chain. Each test is presented in a kit comprised of as few components as possible, along with an easy-to-follow pictorial manual that documents every step from collecting the specimen to interpreting the results. This approach makes it unnecessary to equip new laboratories with sophisticated or expensive equipment. No complex measurements or other difficult technical procedures must be performed, obviating the need for highly skilled technicians. The only thing a lab worker has to measure is time. All test components, including reagents, are part of the kit and are color coded to reduce the possibility of error. Lee's team is developing multiplex dipsticks that permit a number of different pathogens or pathogen subtypes to be detected: one test will be used to screen blood for HIV, hepatitis B, and hepatitis C viruses simultaneously. This approach is invaluable for screening blood for transfusion, particularly in developing countries where unscreened blood, essential for patients with severe malaria, is a major route for transmitting blood-borne HIV and hepatitis.[42]

Most intriguing of all, the combined HIV–hepatitis C–hepatitis B virus test, like Lee's earlier inventions, is a molecular one. Lee and her co-workers have successfully overcome resource constraints for molecular testing. Many molecular tests aim to detect the pathogen's DNA or RNA in clinical specimens. To do so, they use probes that are complementary to and specific for pathogen DNA or RNA. The first step in these nucleic acid tests is isolation of both pathogen and patient DNA/RNA from clinical specimens such as swabs or body fluids. For body fluids, some concentration may be necessary. Next, the sample is enriched for pathogen DNA by amplification. Specific probes are applied, which "stick" if the complementary sequence from the pathogen is present. Finally, a means to detect stuck probes is needed. Conventionally, radioactive or fluorescent methods are used, all of which require expensive equipment. Lee's group has developed sensitive and specific color tests on dipsticks, taking advantage of modern technology to amplify DNA but precluding the need for expensive detection systems. Using innovative isothermal amplification as an alternative to more traditional amplification by thermocycling, and including a signal amplification system to increase the sensitivity of detection, makes it possible to dispense with expensive electronic thermocyclers. Innovation was even applied at the level of collection. For their chlamydial test, Lee's group invented a device to capture the first 3–4 ml of urine, the part of the specimen that contains the highest concentration of pathogens, which increases the sensitivity of direct tests without the need for expensive equipment to concentrate the sample.

Lee's laboratory and company are developing just the sort of tests that Africa needs. Their projects demonstrate that test sensitivity and specificity are not inconsistent with low cost and ease of use. Lee's rapid test for chlamydia, a widely prevalent sexually transmitted infection that is impossible to reliably diagnose clinically, is the best in its class. It has comparable specificity to the next best test and superior sensitivity, speed, and ease of performance. Lee even has an answer to the question of how her strategy will remain economically viable. She plans to use a two-tiered system to market diagnostics for chlamydia, so that higher pricing of home-based individual tests in developed countries will permit her to sell bulk packages at or below cost to health institutions in developing countries.[43] The chlamydial dipstick test will be invaluable for diagnosing this often symptomless but damaging disease, which is dangerous to the fetuses of infected mothers. Profits will also be devoted to enhancing the detection of *Chlamydia trachomatis,* the etiologic agent of trachoma, which is the most common cause of blindness in the developing world.

Lee is no longer alone in her effort to develop diagnostics "for the real world." The dawning recognition of the need for simple, rapid diagnostic tests has resulted in recent development of new tests for diseases as diverse as malaria, meningococcal meningitis, leishmaniasis, and plague.[44] These tests have been field tested in remote parts of Africa and their initial success offers promise for their use in facilities that do not have highly skilled technicians, a stable electric supply, or biomedical equipment. A test for schistomiasis was recently developed in Ghana by professor Kwabena Bosompem's research group at the Noguchi Research Institute in Accra.[45] With the right motivation and very basic molecular biology facilities, tests for other diseases endemic in Africa could be developed by other scientists on the continent. The cost of developing many tests is not high. Medécins Sans Frontières (MSF, Doctors without Borders) claims that the development costs for a rapid point-of-care malaria test were as little as $100,000.[46] Why diagnostic test development for Africa has not been prioritized is a large question, and high cost is only one of several myths standing in the way.

CONCLUSION

The Feasibility of Laboratory Diagnosis in African Settings

> We have the research knowledge, but it is a question of getting it into the field and actually doing something about the problem.
>
> —Tony Jordan, 2001

In May 2009, the *Annals of Tropical Medicine and Hygiene* published an audit of diagnostic services in the Tanga region of Tanzania. The audit was performed roughly five years after Tanzania had committed to an ambitious health care reform program, which commendably included a stated intention of ensuring access to high-quality and effective laboratory services whenever these were required for diagnosis. The findings were, as described by the report's Tanzanian authors, "depressing":[1] most of the labs failed to meet the Tanzanian national recommendations. As few as eighty-four personnel staffed thirty-seven health laboratories, most of whom lacked training in diagnostic laboratory services and were working without supervision. Essential protocols such as culture—for diagnosing life-threatening bacteremia and meningitis—could not be performed at any laboratory. HIV and tuberculosis testing was available at less than half of them, and although most reported that they performed blood smears for malaria, microscopes were often defective so that the quality of these tests, and many others, could not be assured. Whenever only limited testing is available, the priority should be highly prevalent diseases or those where a precise diagnosis would alter the course of treatment. Instead, the researchers observed that resources available at laboratory facilities in the Tanga region were not reflective of health care needs or the burden of disease.

The Tanzanian laboratory audit cited Ghana as a model of diagnostic development but even there, regional laboratories are often not equipped to respond to local health needs.[2] However, Ghana's first two teaching hospitals do have reasonably well-equipped and staffed laboratories. Laboratory capacity at one of these hospitals was formally assessed in 2005, revealing that blood, cerebrospinal fluid, urine, and stool were routinely cultured for bacterial pathogens. Sputum smear microscopy was available for tuberculosis diagnosis, and malaria could be diagnosed by microscopy. Eleven of the twenty lab staff members had a bachelor's degree in medical laboratory sciences, and five others were qualified laboratory technicians. Four of the five laboratories in the twelve-hundred-bed institution used appropriate internal quality control methods. Even though problems with data management and physician attitudes were recorded, the laboratory was equipped for the task of diagnosing the most common endemic infections that can be cheaply identified with present-day technology.[3]

Ghanaian teaching hospital laboratories are attached to local tertiary-care hospitals. Although they do participate in international research projects and clinical trials, their primary function is to support patient care. They are answerable to the Ghanaian health system and in some cases oversee services at district laboratories. They demonstrate that integrated laboratory services can and do work. At a time when health care development on the continent is of global interest, the rarity of such establishments raises the question of why laboratory services in many more parts of Africa, as illustrated by the Tanga evaluation, are suboptimal or derelict. The failure to imagine a different mode of health care delivery for Africa is so widespread and of such long standing that many people inside as well as outside the health care sector, incognizant of or ignoring the important exceptions, assume the situation is intractable. Long-standing arguments against providing diagnostic laboratory services at all levels of medical practice in developing countries are repeatedly echoed, even in association with the most well-meaning health initiatives. These paralyzing arguments are grounded on unsupported presumptions that must be unpacked and critically examined.

Many adamantly argue that laboratory testing is not feasible under African conditions. This, in turn, is accompanied by the notion that diagnostic testing necessarily requires more time than clinical practice allows. Then there is the belief that the cost of microbiological diagnostics would simply be untenable given resource constraints. Finally, many presume that there is, and always will be, an insurmountable lack of the kind of expertise required to use appropriate diagnostics. All of this is amplified by the misconception that diagnostic testing is not really necessary. Justifying diagnostic development in Africa requires us to debunk the six most prevalent myths.

Diagnostic Mythology

Too Many Patients, Too Little Time

Government hospitals in developing countries are among the most crowded health facilities in the world and are staffed by woefully overworked health professionals. The seemingly unending stream of patients makes it impossible for them to devote more than a few minutes to each one.[4] Even the most rapid laboratory tests take a few minutes, and often outpatients must come back for their results to be read. The idea that ordering, performing, reporting, and interpreting diagnostic tests could slow down long lines is a valid concern. Eliminating necessary diagnostic tests does not make patient care more efficient, however, because every misdiagnosis incurs costs in time and money for patients as well as for health care systems. Incorrectly treated outpatients return, or go elsewhere; they spread the disease to others, who must then seek care. Misdiagnosed outpatients often end up as inpatients, who more easily overwhelm resource-constrained health systems.

It is no coincidence that Sir Arthur Conan Doyle, author of the popular Sherlock Holmes detective tales, was a medical doctor. Medical diagnosis is a sophisticated and often time-consuming process of careful observation and deductive reasoning. Research has repeatedly shown that, even with diagnostic flowcharts and other aids, health workers, particularly when they are not qualified doctors or nurse practitioners, are imperfect clinical diagnosticians.[5] Incorporating objective information from laboratory tests increases diagnostic precision. Laboratory testing is especially important when health workers are overtaxed or semitrained, and when consulting time is short.

Today, rapid malaria tests can be performed during a single outpatient visit. Laboratory diagnosis of many other infections takes longer, but the technology to develop rapid tests for other common infections exists. In the most overcrowded health facilities, the time that outpatients spend sitting or standing in line is often used for prescreening by a nurse or aide who looks for clinical signs of disease. Rapid diagnostic tests for one or more highly prevalent diseases could be performed as part of the screening process so that results are available to the prescriber and no time is lost. Less rapid and more expensive tests, if required, could be ordered by the consulting health worker. It is unfortunate that patients must wait at all, or, when unavoidable, return for the interpretation of the results, but the gains in terms of diagnostic accuracy, appropriate prescription, and the avoidance of therapeutic failure far outweigh the inconvenience.

A critical examination of the "inconvenience" that routine testing might entail is worthwhile. In many parts of Africa, a culture of treating patients as aggregates is a legacy from colonial medicine, where the health of the individual African was not of interest and patients were processed in a conveyor belt mode.[6] It may be the baneful influence of this construct on medical practice, rather than the nature of biomedical science per se, that occasions the prevalent criticisms of biomedical neglect of the whole person and alienation of the patient.[7] Patients are less likely to be suspicious of a system that views them as individuals rather than as faceless members of an aggregate. Diagnostic development will force a level of individualization in healthcare delivery that could also improve patients' attitudes toward health services.

Laboratory Facilities Are Too Expensive

The largest share of health expenditure in Africa, from colonial times until today, has gone to medicines. A long-standing misperception that is prevalent world-wide is that diagnostics are of lower value than drugs.[8] Diagnostics inform drug development and they are key to ensuring that existing drugs are appropriately used. Diagnostics are not cheap, but their direct costs should not be the primary factor in deciding their use and development; to authentically assess costs, the savings that diagnostics provide must be deducted from their price. Recent studies in resource-poor settings, as well as mathematical models, show that for malaria, sexually transmitted diseases, and other infections, diagnostic testing is almost always cost effective, even when testing is not optimal.[9] In some cases, the cost-effectiveness of diagnostic testing has been compromised by prescribers failing to utilize test results to inform care. But this points to the need for prescriber education rather than toward abolishing testing.

Add-ons to the real cost of materials inflate the cost of biomedical science, including testing in many parts of Africa. Converters and other supporting equipment must be purchased to utilize machines that are designed to operate in other countries. Present-day prohibitive maintenance costs arise because "gadgetry [is] simply too scarce to support a domestic service economy."[10] In the West, a substantial proportion of the cost of a test covers the time spent by technicians and consultants to perform and interpret it. As the absolute value of salaries in Africa is lower, this component of the cost will also be lower.

Another common miscalculation arises from the fact that diagnostic services are much more expensive on a case-by-case basis when used rarely than when used routinely. Because it often costs as much to run five samples through laboratory tests as it does two dozen, the cost of each test falls dramatically when more patients in need of testing are screened. Currently, where available at all, laboratory diagnostics in Africa are often reserved for complicated or refractory cases and available at tertiary care and research centers. Were they used routinely, economies of scale could sustain a market for equipment and reagents. Competition should encourage lower markups as well as local manufacture and distribution.[11]

A global economic crisis that became apparent in 2008 overlapped with health care crises of emerging infections and drug resistance. All of these threats must be addressed by careful investment of resources and in a manner that guarantees successes and minimizes waste. For infectious diseases, this includes adequate preventive measures and the efficient diagnosis of common infections so that they are treated with the cheapest appropriate medicines before they are allowed to spread. Resource-poor health systems that are weighed down by the needless disease transmission that accompanies misdiagnosis have a greater need for diagnostic precision than their more affluent counterparts. It behooves us to be wary of naysayers who cite prohibitive cost as the excuse for avoiding any effective health intervention. Almost every time someone has bothered to check the figures, the indirect cost of doing nothing, or doing the improper, exceeds that of the direct cost of administering appropriate care. Still, cries of "cost-ineffectiveness" continue to undermine health care delivery in the poorest countries, very often masking less easily justified reasons for inaction.[12]

The Ideal Tests for Africa Have Not Been Invented Yet

Interest in diagnostics has increased in recent years. However, as clinical microbiologist Keith Klugman lamented in 2010, the revolution in diagnostics is a slow one. Some of the sluggishness arises because current resources are underutilized. A tuberculosis laboratory capacity building program in Lesotho has demonstrated that we do not need to wait for improvements before implementing currently available tests in African health clinics. However, it must be acknowledged that the age-old scourges of tuberculosis, typhoid fever, and other bacterial infections—and malaria until recently—are all diagnosed with tests that are approximately a century old. Many of these tests are too slow, too complex, or too expensive to be used at the point of care. By contrast, HIV, a "new" virus of global significance, has seen four cycles of diagnostic test development within a quarter of a century. Why is there such a small knowledge base for appropriate primary-care diagnostics for Africa? The answer is connected to profit motivation because most common infectious agents are known and can be detected, many of them simply and rapidly. For many tropical diseases where a useable test is yet to reach the clinical laboratory bench, we know development is possible because diagnostic tests are available for similar organisms that are prevalent in Western countries.[13]

Vaccine and drug development are driven by the needs of patients in the richest countries in the world. The same is true for diagnostics. Multiplex tests, which could detect more than one pathogen in a single specimen, would have inestimable value for many syndromes common in Africa, but they do not yet exist. However, veterinary diagnostics that can detect up to five different pathogens in a stool sample from a calf with diarrhea are routinely used in industrialized countries. One of these tests screens for two common viral, one protozoal, and two bacterial targets. The test is performed without any equipment, can be run outdoors on a farm, and the results are ready in fifteen minutes.[14] An outbreak of calf diarrhea can have tremendous financial implications for a farm and even a national food program, which is what motivated the development and use of the test.

Until very recently, there were few financial incentives for developing vaccines or drugs specifically designed for people who cannot pay for them, and even fewer for developing diagnostic tests. But today, economists and policymakers are beginning to put forward ideas to incentivize innovation that could improve the health of the poor. These include public-private initiatives, such as the suggestion that donors offer to pay for drugs when they are developed.[15] Similar stimuli would apply to diagnostics so that the estimated one hundred million rapid diagnostic tests for TB required each year will be paid for when they become available.[16]

We have the technical expertise to develop tests de novo in areas of need. Diagnostic development has yet to receive the same attention or lobbying effort as medicines, but, with the right stimulus, the ongoing genomic and nanotechnology revolutions make it relatively simple to identify diagnostic candidates and make them the basis for point-of-care tests. Veterinarians performing molecular tests out in the field, under conditions that are much worse than in an African clinic, do not need to understand molecular biology to accurately perform and interpret the tests, nor do they need temperamental electronic equipment.[17] The chlamydial rapid test developed by Helen Lee's group is as sensitive as conventional nucleic acid amplification tests but lacks their technical complexity and instrumentation requirements. This thirty-minute test can be performed while a patient visits any health provider, and the test is so simple that a version has been developed for home use. Blood tests for estimating blood cell counts and hemoglobin levels traditionally required microscopes and skilled technicians. Today they can be performed with a portable instrument that provides a digital readout when blood collected from a pinprick is applied. This type of test has been used to assist diagnoses of very sick children in Tanzania.[18] Recently, an isothermal amplification test for drug-resistant tuberculosis was developed and tested in Peru, Bangladesh, and Tanzania. Although the test has a molecular basis, it is simple and safe to perform and is rapid and robust.[19]

WHO has suggested that diagnostic tests for use in resource-poor areas must be "ASSURED": affordable, sensitive, specific, user-friendly, robust and rapid, equipment-free, and deliverable to areas of need.[20] The aforementioned examples meet most or all of these important criteria. Incentives to develop, validate, and deploy diagnostic tests for Africa's infectious diseases exist primarily in Africa's health and research sectors. The tardy and slow entry of molecular biology and nanoscale chemistry into the underexploited local scientific community is one of several factors limiting diagnostic development.[21] Africa's scientific community is small, but a relatively high proportion is studying endemic infectious diseases, with a handful of scientists focusing on diagnostics. Some are making good progress and beginning to generate global interest. A research group in Ghana has developed and field tested a point-of-care urine test for schistosomiasis. The test has greater sensitivity than microscopy, the currently advocated method of diagnosis, but is easier to perform. Similarly, researchers at the Kenya Medical Research Institute (KEMRI) have developed tests for hepatitis B and HIV, and a Nigerian working in South Africa is the innovator for a promising new tuberculosis diagnostic platform.[22] With the right support,[23] African scientists could drive the development of diagnostics, as well as control measures and treatments, and their innovations could improve health care delivery in their own countries.

New diagnostics offer great promise, but even currently available tests are underutilized across Africa. Lack of infrastructure is often cited as the reason for dispensing with even the most basic tests. But microscopy can be performed without electricity, using a mirror and sunlight, and even bacterial culture can be performed in laboratories equipped with sterilizers that use alternate fuels, kerosene-fueled refrigerators, and phase-change incubators.[24] Most existing tests are less complex than mobile phone technology, which was unheard of when bacteriology tests were developed, but which, unlike microbial diagnostics, has invaded the most remote African villages in the last twenty years. In short, tests that were developed a hundred years ago typically don't require expensive or sophisticated infrastructure, and newer rapid diagnostic tests can be used with no equipment at all. Even without new developments, it is possible to offer many effective tests in today's health clinics.

Local Technical Expertise Cannot Support Diagnostic Testing

From the late colonial era, African doctors, nurses, engineers, and teachers were produced in specially targeted training programs, modeled on European systems, with the specific goal of creating a professional cadre that could build Africa from independence and teach later generations. The real and the perceived shortage of technical expertise for diagnostic testing is as much the consequence as the cause of diagnostic insufficiency. Failure to prioritize the development of diagnostic capacity in the hospital and public health infrastructure has been coupled with the collapse of educational facilities for laboratory scientists and pathologists. Laboratory specialties were included in Africa's first medical schools, such as the University of Ibadan and University of Ghana Medical Schools but in 2004

'Ṣegun Ojo, a Nigerian professor of pathology, noted that many newer medical schools in his country did not have a pathologist on the faculty. Similarly, in Malawi, medical schools train too few students in laboratory medicine.[25]

Diagnostic laboratory services are best overseen by consultant pathologists and are appropriately staffed by clinical scientists who have received training and certification in biochemistry, microbiology, or related sciences. A college degree in the sciences or, at the very minimum, two years of postsecondary education with compensatory experience is optimal for reliably implementing all but point-of-care diagnostic tests. In developing countries, the shortage of people with higher education is felt intensely in the health sector. It would be a real challenge for several countries to staff fully functional diagnostic laboratories in every secondary and tertiary care health facility. However, highly skilled workers are not required for all tasks in a diagnostic laboratory, and diagnostic services can be structured to make the most of staff with less formal training. Moreover, technical training programs are less expensive and difficult to mount than programs to train clinical professionals. However, Nigeria, the African country with the most medical schools, trains more doctors and pharmacists than medical laboratory technologists.

Were every patient with relevant symptoms to gain access to as few as eight diagnostic tests, including point-of-care tests for malaria, sexually transmitted infections, and tuberculosis, as well as blood tests for endemic parasites and bacteria, medical care in Africa would be revolutionized. Modern point-of-care tests are often simpler than the highly technical tests of yesteryear and could be performed by trained semiskilled workers at the primary care level with local or regional supervision. Laboratory scientists at Zambia's University Teaching Hospital effectively supervise sputum smear microscopy for tuberculosis diagnosis at several health centers in and around Lusaka and the Lesotho national TB lab was recently equipped to perform a similar function. Ongoing boosts to information technology and communications across Africa offer attractive possibilities for even more remote supervision. For example, microscopy slide data can now be transmitted via the Internet or mobile phones.[26]

Currently, even in the face of a shortage of laboratory technologists, there are very few career opportunities for graduate biochemists, biologists, chemists, and microbiologists in much of Africa. A significant proportion of graduates working in the banking and insurance industries hold bachelor's degrees in scientific disciplines, and biomedical laboratories struggle to retain highly skilled staff.[27] Attrition of the potential laboratory workforce begins even earlier as concerns about poor employment prospects lead the strongest biology and chemistry students to enter undergraduate programs in medicine, pharmacy, or engineering, so that potential biomedical scientists are diverted to other professional fields.

Medical doctors who choose to specialize are unlikely to select pathology or laboratory medicine, as these specialties offer few opportunities to augment income through private practice. Adjustments in compensation and working conditions for laboratory technologists could address many of these problems.

Any diagnostic development initiative must seek to address the root causes of the laboratory workforce shortage but should also provide training for existing laboratory staff, many of whom have never performed some tests for the most prevalent diseases in their countries. In 2005, the American Society for Microbiology began its International Laboratory Capacity Building Program, or "LabCap," which solicits scientists from its forty-thousand-strong membership (five thousand of whom are certified clinical microbiologists) to assist in developing laboratory capacity in Africa. In less than three years, volunteers had built significant capacity for tuberculosis diagnosis in Namibia, Zambia, and Nigeria, training local personnel in sustainable methods. By 2009, programs in those countries had begun to have spillover effects on other laboratories in those countries while "LabCap" programs were also established in Tanzania, Botswana, Kenya, Cote D'Ivoire, Rwanda, Mozambique, and South Africa. The Society estimates that at least ten thousand technicians will need to be trained for about two thousand African laboratories. It is far from this goal, but the initial successes demonstrate that developing the necessary human resource is feasible.

Diagnostic Tests Are Superfluous

Many argue that if intensive use of laboratory diagnostics were best practice in medicine, this would be the norm in the developed countries. People who state this position do not take the African disease landscape and differences in resource availability and access to care into consideration. Sadly, both Western and African physicians and public health professionals are guilty of attempting, or at least wishing, to model health care delivery in Africa after that in Europe or North America. This misguided aspiration is due not only to the absence of other models but also to practitioners' efforts to make the practice of medicine more uniform around the globe.[28]

The differences in the need for laboratory diagnostics in these two settings can be easily explained. First, most outpatient visits in the West are for irritating but self-resolving infections, such as the common cold, ear infections, and benign food poisoning, or for conditions with noninfectious etiologies. If there is a chance that symptoms are masking a more serious infection, patients are given supporting therapy and told to "come back if things do not improve." In tropical Africa, most patients coming to an outpatient clinic have life-threatening infections such as malaria or pneumonia. A good number present for the first time only days before they might be dead or disabled by the infection. Many cannot afford to return for a reevaluation if the first course of therapy fails. If they receive the correct diagnosis promptly, most patients can be given medicine that will cure them. The proportion of patients with relatively mild, self-resolving illnesses is smaller and less likely to reach the clinic. These differences in acuity and the prevalence of infectious diseases mean that initial microbiological diagnosis is more important and more cost effective in Africa than in the West.

Those who insist on applying Western standards of care in Africa seem unaware that patients in the West who present with symptoms of fever and a travel history to a malaria-endemic area are invariably tested.[29] So are patients who present with signs that suggest life-threatening infections, including medium-grade fevers. The idea that medical institutions in Africa can or should be less well equipped than those in the West that address diseases common or endemic in Africa is one piece of unpacked colonial baggage.

Even more important, the impression that diagnostic tests are rarely used in the West is erroneous and outdated. It is true that a 1975 British study reported that 85 percent of final diagnoses were based on information that the physician obtained during consultation in the course of taking a history and 7 percent on physical examination, while only 8 percent of diagnoses required a laboratory test or other diagnostic procedure such as an X-ray.[30] However, since that time, more, faster, and better diagnostic tests have become available. At the same time, diseases that present with macroscopical diagnostic features, such as measles, mumps, whooping cough, and chickenpox, have become less common. Importantly, the need to make diagnosis more precise in order to use antimicrobials prudently and avoid promoting resistance has recently been acknowledged. As a result, laboratory diagnosis has increased severalfold.

In the United States, 170,102 diagnostic laboratories were documented in 2000.[31] A tenth as many laboratories could solve the problems of TB diagnostic delay in Africa. Well over half of the U.S. labs (62%) were in physicians' offices, undertaking simple tests for conditions such as strep throat at the point of care. Other tests, often forgotten by the patient, are sent away to laboratories by the physician's office. In the Netherlands, a 2006 study recorded that 12 percent of patients with diarrheal disease were tested.[32] Testing is recommended when the patient has protracted diarrhea, bloody diarrhea, acute pain, or a history of foreign travel—particularly to Africa. In U.K. (2000) and U.S. (2004) studies, rates of testing were even higher (27% and 44%).[33] Outbreak identification for *Shigella* and O157 and other enterohemorrhagic *E. coli* in Western countries depends on analysis of specimens from patients visiting their primary care providers.[34] Testing and surveillance are routine in spite of the fact that diarrheal disease, a major but silent killer in Africa, kills or permanently disables relatively few Americans and Europeans.

The microbiology laboratory in a Nigerian teaching hospital that attends over two hundred thousand patients annually, over half of whom have an infectious disease, processes only fifteen thousand specimens each year. In a recent Swedish study, half of children presenting with symptoms suggestive of an infection, including the common cold, were referred for laboratory testing.[35] Authors of the report, who found that test results promoted rational drug use, advocated even more testing. This point underscores an important consideration. Although laboratory tests are regularly used in the West, their use is still insufficient to inform rational prescribing; in this sense, diagnostic insufficiency exists even there.

The response to the accusation that patients in Western countries do not get tested very often is that, compared with patients in sub-Saharan Africa, they need testing less, receive it more, and will be subjected to even more testing in a future of increasingly personalized care.[36] Diagnostic tests are not just nice to have, they are essential for health care delivery, and their deployment in resource-limited settings would have a significant and measurable impact on the major causes of death in developing countries.[37]

Laboratory Diagnostics Make No Contribution to Disease Prevention

Many preventive interventions can be implemented without laboratories. For example, barriers against biting insects, safe drinking water supplies, good sanitation, and improved nutrition do not require laboratory testing. Diagnostic development will have its greatest impact on curative medicine, but it will make important contributions to preventive medicine and public health such as supporting prioritization and assessment of costly but high impact interventions.

At the very least, diagnostic support for curative medicine contains infectious diseases. Safe water prevents cholera, which continues to plague African societies without access to potable water supplies. If rapidly and adequately rehydrated, cholera patients will recover from this dreaded and deadly disease without antimicrobial drugs. However, when appropriate antimicrobials are not used in a cholera outbreak, the disease spreads rapidly and the size of the outbreak is increased severalfold. Identifying a cholera outbreak early, and determining the susceptibility pattern of the causative strain, can prevent thousands of illnesses and deaths. In the last fifteen years, documented outbreaks that were amplified by diagnostic insufficiency have occurred almost exclusively in sub-Saharan Africa.[38] Similarly, as discussed in chapter 7, diagnostic delay is driving drug-resistant tuberculosis epidemics.

Disease-specific interventions, such as new vaccines against the causes of deadly pneumonia and diarrhea in children, would be helped by information that a diagnostic infrastructure and surveillance systems could provide. Researchers developing vaccines for typhoid and tests for schistosomiasis all agree that preventive and curative interventions for both diseases are underimplemented because of epidemiological blindness arising from diagnostic insufficiency. Epidemiological data also assists scientists in developing life-saving vaccines and convincing countries to adopt new vaccines and donors to pay for them.[39]

Diagnostic facilities are essential to identify and contain new diseases and to disburse health assistance to the areas of greatest need. Emerging infectious diseases are carefully mapped in Europe, Oceania, and North America, less robustly documented in Asia and South America, and rarely documented in Africa.[40] As a consequence, interventions that could prevent or halt epidemics in Africa are often delayed.

The Real Roadblock: Lack of Sustained Commitment

In Lesotho, efforts to increase the speed of diagnosis and introduce diagnostic capacity for multidrug-resistant tuberculosis required the revolutionizing of the national laboratory. Authors of a technical paper describing the two-year initiative attributed its success to strong collaborations—between the national reference laboratory, WHO, and international foundations devoted to global health and diagnostic development—and to political commitment.[41] Diagnostic development lies within the realm of science, but diagnostic insufficiency is also a political and socioeconomic problem. More than funds, expertise, or knowledge, what is needed to spur diagnostic development is a long-term commitment from all stakeholders. This includes health workers and policymakers as well as those that bear the ultimate costs of diagnostic inadequacies—patients and others that pay for health care such as governments and donors.

Local initiative and partnering is as crucial as external support in developing lasting laboratory services because temporary diagnostic proficiency can be attained even without diagnostic development. An illustrative example is the deployment of military diagnostic personnel and resources during the post–September 11, 2001 war in Iraq. Following a report of severe acute pneumonitis as the cause of two deaths, the military recognized the need for on-site clinical diagnostic support and promptly set up microbiology laboratories in Iraq.[42] Although the U.S. military claimed that since ailing soldiers are often repatriated, the long-term beneficiaries of these services were Iraqis, that claim is questionable. The laboratories were rapidly stocked with highly specific and sensitive imported and kit-based test reagents. In most cases, although cheaper, more rugged protocols were available, the army opted for those tests that could be performed with minimal on-site pre-preparation. Most of the selected reagents were more expensive than those that would be employed by diagnostic laboratories in the United States. Specimens for essential tests that could not be performed on-site were shipped by the Air Force to a reference laboratory in Germany.[43] The diagnostic facilities developed to serve the base during the war did help treat Iraqi civilians as well as military patients but are unlikely to assist in diagnostic development in postwar Iraq.

The purpose of the military diagnostic initiative was to serve U.S. interests while the country was at war, but it is an illustrative model of unsustainable diagnostic aid, which has been offered innumerable times in response to epidemics and other health needs in Africa. Upon exacerbation of mortality due to an outbreak that is amplified by misdiagnoses, a WHO, CDC, or other humanitarian fairy godmother brings a field laboratory or facilitates access to a reference lab to enable accurate diagnosis. The agent is rapidly named, its spread is halted, and the epidemic abates with the wave of a wand. When her task is done, the fairy godmother vanishes, taking with her essential resources for diagnosing and controlling the disease. In the more memorable cases, some disused equipment of ornamental rather than practical value remains as a glass slipper reminder of the efficacy of laboratory diagnostics.

To end the Cinderella cycle, infrastructure needs to be put in place so that diagnostic support can be obtained routinely, not just in visible crises. National and international health policymakers need to acknowledge that medicines should be prescribed for the specific diseases they are designed to treat. The cost of diagnosis must be acknowledged as a necessary component of care that can produce savings in other areas. Allopathic medical doctors must acknowledge that, just as they were taught in medical school, laboratory input is needed to resolve a differential diagnosis. They must view their access to laboratory services as an important and distinctive feature of their practice, and one that delineates them from the practitioners of other schools of medicine. They must then, of course, be granted this access. Finally, patients need to advocate for the best standard of care, including the right to know what is wrong with them at the time they are being treated.

A recent study cataloging emerging infectious disease events identified very few events in Africa, not because they did not occur but because the distribution of documented events mirrors the availability of diagnostic laboratory infrastructure. Like disease eradication, global diagnostic proficiency is a "Weakest Link Public Good,"[44] because all countries are at risk when a particular locality lacks the resources to identify and report dangerous pathogens. (This is true at the level of the individual as well as the collective.) Wealthy countries can gain from assisting in the development of diagnostic capability in less affluent countries, even if they have lower infectious disease burdens, because it will increase the likelihood that a new disease, or a new version of an existing disease, will be contained before it is disseminated internationally.[45]

From the mid-2000s, some actors in richer countries began to recognize this and commenced model initiatives to improve laboratory capacity. For example, the U.S. Clinical Laboratory Standards Institute (CLSI), the WHO, the CDC, the U.S. President's Emergency Plan for AIDS Relief (PEPFAR), and the World Bank all have laboratory capacity-building programs and the Clinton Foundation now negotiates discounted diagnostics, as well as medicines, for HIV patients in Africa. The American Societies for Microbiology and Clinical Pathology are among professional societies that offer human resources to train laboratory personnel in-country. These and other types of international aid can result in maximal gains for primary health care only if they are an adjunct to local efforts. The best outcome would be diagnostic development that improves the management of endemic diseases in African countries and enhances capacity to detect pandemic diseases of global concern. Donors are becoming increasingly aware that the most effective aid is that awarded in response to locally articulated needs and toward measurable outcomes.[46] To achieve cost-effective, sustained, and accountable diagnostic sufficiency, Africa must drive her own diagnostic development.

A Road Map for Africa to Advocate Her Own Diagnosis

Although the benefits in averting high human costs and economic losses would be great, the infrastructural, educational, and financial investments required to attain diagnostic sufficiency in Africa are undeniably large and must be allocated in the face of competing demands such as governance, preventive health, elementary education, food security, general infrastructure, and the eradication of extreme poverty.[47] This must have been on the minds of the "representatives of governments, multilateral agencies, development partners, professional associations and academic institutions" who were signatories of the Maputo Declaration on the Strengthening of Laboratory Systems in January 2008.[48] An awareness of diagnostic needs emerged coincident with a global recession that made it necessary for individuals, countries, banks, and potential donors to tighten their belts. Diagnostic development will not come cheap and must quickly produce detectable results. Reassuringly, unlike many development objectives, diagnostic development increases the quality and precision of measurement, so that implementation enhances assessment.[49]

Ideally, every patient would have access to all the laboratory support necessary to confirm his or her diagnosis. This goal is neither feasible nor cost effective but it is certainly essential and possible to grant most patients lifesaving diagnostic support. High-burden diseases should be the most important targets for diagnostic test development and deployment, particularly when testing would contribute significantly to treatment and disease control.[50] Laboratory support that makes it possible to use inexpensive, first-line drugs instead of expensive, newer therapies, or that preserves the effective life of antimicrobial agents, could pay for itself and should be a priority for diagnostic development. For prevention, diagnostic support for eradication and elimination must be prioritized, as diagnostic precision is indispensable at the tail end of such programs. Finally, as many different diagnostics are needed, it makes sense to begin by developing those that can be easily and cheaply designed.

The case studies in this book have highlighted areas where diagnostic development would easily bring cost savings and significant improvements in the delivery of curative care. Fever management and diagnosis of infections caused by sexually transmitted pathogens and blood-borne viruses are crucial. Malaria diagnostics are reasonably well developed but inadequately deployed and are compromised by the absence of other diagnostics to support a differential diagnosis of fevers. It makes sense to use malaria tests in conjunction with diagnostics for a multitude of common infections, particularly treatable bacterial infections. Multiplexes, that is, single tests that return results for multiple diagnostic queries would be valuable for patients with fever, sexually transmitted diseases, respiratory infections, and persistent diarrhea.

Scientists in Africa need to play a central role in developing and validating diagnostics for endemic diseases. Not only do they have a real incentive to do so, they also have the most familiarity and best access to patients and health systems for which these tests will be used. It is not enough to develop or validate tests locally. They can and should be manufactured on the continent. This will bring production costs down, secure the supply chain, and make it easier to get diagnostics to primary health centers regularly. It also will ensure that diagnostic sufficiency is sustained when Africa weans itself off international aid.

Diagnostic facilities must be decentralized. As of 2006, 80 percent of the seven hundred hospitals and health centers in Tanzania had at least some laboratory facilities, most admittedly in need of development. However, a 2006 audit reported that most Tanzanians sought care at one of 4,679 dispensaries, almost all of which lacked any diagnostic capability.[51] The capacity to transport infectious specimens safely while retaining their diagnostic worth is lacking in most of tropical Africa. The more specimens that can be tested close to the patient's primary health care provider, the more useful information can be obtained in time to influence treatment. In developing countries "primary health care" and "technology" have long been considered oxymorons. However, the 1978 Declaration of Alma-Ata, made at the end of a pivotal international conference on primary health care, requires primary care to have a practical and acceptable *scientific* basis, using accessible *methods and technology*.[52] Such a basis cannot but include diagnostics. When testing becomes a standard and visible part of primary care, patients will come to understand it as an integral part of the diagnostic process. In appreciating how diagnostic tests enhance their therapy, patients will be more inclined to use official rather than unsanctioned health care providers or to self-medicate. An increase in successful treatments at first presentation will engender confidence in allopathic medicine and the distinctions between allopathic and other forms of medicine will become less blurred.

Rapid diagnostic tests, with acceptable sensitivity and specificity, should be performed by nurses or aides at the point of care, or by technicians who have received specialized training. Diagnosis of up to 90 percent of the population 90 percent of the time could very well be performed at the primary care level. Point-of-care tests for malaria and other endemic parasites and common viruses such as HIV, culture and sensitivity testing of common bacteria and, in most cases, tuberculosis testing should be available at, or close to, the primary care level. Although existing technology does not permit $CD4^+$ counting for HIV patients at this level, special equipment that allows samples to be collected for this purpose and relayed to regional diagnostic centers has recently been developed. Remote testing is not sustainable for many infectious diseases, but it is useable for HIV because patients require continuous care and often lifelong drug therapy. Rapid diagnostic tests for some bacterial pathogens could be developed for point-of-care use and would enhance the diagnostic value of the other tests. General hospitals should be given the capacity to assess performance of point-of-care tests, perform expert microscopy for parasitic diseases, and carry out bacterial culture and antimicrobial susceptibility testing.

Regional laboratories with more sophisticated equipment, managed by infectious disease consultants and technicians with advanced training, could test for less prevalent pathogens and oversee local primary care centers.[53] These laboratories would be located at tertiary care centers, or located within secondary-level state hospitals. In this era when infectious disease can spread rapidly, every country requires the capacity to detect all known pathogens and to perform preliminary characterization of new agents. This means that every country needs at least one facility with Biosafety Level 3 or 4 laboratories, to detect the most dangerous pathogens. Although they require the most sophisticated personnel and infrastructure, this aspect of diagnostic development could be more easily established by taking advantage of existing research institutes. African health ministries could work up collaborative agreements to set up national diagnostic laboratories attached to research centers of excellence, which could take advantage of such expensive resources as large equipment and reference libraries.

A real challenge for clinical laboratories is sourcing reagents and equipment. Laboratory equipment is produced by very few companies worldwide and is designed for use in industrialized country laboratories in temperate parts of the world, located in close proximity to manufacturers who provide servicing and technical support. Christoph H. Larsen, Gary M. Cohen, and C. N. "Param" Paramasivan and his colleagues have independently cataloged the challenges that laboratories face when they try to use such equipment in Africa and have proposed possible solutions.[54] Today, African laboratories invariably pay more for equipment but receive less service over a dramatically shortened life span. Service contracts, which are the norm in North American laboratories, are either too expensive or are not offered to African laboratories. When equipment fails, it can take over three weeks to secure what should be a one- or two-day repair job. Many of these challenges arise because there are too few laboratories running such equipment to make local servicing and repair attractive to manufacturers and their agents. Manufacturers should be encouraged to modify equipment so that it is less likely to be susceptible to electricity blackouts and brownouts, and to damage from heat and particulate matter. It is also possible to engineer system components to allow users to effect minor repairs with remote assistance. These sorts of adaptations have been made for sophisticated equipment ranging from automobiles to computers, and they should be applied to laboratory equipment. Heat-stable formulations of reagents also need to be developed where possible to make shipping less dependent on cold chains, and the more that can be manufactured and procured locally, the better. All of these issues can be avoided in all but reference laboratories if equipment-free point-of-care tests are developed.

Many of the laudable recent laboratory capacity building and diagnostic development projects have unfortunately been focused on a single disease. There are now a few excellent laboratories dotted across Africa that focus on diagnosis of tuberculosis alone, or on diagnostic tests needed to detect and manage HIV patients. In remote clinics that have any kind of diagnostics at all, rapid diagnostic tests for malaria introduced after 2006 often comprise the entire diagnostic portfolio. These laboratories, and tests, came to Africa following diagnostic advocacy from researchers and health policymakers focused on those high-burden conditions. However, when they do not build capacity for diagnosing most common infections, they lead to expensive duplication of resources and deprive institutions of more broadly applicable diagnostics. As in the case of rapid diagnostics for malaria, where patients who test negative may still receive antimalarials, disease-specific initiatives that do not address confounders may undermine their own programs. The recent Maputo Declaration on Strengthening of Laboratory Systems calls for integration of laboratories but it does not go far enough in that it still advocates principally for laboratories for HIV, malaria, and TB diagnosis.[55] There are equally pressing diagnostic needs for sexually transmitted diseases other than AIDS, for blood-borne bacteria, and for respiratory and enteric pathogens—to name a few—and these needs are critically neglected. Laboratories can specialize for control programs, research, or surveillance, but they need to be able to offer a broad range of basic diagnostic services.

As with specialist laboratories, it would be valuable to reexamine the way centers of medical research excellence operate in Africa.[56] Some research institutes on the continent do offer diagnostic support for care, but commonly on an informal and ad hoc basis. Although their work demonstrates the urgent need for reliable diagnostics, researchers are often powerless to do anything about the problem in the areas they study. These laboratories are few and far between and must continue to focus on the underaddressed research needs of Africa. However, if health ministries affiliate regional or national diagnostic laboratories with these institutions, they could take advantage of some resources and training that these centers of excellence could offer. Providing auxiliary diagnostic services, or at least diagnostic oversight, from an expanded number of research institutes is one way to stimulate diagnostic development.

It makes sense to support and develop existing diagnostic facilities and technical personnel. Where required, we must improve the quality as well as the breadth of services they offer, and encourage prescribers to use them. Quality assurance is an essential and often neglected aspect of laboratory diagnosis. Without adequate built-in quality assurance, diagnostic tests can be more misleading than if they were not performed at all.[57] Many laboratories supply susceptibility test results but lack control organisms to ensure that their discs are working properly. An unpublished report on "Resistance to Antimicrobial Drugs in Ghana" demonstrated that a 53 percent to 75 percent discrepancy was seen in the susceptibility data reported from seven regional hospitals when the same isolates were tested in a reference laboratory. Some laboratories had improvised rather than followed protocol on small but crucial steps in the key methods used to determine susceptibility. Similar reports have come from Nigeria and Kenya, emphasizing the need for quality control and regional monitoring and supervisory programs.[58] The first step in this direction would be for national ministries of health to establish formal bodies to accredit existing laboratories and ratify testing standards. Such institutions exist in countries on other continents.

Key challenges in the development of diagnostic infrastructure in Africa require development of other sectors. A well-run diagnostic laboratory must be able to procure materials regularly via a secure supply chain. The supply chain and regulatory framework for diagnostics in many African countries is even weaker than the well-documented weak situation for pharmaceuticals. Currently several tests are sold without evidence of effectiveness. Recent initiatives by WHO to precertify rapid diagnostic tests for some conditions such as malaria and syphilis could serve as a model for implementing quality assurance in a cost-effective manner. Predeployment assessments are not enough, however; diagnostics, which are often heat sensitive and moisture labile, must be quality assured at purchase and at point of use. Additionally, laboratory technicians' testing must be continually assessed and supported by external monitors in home-country reference labs. Laboratory safety must also be built in parallel with capacity to assure the well-being of workers, patients, and the wider community.

As evidenced by the cases of malaria and HIV, diagnostic tests can be developed and quality assured in a remarkably short time once a commitment is made. Malaria rapid diagnostic tests were developed and field tested in the early 1990s. Pilot studies revealed problems with quality assurance, which were addressed by a quality evaluation program spearheaded and managed by the WHO with input from the Foundation for Innovative New Diagnostics (FIND) and the U.S. Centers for Disease Control. By 2009, rapid diagnostic tests had been deployed at sentinel sites in many countries and nationally in Madagascar. Uganda, Zambia, and Ethiopia were at the time discussing or designing national programs that would target artemisinin-based combination therapies to malaria patients based on parasite-based diagnosis made with rapid diagnostic tests.[59] Spurred by very recent global interest in the disease, malaria rapid diagnostic tests made it from the laboratory bench to public health impact in Africa in less than two decades. Although more went into product optimization and quality assurance, the estimated cost of the innovation that brought us point-of-care malaria diagnostics was a mere US$100,000.[60] Thus, if other neglected diseases are properly prioritized, with political will and donor interest diagnostic development can be rapid, affordable, and successful.

For malaria diagnostics, scaling up is the remaining challenge. The surreptitious battle against diagnostic development is fought as fiercely within Africa as on the outside. Christopher R. Polage and his co-investigators found that even though diagnostic development has become a priority of the Komo Anokye Teaching Hospital in Kumasi, Ghana, physicians were underutilizing diagnostic resources to the detriment and cost of their patients. Physicians claimed that laboratory tests were underresourced, improperly performed, and prohibitively expensive. Contradicting this misperception, Polage and his co-workers found that the most critical tests were available and implemented to high standard. Patients' medical expenses were unreasonably high because expensive antimicrobials were routinely being used without testing to determine whether they were necessary. Fifty-one of the eighty physicians polled said that they frequently or always diagnosed malaria without laboratory support. However, only 24 percent of malaria smears were positive in the lab. Almost all the physicians expressed the opinion that tests were too costly, but medicine costs far outstripped laboratory testing expenses. The investigators concluded that "perhaps the most significant barrier to laboratory use was physicians' reliance on clinical judgment" and "this attitude is not surprising in resource limited regions where clinical algorithms are often promoted as the diagnostic standard."[61] Promoting diagnosis based on signs and symptoms alone, typically in a non-evidence-based manner, is a principal reason why diagnostic insufficiency is ingrained.

Physicians' insistence on the reliability of their clinical judgment, even in the absence of supporting evidence to this effect, is the product of a century of struggling to provide care without support and the absence of systems to measure the success of treatment programs. As malaria control interventions take root and reduce the incidence of this common febrile disease, the number of misdiagnosed fevers is set to rise. Prolonged illnesses and even the deaths of a "small" proportion of the misdiagnosed are unacceptable. Prescribers provided with reliable laboratory services need to be educated and encouraged to use them.

Shifting attitudes may be the most challenging aspect of diagnostic development and they extend to patients, who tend to regard testing as applicable to research but not to treatment. Blood draws in particular are considered a research activity, and benefits to study participants, including financial compensation, medicines, and other items, are often seen as payment for blood.[62] If the collection of blood and other body fluids is to become integral to health care practice, the use of blood for research might be viewed more positively, for what it actually is—a diagnostic medium.

Patients may be more receptive than we think. In the case of life-threatening diseases, laboratory diagnosis is generally appreciated. During focus group discussions conducted in Malawi, participants associated involvement in research projects and access to quality care, including better diagnosis, with blood and urine tests.[63] Clearly, patients can recognize optimal and suboptimal care even when they rarely encounter best practices. Physicians, other health workers, and those who dictate Africa's health policy have the responsibility of offering more to those receiving care, and more to those who pay for it.

Any sustained effort at diagnostic development for Africa must be spearheaded by Africa's clinicians, scientists, and governments, who are directly responsible for their patients.[64] Pilot projects and new technical initiatives to build diagnostic capacity that were initiated in the mid-2000s must be viewed as key germinating seeds. These programs must be nurtured, grown and then harnessed toward improving the practice of medicine on the continent. Their success will depend first on an appreciation in political circles of the importance of science and technology to medical practice. Second, this appreciation must be translated into practical outcomes. Laudable programs such as the Wellcome Trust–supported African Institutions Initiative, which is directed at the first problem, and the African Network for Drugs and Diagnostic Innovation, focused on the second, have the potential to move African research in these directions as do country-specific initiatives launched by governments sensitive to this need.[65]

Tropical parasitic diseases and bacterial infections are among the easiest to diagnose, as they have been for almost a hundred years. Throughout this time, they have remained the most common causes of death in equatorial Africa. Each syndrome is produced by a specific pathogen, and in most cases it can be eliminated by a specific and often inexpensive treatment. These facts have been known to biomedical science since its importation to Africa. Biomedicine is the dominant form of health care delivered in Africa and commonly the only form sanctioned by the state and the global community. However, poor health remains one of the most important impediments to productivity and quality of life. This situation prevails in spite of the efforts of millions of qualified health workers who are largely focused on disbursing medicines in a manner that is difficult to delineate from the parallel practices of unsanctioned providers. This approach is akin to the "activity without insight" disparaged by German philosopher and writer Johann Wolfgang von Goethe. Only judicious testing will provide the diagnostic insight every infected patient deserves.

Notes

INTRODUCTION

1. Nuland 1989.

2. I remain uncomfortable with current terminology for systems of medical knowledge. This work focuses on what is often referred to as "biomedicine" or "scientific medicine." Since this form of medicine is not practiced scientifically in much of Africa, however, neither term is appropriate. I have settled for "Western" medicine, even though this is a misnomer because the form of medicine that is said to have originated in Greco-Roman cultures drew from cultures across the East, and even from African cultures. "Modern" medicine is also a misnomer, since other systems continue to be practiced. However, since this form of medicine was brought to Africa from Europe and imposed upon the continent by colonialists, the term "Western" is particularly applicable. Present-day medical systems that derive from African culture are frequently referred to as "traditional," and I use this term on occasion. Many of these systems, however, have evolved considerably, and what passes for "tradition" is never static. Terms such as "alternative" or "complementary" medicine suggest that they are cheerfully practiced alongside Western medicine, which is not the case, and they suggest that African medicine is secondary, which is certainly not true for many patients. Because African medical systems have been suppressed, we have insufficient knowledge to determine whether they are complementary with biomedical protocols. I favor the term "indigenous" medicine, although not all nonwestern medicine is indigenous to a single culture. I refer to practitioners who are licensed by the state as "sanctioned" practitioners, borrowing the terminology from Djimde et al. 1998; these include doctors, nurses, pharmacists, and other health personnel trained in Western-type programs, as well as less professional and skilled primary health care workers, village health care workers, and public health officials recognized and trained by the state. Indigenous practitioners are also sanctioned providers. Unsanctioned providers, sometimes disparaged as "quacks," include those who practice any form of medicine—often, Western medicine—without any formal training or state registration. Most African states lack the resources or the will to proscribe and prosecute these illegitimate practitioners.

3. If the time available for the physical examination is short, precision declines sharply. Guyon et al. 1994 recorded a mean of fifty-four seconds consulting time per patient in Bangladesh.

4. See Wootton 2006. Despite the inability of routine diagnostic protocols to provide the correct diagnosis for all conditions, overinvestigation, sometimes referred to as "medical vampirism," is also potentially detrimental (Le Fanu 2000). In some instances, the quantity of blood taken for tests is so great as to cause anemia (Abrams 1979; Burnum 1986). The burden placed on health systems for expensive but useless tests is of concern in some places. So is the performance of tests to stroke the physician's ego or protect from liability, when the results would be obvious ("Reducing Tests" 1981; Showstack, Schroeder, and Matsumoto 1982; Griner and Glaser 1982). There is definitely a balance to be struck between diagnostic sufficiency and diagnostic abuse. A justifiable diagnostic is not an end in itself.

5. The terminology was coined by Chambers 1989. For more on the poverty-disease cycle, see Jeffrey Sachs 2005.

6. Foege 2002.

7. Brock 1999, 1.

CHAPTER 1

1. The University College Hospital is the premier institution for nursing education in Nigeria ("British Contributions to Medical Research and Education in Africa after the Second World War" 1999).

2. Pyrimethamine, a malaria preventative, was marketed as Daraprim and called "Sunday-Sunday medicine" because it was taken once a week.

3. Atta 2005.

4. Although malaria is a serious, even life-threatening, disease, attacks are so frequent and widespread that most West Africans consider malaria a relatively mild illness in adults.

5. Until recently, when its effectiveness was compromised by the emergence of drug resistance, chloramphenicol was the drug of choice for typhoid fever.

6. Porter 1998; Wootton 2006.

7. Such as Andreas Vesalis (1514–64), William Harvey (1578–1657), Giovanni Morgagni (1682–1771), and John Hunter (1728–93), who are chronicled by Nuland (1989) and Porter (1998).

8. Good historical overviews are provided by Nuland 1989 and Porter 1998. Leeuwenhoek is often erroneously given credit for building the first microscope; it was probably Zacharias Janssen (1590) who first peered through a tube in which he had mounted two lenses. Leeuwenhoek pioneered microscopy for biological observation. He was a prolific observer and contributor to the *Philosophical Transactions of the Royal Society* (of Great Britain), authoring 190 letters on microscopy between 1673 and 1723, and was elected a fellow of the Royal Society in 1680. Leeuwenhoek did not, and indeed could not, presuppose that microbes caused disease. He found that "animacules" were ubiquitous. He did not have the discriminatory power that later microbiologists used to delineate different subtypes; he did not even examine the specimens from infections. Koch's tuberculosis paper was published in 1882.

9. Cunningham 1992.

10. At the time, plant biologists were preoccupied with fungi, which were larger and more easily observed than bacteria. In the late 1850s, Anton deBary performed a controlled study to determine the role of the fungus *Phytophthora infestans* in the etiology of potato blight; he succeeded in demonstrating causation earlier than Koch. Other plant biologists questioned this explanation for deBary's data. We now know that the real causative organism was probably a virus carried on the fungal spores, so the skeptics may deserve some credit. The disconnect between the study of the biology of plants and humans as well as between studies on fungi and bacteria did not permit the debate to enter human medicine at that time.

11. Santer 2009; Wootton 2006.

12. The technology needed to move an individual bacterium, to the exclusion of other organisms that may be present, from an infected individual to a healthy one became available only in the last decade. In most cases, more than one bacterium is needed to seed an infection. Nineteenth-century microbiologists needed to be able to produce large numbers of identical bacteria from a mixture in order to inoculate healthy hosts. The production of pure cultures required the scientists to be able to isolate the candidate bacterium and to permit it to reproduce in a bacteria-free environment.

13. For example, Edwin Klebs (1834–1912) used fractional culture methods in his work with anthrax (Koch 1876). Although his results were consistent with later work, the

reproducibility of his experiments was a problem (Brock 1999). In 1878, Joseph Lister, who coined the term "germ theory," probably produced a pure culture by subculturing *Lactobacilli* in very dilute milk samples until he obtained samples that contained one organism. The qualifier "probably" is significant. Current methods of liquid fractionation used in water and milk assessment produce only a "most probable number" of bacteria, an estimate rather than an accurate count of individual bacteria. Lister's methodology was not precise, absolute, reproducible, or practicable.

14. Lister 1878; Schroeter 1875.

15. Koch, the son of an engineer, was born in 1843 in Clausthal, Germany. He studied natural sciences and medicine and was a student of Jacob Henle at Göttingen. After graduation, he practiced medicine and experimented in a private laboratory attached to his office. Koch's postulates were published after his seminal paper on the etiology of tuberculosis, which was the first of his papers to fulfill them rigorously (Koch 1882). Stated in their simplest form by Koch himself, the postulates are designed "to obtain a perfect proof to satisfy oneself that the parasite and the disease are not only correlated, but actually causally related, and that the parasite is the direct cause of the disease. This can only be done by completely separating the parasite from the diseased organism…and then introducing the isolated parasite into healthy organisms and induce the disease anew with all its characteristic symptoms and properties" (Koch 1884, translated by Brock 1999, 116). In order to separate the parasite from the host and all other materials associated with the disease, in vitro pure cultures must be prepared, which makes the study of causation dependent on techniques of microbial culture.

16. Anthrax (Koch 1876), wound fever (Koch 1880), tuberculosis (Koch 1882), and cholera in 1883.

17. In *Wives and Daughters,* a novel published in 1866 by the English novelist and social observer Elizabeth Gaskell, a mother says about her deceased husband and healthy daughter: "Poor dear Mr. Kirkpatrick was consumptive, and Cynthia may have inherited it, and a great sorrow might bring out the latent seeds. At times I am so fearful" (Gaskell 1866, 55).

18. Koch 1884. Daniel Salmon, who was working on causation at the same time as Koch, proposed even more stringent criteria for causation (Salmon 1881). In addition to criteria similar to Koch's postulates, he maintained that in order to establish causation, it must be possible to interrupt the pathogen's transmission cycle and obliterate the disease. Salmon spent years studying hog's cholera. He was able to fulfill Koch's postulates for *Salmonella cholerasius* in pigs, and others accepted this organism as the etiologic agent of the disease. Salmon himself was dissatisfied because he was unable to create a vaccine and thereby fulfill his more stringent criteria. In the final analysis, Salmon's reservations were justified in this case. In 1903, it was shown that a filterable RNA virus causes hog's cholera, and the confounding of *Salmonella cholerasius* was produced by the inability to eliminate the unseen virus from bacterial cultures. Instances similar to hog's cholera are unusual, however, and Koch's postulates have proved sufficient and reliable enough to attribute causation of numerous infectious diseases to specific microbial agents. Were Salmon's more stringent criteria applied, it is unlikely that causation would have been established for so many diseases in the short time after Koch began his work. However, a theory of causation that included a therapeutic intervention might have assisted in linking discovery and control more tightly. The science of virology developed after bacteriology because viruses are hundreds of times smaller than bacteria, so they remain invisible to the light microscope, and, without a cell structure of their own, they cannot be cultured outside of living beings. In the early twentieth century, the invention of tissue culture and electron microscopy allowed for many viruses to be rapidly described and cultured. For reviews, see Oldstone 1998 and Creager and Landecker 2009.

19. Koch 1881, 1882. Thomas Brock writes of Koch's 1881 paper, "Methods for the Study of Pathogenic Organisms": "If I had to choose one paper as most significant for the rise of microbiology, this would be it" (Brock 1999, 108).

20. This invaluable bit of laboratory ware is named for its inventor, Richard J. Petri 1887.

21. Nuland 1989, xvii.

22. See Twumasi 1975.

23. Sofowora 1982.

24. Needham 2000, 130–31; Hughes et al. 1993.

25. Groopman 2007.

26. Nuland 1989.

27. Thomas 1978, 85.

28. Addae 1997, 232.

29. Twumasi 1975; Ogungbamila and Ogundaini 1993.

CHAPTER 2

1. Ogonim's story is told in chapter 4 (Nwapa 1966).

2. Although the Aro confederation resisted British military domination, the Aros conquered many local groups and captured individuals across Ibo-land. They sold their captives into slavery from the eighteenth through the late nineteenth centuries See Acholonu 1999 and Orji 1982.

3. Onyeka Onwenu was educated at Wellesley College and the New School for Social Research in the United States. She returned to Nigeria and worked as a reporter for the Nigerian Television Authority for several years. The *ONOK* incident occurred just after she left journalism for a more lucrative and very successful musical career.

4. Based on data from the Malaria Foundation International, available at www.malaria.org and from Phillips 2001. According to the U.K.'s Department for International Development, Nigeria, like some other African countries, will not meet the Millennium Development Goal to decrease under-five mortality to two-thirds of 1990 levels by 2019. http://www.dfid.gov.uk/Documents/publications/PSA/E_Nigeria.pdf .

5. In his introduction to *Infection and Inequalities,* physician-anthropologist Paul Farmer writes: "I was accustomed to ferreting out accusations of sorcery and had previously spent some years trying to make sense of them. And that, paradoxically, is the primary function of such accusations: to make sense of suffering" (Farmer 1999, 3).

6. Spiritualist churches in modern Nigeria often double as faith healing houses. They do not use, and may even frown on, pharmaceuticals as well as indigenous medicines, sometimes to the detriment of patients (Etuk, Itam, and Asuquo 1999). Faith healers and prayer houses are one of several options used by ill patients in eastern Nigeria and elsewhere on the continent, and are often the venue of choice when a nonbiophysical etiology is suspected (Izugbara and Afangideh 2005).

7. The chance of child's caregiver spotting a fever is quite high and errs on the false-positive side. Therefore, determining the cause of this fever and prescription of effective medicines is the most important intervention (Schapira 1994; WHO 2006c; Wammanda and Onazi 2009). "Fever equals malaria" is a popular twentieth-century adage that advocates for diagnostic testing have begun to work hard to unteach (Hopkins, Asiimwe, and Bell 2009).

8. Needham et al. 2001 found that among the factors contributing to diagnostic delay among tuberculosis patients in Zambia were lower education and visiting a private doctor or traditional healer instead of a government clinic or hospital; women also were less likely to secure a timely diagnosis.

9. WHO 1996; Hopkins, Asiimwe, and Bell 2009.

10. According to Murphy and Breman 2001, approximately 2% of children who recover from cerebral malaria suffer brain damage that results in detectable learning disabilities.

11. Sachs 2005, 115.

12. Ross reputedly compared the significance of his discovery to that of Columbus's discovery of the American hemisphere. See the Nobel Prize citation at http://nobelprize.org/nobel_prizes/medicine/laureates/1902/, © The Nobel Foundation 1902.

13. In 2008, malaria infections and deaths in Africa respectively accounted for 85% and 89% of those worldwide (WHO 2009b).

14. Reviewed by Arrow, Panosian, and Gelband 2004.

15. *Plasmodium ovale* and *P. vivax,* two other species, also have a dormant hypnozoite stage. Hypnozoites can persist in an infected person for years, convert to the merozoitic form in the liver at an unexpected time, and resume an infectious cycle. However, *P. ovale* and *P. vivax* are relatively uncommon in Africa. Most infections in Africa are caused by *P. falciparum,* the most efficiently transmitted and deadliest species; the infection can be completely eliminated if treated with the right medicine, at the right time.

16. The predilection and, indeed, the imperative to self-medicate assumes that patients and their caregivers are competent to assess when they are ill. Whereas severely ill patients are easily identified, in mild illnesses the reliability of even this most basic premise is open to question. A history of fever is likely to bias a patient toward believing that their temperature is elevated, so that if clinical measurements are used to the exclusion of patient complaints, intermittent fevers would be missed. The problem with basing diagnosis on clinical signs and symptoms alone is that, in all but textbook cases, these criteria are unavoidably subjective. There are some important exceptions; for example, many conditions produce a characteristic rash. As more of these vaccine-preventable conditions, such as measles, become controlled, the ease with which infections can be delineated without diagnostic tests will continue to fall.

17. WHO 2006c, 8.

18. Ibid.

19. Reyburn et al. 2004; Gwer, Newton, and Berkley 2007.

20. Farmer 1999.

21. According to Millennium Development Goal evaluation estimates, African countries typically record between 40 and 260 deaths per 1,000 live births in children under five; in almost all African countries, infant mortality estimates remained the same or rose between 1990 and 2004. The Millennium Development Goal is to halve these deaths by 2015. http://millenniumindicators.un.org/unsd/mdg/SeriesDetail.aspx?srid=561&crid=.

22. It is easier to identify parasites in thin blood smears, but at low parasitemia, parasites are more likely to be visible in thick smears, so both thick and thin smears are advocated for diagnosis. A qualified laboratory practitioner can determine which *Plasmodium* species is present to delineate malignant tertian malaria from the more benign form of the disease. When properly conducted, the probability of false positives is small. The chief barriers to the routine use of this method are the high level of test-specific technical expertise required and the labor-intensity of the process. A skilled technician can typically read sixty slides a day (Durrhelm et al. 1997; Cheesebrough 1984; Barker et al. 1986; Zurovac, Midia, et al. 2006; Wongsrichanalai et al. 2007).

23. Assuming eight thousand white blood cells per milliliter of blood, the number of parasites per two hundred white blood cells multiplied by forty will yield the number of parasites per milliliter (Makler, Palmer, and Ager 1998). This method is best used when a white cell count is taken, as patients' white blood counts vary.

24. Durrhelm et al. 1997; Cheesebrough 1984.

25. Microscopists with very little basic education have successfully been employed for malaria diagnosis but high-quality on-the-job training and quality assurance are needed to ensure that smears are prepared and read correctly. In Ethiopia, where malaria is not hyperendemic but epidemics carry a potential for high mortality, diagnostic strength is a major asset. One assessment of the northern Gondar region of Ethiopia found that when a certified reference reader was asked to review slides processed by an operational diagnostic lab technician, the results concurred only 75% of the time, and up to 63% of diagnoses could represent false positives (Mitiku, Mengistu, and Gelaw 2003).

26. Okeke 2006.

27. Zurovac, Larson, et al. 2006.

28. For reviews of recently developed tests, see Makler, Palmer, and Ager 1998 and Bell, Wongsrichanalai, and Barnwell 2006. The sensitivity and specificity of today's rapid diagnostic tests for malaria approach that of microscopy, and in health centers where skilled technicians are not available to prepare and read stained slide smears, rapid diagnostic tests offer superior reliability (de Oliveira et al. 2009).

29. Unlike bacteria, malaria parasites cannot be routinely cultured. When detecting a pathogen is complex or expensive, detecting an immune response in the infected patient can serve as a useful surrogate. The presence of detectable antibody against a specific pathogen is usually indicative that the pathogen is, or was, in the body of the patient. In malaria-endemic areas, most people are exposed to *Plasmodia* several times a month and almost everyone has antibodies, regardless of whether they are currently ill. Some harbor low numbers of parasites that can be detected by molecular tests, some of which are actually too sensitive to employ for clinical diagnosis. Molecular tests may also require reagents that are presently difficult to source in developing countries, such as radioactive probes (Barker et al. 1986).

30. Makler, Palmer, and Ager 1998; Mitiku, Mengistu, and Gelaw 2003; Wongsrichanalai et al. 2007; WHO (2009a).

31. WHO 2008.

32. Costs of antimalarial drugs at the time of the 2003 Africa Malaria Report (WHO and UNICEF 2003) were (in US$) .13 for chloroquine, .14 for sulfadoxine-pyrimethamine (Fansidar), .20 for amodiaquine, and 1.00–3.00 for artemisinin-based combinations. More recent pricing comes from parameters used in cost-effectiveness assessment five years later by the WHO (Shillcutt et al. 2008).

33. WHO 2009a

34. Lubell et al. 2007. Bell and Perkins 2008 point out factors contributing to this problem and how it might be addressed.

35. Nabarro and Tayler 1998. See also http://www.rollbackmalaria.org/. Halting and reversing the incidence of malaria by 2015 is also Millennium Development Goal 6c http://www.undp.org/mdg/basics.shtml.

36. For example, a manufacturer donation program supplies the antifungal drug to many African countries, but fungal diagnostics are almost universally unavailable.

37. The Zambian Ministry of Health's policy (CBoH 2003) followed the international "Roll Back Malaria" proposal (WHO, RBM, 2001). In 2003, malaria was the greatest contributor to the disease burden in Zambia, with fifty thousand deaths from malaria each year and four million people, roughly a third of the population, sickened annually (Masiye and Rehnberg 2005). Zambia's program is consistent with the global plan to roll back malaria and has been proposed as a model for other African countries (Singer 2005). It advocates the use of insecticide-treated bed nets and access to treatment. Both interventions have been proven to be effective. The proposal to boost effectiveness with diagnostics only

came in 2006 (CBoH 2006). Challenges associated with artemether-lumefantrine rollout in Kenya are described by Amin et al. (2007). The study that evaluated testing in Kenyan health institutions and also provides an overview of malaria policy in that country is by Zurovac et al. 2008.

38. Phillips, Kumate-Rodriguez, and Mota-Hernández 1989.

39. de Vries, Kager, and Borgdorff 2004, 1161.

40. AMFm 2007.

41. Snow et al. 2003 present rough estimates of antimalarial use, and the cost estimate for antimalarials dispensed to patients with other infection is provided by Hopkins, Asiimwe, and Bell 2009. Thwing et al. 2009 reported that although approximately half of patients attending primary health care centers typically receive antimalarials, less than 5% of 864 laboratory-evaluated patients tested positive.

42. Chandler et al. 2008; Drakeley, Gosling, and Reyburn 2005; Lubell et al. 2007, 2008; Reyburn et al. 2004, 2006, 2007, 2008; Shillcutt et al. 2008; de Oliveira et al. 2009; Uzochukwu et al. 2009; Hamer et al. 2007; Msellem et al. 2009.

43. Reviewed by Perkins and Bell 2008 and Hopkins, Asiimwe, and Bell 2009. Following recent technical consultation, WHO recommended parasite-based diagnosis for all patients in highly endemic areas except young children, for whom a false-negative test could be fatal (WHO 2006d). The 2009 recommendation was for parasitological diagnosis in all patients (WHO 2009b). See D'Acremont et al. 2009 and English et al. 2009 for perspectives on the ongoing debate on the use of diagnostics for the very young.

44. Only 12 African countries has a policy recommending testing at the community level in 2008 (WHO 2009b). Initial evaluations of rapid diagnostic tests for malaria have proved unreliable when used by patients (Jelinek, Grobusch, and Harms 2001; Jelinek et al. 1999). Further development will be needed before a home-based test, or even one that can be used by every village health worker, becomes available. Present-day tests have almost overcome the challenge of making tests technically accessible, but sample collection remains a major roadblock. Collecting blood comes with some risks for patient and health worker and safely collecting the right amount of blood without contaminating it can be tricky (Luchavez et al. 2007).

45. The subhead title is from Grabowsky 2008, 1052). Barker et al. 1986; de Vries, Kager, and Borgdorff 2004; Zurovac, Larson, et al. 2006; WHO 2006d.

46. Editors, PLoS Medicine 2006.

47. Zambia's progress was recently reviewed by Steketee et al. 2008; WHO 2008 and 2009b summarize continent-wide progress in the Roll Back Malaria campaign.

48. Bohannon 2006, 599.

49. Carson 2002; Towner et al. 1980. See also chapter 6.

50. Nabarro 1999; Balter 2000; Nabarro and Tayler 1998. For information about the more recently proposed campaign to eradicate malaria, see chapter 7 and the Gates Foundation's website: http://www.gatesfoundation.org/GlobalHealth/Pri_Diseases/Malaria/default.htm.

51. See "the Abuja Declaration and the Plan of Action" 2000. Support for the initiative is largely disbursed through the Global Fund (Campbell 2008).

52. Snow et al. 2005, 214.

53. Nahlen et al. 2005, e3; Bell et al. 2005.

54. Mwanziva et al. 2008.

55. Snow et al. 2005, 216.

56. Mboera, Makundi, and Kitua 2007; Makundi et al. 2007; Okiro et al. 2007; Steketee et al. 2008.

57. Breman and Holloway 2007.

58. van Riet et al. 2007. Based on their research on malaria epidemiology in Angola, Thwing et al. 2009 recommend that resources for preventing, diagnosing, and treating malaria be focused on areas that are fifteen kilometers or more away from the city of Luanda.

59. Goodman et al. 2007.

CHAPTER 3

1. (1844, 25), quoted in Carter 2003.

2. Snow et al. 2003; Snow et al. 2005; Snow, Korenromp, and Gouws 2004.

3. Untreated severe malaria is invariably fatal. Mortality rates for treated severe malaria are from WHO 2006c. Patients with severe malaria can present with severe malarial anemia or cerebral malaria. Severe malarial anemia is defined as having less than five grams of hemoglobin per deciliter of blood with *Plasmodium falciparum* levels of over 10,000 per ml (McElroy et al. 1999). The signs of severe malaria described here commonly manifest in children; in adults, pulmonary and renal failure are more common (Planche and Krishna 2005; Arrow, Panosian, and Gelband 2004).

4. Evans et al. 2004 reported the Ghanaian study, the 2000 Tanzania study was published by Reyburn et al. 2004, and the other Kenya, Malawi, and Tanzania studies were respectively authored by Berkley et al. 2005, Peters et al. 2004, and Blomberg et al. 2007.

5. Mtove et al. 2010.

6. In a recent study, most Gabonese children evaluated had high prevaccination titers of antibody specific for one or more influenza viruses, suggesting that they had been exposed to these viruses before the study. The researchers hypothesize that influenza occurred routinely in Gabon but was probably misdiagnosed as malaria (van Riet et al. 2007, 7035). Relapsing fever or Lyme disease was recently reported as being misdiagnosed as malaria in Togo (Nordstrand et al. 2007).

7. This is one of many examples that demonstrates that testing is more useful as a first rather than as a last resort. Cheesebrough 1984 describes existing diagnostic tests for typhoid.

8. Olopoenia and King 2000; Mirza 1995; Baker, Favorov, and Dougan 2010.

9. Ibadin and Ogbimi 2004.

10. Osler 1892; Cox 1996.

11. Nsutebu, Martins, and Adiogo 2003; Nsutebu, Ndumbe, and Adiogo 2002; Nsutebu, Ndumbe, and Koulla 2002.

12. Mensah et al. 2000, 69.

13. Personal communication. Baker, Favorov, and Dougan 2010 have coauthored an informative review on the limitations of current tests and the challenges associated with developing diagnostics for typhoid. Two more recently developed typhoid tests are Tubex and Typhidot. Both have been employed in parts of Asia where typhoid is highly endemic but, like the Widal test, the sensitivity, specificity, and positive predictivity of these tests is too low. Efforts to develop typhoid tests that could be used at the point of care are few, and in very early stages of development. Preliminary efforts demonstrate that, although they would be challenging to develop, such tests are feasible (Fadeel et al. 2004; Hatta and Smits 2007; Naheed et al. 2008; Thompson et al. 2009; Baker, Favorov, and Dougan 2010; Helen Lee, personal communication).

14. Neil et al. 2009; O-tipo et al. 2009.

15. Chanteau et al. 2003; Bertherat et al. 2007.

16. Lin et al. 2005; Basnyat et al. 2005; Basnyat 2005; Tankhiwale, Agrawal, and Jalgaonkar 2003.

17. Baker, Favorov, and Dougan 2010.

18. Leavitt 1996.

19. Feglo, Frimpong, and Essel-Ahun 2004 published the Ghana study. The Gambian situation was learned from a personal communication with staff at the Royal Victoria Teaching Hospital, Banjul, in 2006.

20. Kariuki et al. 2006; Berkley et al. 2005; Mtove et al. 2010. There are convincing, if few, studies that focus on this problem, largely from Kenya, Tanzania, The Gambia, and Malawi. Almost nothing is known about the epidemiology of this important pathogen in much of central Africa and West Africa where there are few published reports on bacteremia etiology.

CHAPTER 4

1. Korenromp et al. 2003; Levine 2004.

2. Roper et al. 2004; Wongsrichanalai et al. 2002.

3. Trape 2001; Arrow, Panosian, and Gelband 2004; WHO and UNICEF 2003.

4. "Antimicrobials" include antibacterials, antivirals, antifungals, and antiprotozoals, including antimalarials. Antimicrobials may be synthetic or obtained from natural sources. Quinine, from cinchona bark, and artemisinin, from the Chinese medicinal plant Qinghaosu (*Artemisia annua*), are antimalarials from natural sources. Chloroquine and sulfadoxine-pyrimethamine (Fansidar) are synthetic antimalarials. "Antibiotic" refers to antimicrobials derived from microorganisms, which likely represent defense systems for the source organism. Like penicillin, the first antibiotic discovered and developed for therapeutic use, most (but not all) antibiotics are antibacterials and obtained from fungi or bacteria.

5. For a more comprehensive explanation of the biological basis and clinical consequences of resistance that is accessible to nonscientists, see Levy 2002. A more detailed and technical focus on the problem in developing countries is documented in Sosa et al. 2009.

6. Sokoloff 1954.

7. Paul Ehrlich, the acknowledged pioneer of chemotherapy, first used the term "magic bullet" to refer to the body's own immune system, not to antimicrobial drugs. Antibodies, agglutinating proteins produced by the immune system, have specific targets: "The protective materials which are present in the antiserums whether they be of the ambiceptor or opsonin type, find in infected organisms their point of attach only and exclusively in the bacteria not in the tissues. These antibodies are exclusively 'parasitotrophic' and not 'organotrophic' and so it is not surprising that they seek out their targets like magic bullets" (Ehrlich 1908, translated by Brock 1999, 177). Ehrlich is clearly describing a guided missile, not a targetless weapon. Later uses of the term have lacked this precision.

8. Ehrlich 1909.

9. Domagk 1935; Fleming 1929; and Chain et al. 1940.

10. "Flesh-eating bacteria" are usually Group A hemolytic streptococci. These reports are reviewed by Miller and Bohnhoff 1950.

11. Norrby 2005; Norrby, Nord, and Finch 2005; Talbot et al. 2006; Payne et al. 2007.

12. Talbot et al. 2006; Payne et al. 2007.

13. WHO published the statement, as well as a synthesis of expert recommendations and recommendations for resistance containment in developing countries (WHO 2001b; APUA 2001).

14. Leach et al. 1999; Mulholland et al. 1999; Palmer et al. 1999; Adegbola et al. 2005.

15. Enwere et al. 2006; Hill et al. 2007.

16. Lawn, Cousens, and Zupan 2005.

17. Ishengoma et al. 2009; Tegbaru et al. 2004.

18. Blomberg et al. 2007, 3. There are WHO guidelines for empiric treatment but these should be fine-tuned in response to local susceptibility patterns, something that rarely happens in resource-limited health systems (Graham and English 2009).

19. Bryce et al. 2005.

20. Ypres papyrus, 1600 BCE, quoted by Minot and Murphy 1983.

21. Brown 1996, 952.

22. Mabey et al. 2004, 235.

23. "The Right Tools Can Save Lives" 2006.

24. Palumbi 2001; Lundqvist et al. 2007.

25. Sofowora 1982.

26. Opintan and Newman 2007; Vila et al. 1994.

27. Fleming 1929; Poupard, Rittenhouse, and Walsh 1994; NCCLS 2003. George F. Reddish modified Fleming's diffusion method by cutting circular wells so that many different agents could be evaluated against a single organism seeded throughout the plate. This approach was increasingly used as more antibiotics were discovered and resistance became more commonplace. The Reddish "cup-plate" or "hole-in-the-plate" method is still used today in the preliminarily assessment of natural products. Antibiotic-containing cylinders and tablets also have been used, to reduce variability associated with uneven boring. Subsequently, paper discs impregnated with test agent became the standard and represent the method of choice of most laboratories worldwide. Although there were earlier experiments employing antimicrobial agents in broth, Fleming should also be given credit for originating the broth-dilution method in 1929, which later provided a means for directly measuring the minimum inhibitory concentration (MIC).

28. NCCLS 2003.

29. NCCLS 1990.

30. As more agents were introduced, S. D. Garrett proposed testing only critical concentrations (so-called "breakpoint" concentrations) so that more agents could be evaluated in a single dilution experiment (Ericsson and Sherris 1971). Multipoint inoculators permit several isolates to be printed in spots on a single agar plate. Tests can be automated or accelerated to yield results from some isolates after as little as six hours' incubation, as compared to overnight incubation for traditional methods. Because disc testing uses manufacturer-assured antimicrobial discs and media, the on-site requirements for quality assurance are fewer than for dilution tests. The E-test allows MICs to be determined with a method no more complicated or labor intensive than a disc test, but it remains very expensive. Although many of the additional quality assurance requirements for dilution tests can be avoided, the E-test requires quality assurance that is equivalent to disc testing, and insufficient attention to this matter has led to inaccuracies in their use in parts of Africa (Daly et al. 1997).

31. Tegbaru et al. 2004.

32. Polage et al. 2006.

33. Ukwuoma 2004.

34. Ukwuoma 2006. Additionally, a survey of seven regional hospitals in Ghana revealed that, while culture and identification data for test isolates agreed with results obtained at the University of Ghana Teaching Hospital's Central Laboratory in Accra, discrepancies in susceptibility data were seen in between 53% and 75% of isolates that were tested separately at both locations. In the private laboratories that perform most of the continent's susceptibility testing, external quality regulation is difficult or impossible (Newman et al. 2004).

35. Brown 1996; Newman et al. 2004; Ishengoma et al. 2009.

36. WHO 1973, 1996.

37. Plowe and Wellems 1995; Wilson et al. 2005; Magnaval et al. 2006.

38. Farcas et al. 2006.

39. Attaran et al. 2004.

40. D'Alessandro, Talisuna, and Boelaert 2005.

41. Researchers and hospital laboratories can often obtain free antimicrobial discs for susceptibility testing of new antimicrobials from the manufacturing pharmaceutical company. Often, the only discs donated in this manner to public hospital labs are for antimicrobials that are not in stock at the pharmacy because they are too expensive (Okeke et al. 2007).

42. Hardin 1968; Baquero and Campos 2003; Foster and Grundmann 2005; Okeke 2009.

43. Okeke and Lamikanra 1995, 2001.

44. Alubo 2001.

45. Peeling 2007, 83; Chappuis et al. 2007.

46. "Two Accused over 'Fake' HIV Tests" 2006.

CHAPTER 5

1. Doctors accept the responsibility of providing a cure; many urban physicians simply lack the resources to deliver it. Early in the history of medicine in Nigeria, some physicians worked in communities where they could follow their patients very closely (Colonial Office 1948). In 1888, the "Adeola scandal," in which an incompletely treated woman was discharged from a colonial hospital in Lagos, Nigeria, resulted in the dismissal of three doctors at a time when there were less than fifty allopathic doctors in the entire country (Schram 1971).

2. The WHO constitution defines health as "a state of complete physical, mental and social well-being and not merely the absence of disease or infirmity" (WHO 1948).

3. Bank-Anthony, a businessman and investor, was born in 1907 in Kinshasa and educated at the prestigious Methodist Boys' high and Christian Missionary Service grammar schools in Lagos. The "Black Englishman," who was as well known for his charm as for his wealth, was awarded the Order of the British Empire (OBE) in 1958 and knighted by Queen Elizabeth II in 1962 for services to Nigeria. He was spotlighted by *Time Magazine* in 1965 (http://www.time.com/time/magazine/article/0,9171,842145,00.html). Bank-Anthony died in 1991 and was buried in a tomb at Ayinke House. The maternity center was named for his mother.

4. After I left Ikeja General Hospital in 1991, it was upgraded to a teaching hospital for Lagos State University, so practice there is no longer representative of a secondary care center. The hospital has not achieved the capabilities of a tertiary care center such as the Lagos University Teaching Hospital, however.

5. This facility has since been closed and replaced by a new facility with amenities that approach those at Ayinke House.

6. Patients may view the hospital as a place where sick people go to die as well as to be cured. This experience is poignantly illustrated in chapter 6 of Flora Nwapa's 1966 novel, *Efuru*. Ralph Schram (1971) also describes people's mistrust of hospitals during their development in Nigeria.

7. http://www.msf.org/msfinternational/invoke.cfm?component=article&method=full_html&objectid=2E1DE387-E018-0C72-09DC38F9F6E3DBA7.

8. For more on the Angola Marburg outbreak, see "Marburg Hemorrhagic Fever—Angola (46)" (2005). The 2007 Ebola outbreak in Uganda is described by Mason 2008 and Alsop 2007.

9. Other well-known hemorrhagic viruses are Lassa fever (discussed later in this chapter) and Rift Valley fever. Crimean-Congo hemorrhagic fever virus, hantavirus, and dengue virus produce hemorrhagic fevers, although their endemic foci are largely outside of sub-Saharan Africa.

10. Max Theiler was awarded the 1951 Nobel Prize in medicine for his work on the yellow fever virus and its control. A concise review of the path to the discovery of yellow fever virus, the vectors, and an effective vaccine is provided by Oldstone 1998, 45–72.

11. Mosquitoes are traditionally controlled by destruction of their habitats, by preventing contact with humans, or by chemical killing with insecticides. Because resistance inevitably emerges, chemical control is the least viable means for containing insect vectors in the long term, but it is the means that has been most widely applied. There is increasing interest in enhancing the other two methods, applying newer technologies such as biological control, and using multipronged strategies, such as insecticide-impregnated bed nets, which add a chemical to a barrier mechanism.

12. Schram 1971; Addae 1997.

13. For example, Close 1995; Fuller 1974; Preston 1995.

14. Oldstone 1998, 199.

15. For more on the hypothesis that Ebola has an ancient origin hypothesis, see Monath 1999 and Peterson et al. 2004. The alternative hypothesis, that Ebola is a new virus, is supported by data from Walsh, Biek, and Real 2005 and Suzuki and Gojobori 1997.

16. Most documented outbreaks have affected humans, but these viruses are also deadly for nonhuman primates. Ebola virus presently represents one of the greatest threats to primate populations. The lethality of the virus for chimpanzees and other primates suggests that they are not the viral reservoir, but are incidental hosts just as humans are (Leroy, Rouquet, et al. 2004; Walsh et al. 2003).

17. It is likely that the case-free periods are shorter than is commonly thought. A small human Ebola outbreak in a remote area can easily be missed due to population isolation or diagnostic insufficiency. Exposure to the Ebola virus (detected via antibodies) has been documented among populations in which an outbreak has never been reported (Teepe et al. 1983). It is even more likely that an ape outbreak will be overlooked.

18. Preston 1995.

19. The first documented human Marburg virus infection affected a German laboratory technician who was infected by an African green monkey (*Cercopithecus aethiops*) in 1967. This lab-focused outbreak was traced to monkeys imported from Uganda. Almost a decade later, the first of many Ebola hemorrhagic fever epidemics broke out in southern Sudan and northern Zaire.

20. The course and investigation of these outbreaks is reviewed by Garrett (1994, 100–152). See also Breman et al. 1977.

21. "Ebola Haemorrhagic Fever in Zaire, 1976" (1978, 273).

22. Lapses in infection control, including needle sharing, have been seen with fully trained medical practitioners and those they supervise (Fisher-Hoch et al. 1995). Needle reuse and other unsafe practices arising from shortages of essential supplies have declined but have not been entirely eliminated. The contributions of needle reuse to the dissemination of blood-borne diseases, including HIV, in Africa remain largely open to question (Priddy et al. 2005; Gisselquist et al. 2002; Schmid et al. 2004; Kernéis et al. 2009).

23. Among the many Medline-indexed scientific papers describing the outbreak, the most detailed account is that coauthored by Idris himself, which was published in the *Sudanese Journal of Public Health* (Idris and Idris 2006).

24. Maridi fared better than Yambuku, but Sudanese epidemiologists who investigated and contained the epidemic have listed five factors that constrained its control: inadequacies of transport, communications, and health personnel; fleeing contacts; and the absence of routine or scientific testing facilities (Idris and Idris 2006).

25. The other transmission route with similarly poor prognosis is through indigenous surgical burial rites, which include cleansing of the bodies and surgical evacuation of the internal organs of the deceased, typically performed by female relatives.

26. Khan et al. 1999.

27. For the Zairian dilemma, see Guimard et al. 1999 and *Ebola—The Plague Fighters* (1996). The use of plasma therapy in Yambuku is reported in "Ebola Haemorrhagic Fever in Zaire, 1976" (1978).

28. All cases of Ebola in the outbreak were confirmed retrospectively at the CDC in Atlanta.

29. Khan, Sanchez, and Pflieger 1998.

30. "Ebola Haemorrhagic Fever in Zaire, 1976" (1978);

Garrett 1994, 127–28; Johnson, Webb, and Heymann 1978; *Ebola—the Plague Fighters* (1996).

31. In polymerase chain reaction (PCR) tests, the principle involves the use of short but specific primers to amplify a known sequence in the presence of contaminating DNA from other living organisms, including the infected human host. In a reverse-transcriptase-PCR test, nucleic acid from the virus in the form of RNA is first converted to DNA and then subjected to virus-specific PCR amplification. Sequences specific to the target virus are amplified to a level that can be stained and detected with the naked eye. The degree of amplification is proportional to the initial amount of viral RNA so that the number of viruses, or viral load, can be estimated. Because RNA can be isolated from dead viruses, samples can be shipped and test specimens can be inactivated to protect laboratory technologists. This test is sensitive and rapid enough to identify infected patients early and inform treatment.

32. Towner et al. 2004. Other RT-PCR methods have similar promise (Drosten et al. 2002; Leroy et al. 2000).

33. Muyembe-Tamfum et al. 1999.

34. Holmes 1998, 535. Other accounts suggest that a diagnosis of Ebola virus was actually confirmed within twenty-four hours (Muyembe-Tamfum et al. 1999).

35. Holmes 1998, 534. The diagnostic timeline of the hospital-amplified Ebola outbreak in Kikwit, Zaire (now Democratic Republic of the Congo) and the consequences of delay in new cases were constructed from data documented by Muyembe-Tamfum et al. 1999 and Roels et al. 1999. There were 317 documented cases of Ebola virus infection in Kikwit in 1995; 245 of these died. The epidemic peaked during the week beginning April 30 and began to decline as soon as the disease was named (Roels et al. 1999).

36. See http://www.pbs.org/wgbh/nova/teachers/programs/2304_ebola.html. Press coverage of the epidemic was unprecedented; the virus and the previously unknown town of Kikwit became known across the globe (Garrett 2001).

37. The time between documentation of the first case reporting to an allopathic health center and processing of the first blood specimens was four and a half weeks for the 1995 Ebola outbreak in Kikwit. A satellite outbreak at Mosango General Hospital was only identified retrospectively (Bonnet, Akamituna, and Mazaya 1998).

38. Antibodies against Ebola have been found in humans and other primates as far away from the central African focus of disease as Cameroon (Leroy, Telfer, et al. 2004). Data from eastern Uganda have been available since 1983 (Teepe et al. 1983). Most countries in and around central Africa should have a strategy in place for dealing with outbreaks of Ebola and other hemorrhagic viruses, since there is a reasonable chance that they could occur in the future.

39. El Tahir 1977.

40. WHO and CDC 1998, http://www.cdc.gov/ncidod/dvrd/spb/mnpages/vhfmanual/entire.pdf.

41. Cohen 2004.

42. Ibid, e59.

43. SARS, then a new virus, was essentially identified by exclusion, but ruling out known diseases with similar symptoms was only possible with laboratory and radiological testing (Zhong and Zeng 2003). See also http://www.who.int/csr/sars/casedefinition/en/.

44. Groopman 2007.
45. "Outbreak News: Ebola Haemorrhagic Fever, Uganda—End of the Outbreak" (2008); Mason 2008.
46. Diamond 2002; Woolhouse 2002; Woolhouse and Gowtage-Sequeria 2005.
47. Mason 2008; Towner et al. 2008.
48. Mason 2008.
49. Holmes et al. 1990; Paweska 2007.
50. Arthur 2002.
51. Addae 1997; Mengara 2005; Twumasi 1975.
52. Garrett 1994, 123.
53. Obadare 2005; Leader and Snyder 2006.
54. In 2005, WHO expanded the repertoire of internationally notifiable diseases from cholera, the plague, and yellow fever to include all disease epidemics that could be classified as major public health events (WHO 2005). The longer list includes potentially pandemic influenza, Ebola, and Marburg disease, even though most African caregivers lack the access to local laboratories that could confirm any of these diagnoses.
55. A focus on infection control was justified here. The Gulu outbreak was noteworthy in that health-worker infections continued after the introduction of barrier nursing (Arthur 2002), suggesting that investments in training and facilities were needed in this area. The point is not that these changes were unnecessary but that they should have been accompanied by diagnostic development.
56. Lamunu et al. 2002, 9–10.
57. Khan et al. 1999, S76.
58. Arthur 2002.
59. Mason 2008.
60. Paweska 2007.
61. Frame et al. 1970; Fuller 1974; Fisher-Hoch et al. 1995; Wright 2004; Mellor 2004; Richmond and Baglole 2003; Bausch, Sesay, and Oshin 2004.
62. In Latin, *filo* means thread, and *arena* means sand. The only other arenavirus that infects humans is the recently described Lujo virus from southern Africa (Briese et al. 2009).
63. Troup et al. 1970.
64. There have been several chronicles of the first few outbreaks of Lassa fever and early investigations surrounding them; see, for example, Garrett 1994 and Fuller 1974.
65. Frame et al. 1970.
66. Richmond and Baglole 2003; Khan et al. 2008; Fichet-Calvet and Rogers 2009.
67. Monath 1975.
68. Guerrant et al. 2005.
69. In one case, in the Nigerian city of Jos, although there was some diagnostic delay, no patients or health workers were infected (Cooper et al. 1982).
70. Fisher-Hoch et al. 1995, 859.
71. See Bausch et al. 2001; Richmond and Baglole 2003. Khan et al. 2008 listed twenty-seven potential confounders, including systemic bacterial infections and parasitemias such as malaria. According to Carlos "Kent" Campbell, a malaria and Lassa researcher and Lassa fever survivor, "If you weren't paying close attention, you wouldn't be able to distinguish Lassa from malaria. They look exactly the same until the tail end of Lassa when the hemorrhaging starts" (Garrett 1994, 93).
72. Mortality rates from Khan et al. 2008. State of diagnostic facilities in Nigeria quoted in "Lassa Fever—Nigeria (05)" (2009). According to Inegbenebor, Okosun, and Inegbenebor 2010, "Irrua Specialist Teaching Hospital [in midwestern Nigeria]...was designated a special center for the treatment of Lassa fever....Because of late presentation, a number of people still die even when treatment is offered."

73. Sierra Leone: quote from Richmond and Baglole 2003, 1273; Nigeria: Inegbenebor, Okosun, and Inegbenebor 2010.

74. Khan et al. 2008. Per capita expenditure on health from the WHO statistical information system at http://www.who.int/whosis/en/index.html.

75. Garrett 1994; Alibek and Handelman 1999.

76. According to Laurie Garrett (1994), "For years separate and often isolated research was conducted, and both superpowers [the United States and the Soviet Union] would eventually shut down their West African Lassa laboratories, leaving the Africans the ultimate losers" (1994, 194). A considerable body of U.S. data is published, and there is continuing evidence in the scientific literature of American efforts to understand the disease. Less is known about the USSR's research program. Neither of these initiatives resulted in a lasting diagnostic service for Kenema.

77. Positive predictive value of 0.81/1.00 based on fever, pharyngitis, retrosternal pain, and proteinuria (McCormick et al. 1987).

78. Ibid.

79. Mellor 2004.

80. Paweska 2007.

81. Bausch et al. 2000.

82. Mellor 2004; Bausch, Sesay, and Oshin 2004; Wright 2004.

83. Khan et al. 2008.

84. Richmond and Baglole 2003.

85. In 1957, there were international yellow fever vaccine laboratories in Yaba, Lagos, Nigeria; Dakar, Senegal; and Johannesburg, South Africa (Schram 1971). Yellow fever research was also conducted in Ghana.

86. Kirkland 2003, 6.

87. Harrison, Simonsen, and Waldman 2008.

88. Guimard et al. 1999.

89. Rouquet et al. 2005.

90. Leroy et al. 2005; Towner et al. 2007.

91. "Outbreak of Ebola Haemorrhagic Fever in Yambio, South Sudan, April–June 2004" (2005, 374).

92. Khan et al. 2008; "Lassa Fever—Nigeria (05)" (2009); Beatty et al. 2008.

CHAPTER 6

1. *Guardian* (Nigeria), 19 February 2005; Ojo 2004.

2. Ojo 2004.

3. Syphilis diagnosis in pregnant women (Terris-Prestholt et al. 2003; Watson-Jones et al. 2005); other publications detailing the need for and challenges facing diagnosis of diseases caused by sexually transmitted bacteria (Aledort et al. 2006; Peeling et al. 2006); bacterial sexually transmitted diseases and HIV susceptibility (White et al. 2008).

4. According to Chigwedere et al. 2008, who measured lives saved in nearby Botswana and Namibia, over three hundred thousand South African deaths can be attributed to denialism by the Mbeki government.

5. The phrase "lies, damned lies and statistics" was attributed to the British politician Benjamin Disraeli by the American writer Mark Twain (Samuel Clemens) in 1907. In that context, Twain/Disraeli listed three kinds of lies, among which statistics was the worst because it was the most deceptive. Other sources for the phrase are documented: in 1894, a physician named Pierce gave a paper to the Philadelphia Medical Society in which he characterized this triad of lies as a "proverbial" phrase.

6. Vaughan 1991; Hunt 1999.

7. See Vaughan 1991.

8. Davies 1956.

9. See Vaughan 1991, 132–44. Vaughan also describes the career of Albert Cook, a government-appointed crusader against "diseases of immorality" in the 1920s (1991, 137). Cook's retraction of his earlier conclusions only appeared in "grey" literature that is not listed in the principal medical indexes, such as Medline, and therefore unlikely to be read. A detailed reanalysis of the "epidemic" was presented by J. N. Davies (1956), years after most of the major players and their readers had died. Yaws is a skin disease caused by *Treponema pallidum* subspecies *pertenue*. *T. pallidum* subspecies *pallidum* is the causative organism of syphilis, the sexually transmitted disease. The two organisms are remarkably similar and challenging to delineate, even with present-day technology. It is possible that the Buganda epidemic was yaws, rather than syphilis. Another prevailing hypothesis is that, because yaws was well understood at the turn of the century, the Buganda epidemic must have been a treponemal disease that is different from syphilis and yaws but not sexually transmitted. Either way, it is clear that sexual intercourse was not the transmission mechanism, as the original chroniclers assumed. In a possible attempt to exonerate them, it has been claimed that "the pioneers of medicine in Uganda…worked under difficult and often disheartening conditions with courage and enthusiasm" (Davies 1956). The entire episode is unfortunate on many counts. Had the physicians been willing to acknowledge that the sick Baganda were possibly infected with a less virulent form of *T. palladium*, years later biological scientists might have used the causative organisms as a means to understand the pathogenesis of syphilis or even as the basis for a syphilis vaccine.

10. Murru 2004.

11. Ogunbodede 2005.

12. Nonspecificity of early tests has been studied by Lantin, Peitrequin, and Frei 1987 and Biggar et al. 1985. Newer tests have been developed as a result but second-, third-, and even fourth-generation antibody-based tests have been shown to underperform in Africa, making confirmatory testing essential. Cross-reacting antigens come from infective agents that are common in Africa, such as malaria and schistosomiasis (Biggar et al. 1985; Behets et al. 1991; Everett et al. 2010).

13. Alikor and Erhabor 2006.

14. Different African countries appear to have sustained very different AIDS epidemics, as summarized by Iliffe 2006. Extrapolation from the worst single-country data to the entire continent has exacerbated the myths surrounding AIDS.

15. Meda et al. 1999.

16. Chigwedere and Essex 2010.

17. Granich et al. 2009.

18. Pincock 2006; Olukoya and Ferguson 2003.

19. Schoofs 1999.

20. Oshisada 2006.

21. Adio 2004.

22. "Progress toward Strengthening Blood Transfusion Services—14 Countries, 2003–2007" (2008).

23. Iliffe 2006; Miles 2003; Gisselquist et al. 2004; Schmid et al. 2004.

24. Spurious treatments were also widely touted and eagerly patronized by AIDS patients in California in the 1980s. Then, as in West Africa today, diagnostic insufficiency and the absence of effective treatments allowed many to prey on the terminally ill (Shilts 1988).

25. Sources of information for traditional medical practitioners who treat patients with sexually transmitted diseases (adapted from Elujoba, Fadairo, and Irinoye 2002): the practitioners generally had local names for sexually transmitted syndromes and twenty-eight (54%) had a Yoruba term for AIDS. These terms included *Atosi egbe* (sexually transmitted disease with weight loss), *Arun igbalode* (disease of the times), and *Eedi* (the curse).

26. Elujoba, Fadairo, and Irinoye 2002.

27. Dodd 1996; Kwena 2004; Bateman 2006.

28. Ebenezer Obadare and Iruka Okeke have studied Abalaka's claim and its socio-political and biomedical significance. This analysis will be published in the scholarly literature.

29. Abalaka 2004. What appears to be a duplicate publication appeared in a Chinese journal, *Zhonghua Nan Ke Xue* (Abalaka 2005), three months later, again accompanied by an editorial (Huang and Lu 2005).

30. Abalaka 2004, 3820.

31. "Progress toward Strengthening Blood Transfusion Services—14 Countries, 2003–2007" (2008).

32. Kim and Gilks 2005.

33. Bizuwork et al. 2007; Cohen 2007; Mugyenyi et al. 2010. For more on the causes and consequences of slow antiretroviral roll-out across Africa, see Ford, Mills, and Calmy 2009.

34. WHO 1988; Amirali, Moshiro, and Ramaiya 2004. Patients with less common AIDS-related syndromes such as HIV-associated dementia are very likely to be missed, particularly when nonspecialists perform the diagnosis (Kvalsund et al. 2009).

35. Rapatski, Suppe, and Yorke 2005.

36. Araya et al. 2004.

CHAPTER 7

1. Berhane 2004.

2. For example, eleven West African countries have halted the transmission of river blindness, preventing six hundred thousand cases of blindness and reclaiming twenty-five million hectares of previously infested and now arable land (Levine 2004).

3. Unfortunately, in many parts of Africa, vaccines and chemicals have been used instead of broad-based prevention strategies, rather than in coordination with them.

4. Aylward et al. 2000; Aylward and Birmingham 2005.

5. Stetten 1978; even within the fiber matrix of human scabs, the virus cannot survive longer than two or three years.

6. Oldstone 1998.

7. Quoted in Robottom 1991, 8.

8. Adebayo Lamikanra, personal communication; Vaughan 1991; Oldstone 1998; Schram 1971, 159.

9. Jenner 1798. Jenner was not the first to make this observation. At least two prior examples of people who administered vaccinia to people because they hypothesized that it was protective are known in the United Kingdom: Benjamin Jetsy (1774), a British farmer, and Peter Plett, a schoolmaster from Holstein (1792) (Stetten 1978). Jenner was the first to investigate this idea experimentally and generate supporting data. For this reason, he is given credit for the discovery. Jenner also made his vaccine available for widespread evaluation.

10. Stetten 1978; Oldstone 1998.

11. Commentators called 1965 the "international cooperation year" (Levine 2004).

12. See Stetten 1978 for a smallpox eradication timeline.

13. A laboratory infection occurred in Birmingham, United Kingdom, in 1978.

14. Barrett 2004.

15. Stetten 1978.

16. Malian epithet for guinea worm (Levine 2004).

17. In 1991, the World Health Assembly passed a resolution supporting eradication: "Encouraged by the considerable progress achieved in many countries towards elimination of the disease; Aware that country-by-country elimination of dracunculiasis is considered to be the last step before global eradication can be declared...URGES the

director general [of WHO]…to support global efforts to eradicate dracunculiasis during the 1990s" (Forty-fourth World Health Assembly, Agenda item 17.2: Eradication of Dracunculiasis, Resolution WHA44.5, 13 May 1991, http://www.who.int/dracunculiasis/eradication/WHA44.5.pdf).

18. Sam-Abbenyi et al. 1999.

19. Iriemenam, Oyibo, and Fagbenro-Beyioku 2008; CDC 2010.

20. For historical overviews, see Oldstone 1998 and Oshinsky 2005.

21. Marx, Glass, and Sutter 2000; Minor 2004.

22. "Laboratory Support for Poliomyelitis Eradication: Memorandum from a WHO Meeting" (1989). The network has strengthened surveillance for other viruses and will need to continue to track polio viruses after polio vaccination is discontinued because immunocompromised patients can shed vaccine strains, that can on rare occasions mutate to disease-causing forms (Hull and Aylward 1999; Nsubuga et al. 2002).

23. http://www.cdc.gov/mmwR/preview/mmwrhtml/mm4908a3.htm. Appropriately designed eradication campaigns can build diagnostic infrastructure that has significant impact on the control and treatment of other diseases (Levine 2004).

24. Roberts 2009a, 2009b.

25. Oldstone 1998.

26. Scott et al. 2007; Helfand et al. 2005. Some studies suggest that other subpopulations may need to be vaccinated before nine months, although data are few (Tapia et al. 2005).

27. "Progress in Reducing Global Measles Deaths, 1999–2004" (2006); "Effects of Measles Control Activities, African Region, 1999–2005,"*MMWR* weekly 55 (37): 1017–21; http://www.cdc.gov/mmwr/preview/mmwrhtml/mm5537a3.htm?s_cid=mm5537a3_e.

28. These did not include a few high population countries such as the Democratic Republic of Congo and Nigeria. See data at http://www.cdc.gov/mmwr/preview/mmwrhtml/mm5537a3.htm?s_cid=mm5537a3_e#fig.

29. Hopkins 1976; Zahra 1956.

30. Agadzi et al. 1983, 1985.

31. McLean 1998; Aylward et al. 2000; Aylward 2006; "Update: International Task Force for Disease Eradication, 1990 and 1991" (1992).

32. Molyneux, Hopkins, and Zagaria 2004, 347.

33. Adegbola et al. 2005; Howie et al. 2007.

34. Sow et al. 2005.

35. Shearer et al. 2010 identified proximity to a country that has introduced the vaccine as a principal determinant of Hib adoption. I made the link to surveillance by comparing data on one year olds vaccinated against Hib between 1999 and 2007 (from the WHO statistical database at www.who.int/whosis), with published studies on Hib surveillance indexed by Medline.

36. Tan 2003; Musher 2006.

37. Gordon et al. 2003; Antonio et al. 2008; Adegbola et al. 2006.

38. Musher 2006; Pelton, Loughlin, and Marchant 2004; Moore et al. 2008.

39. The list of artists who fell victim to tuberculosis includes Frederic Chopin at age thirty-nine in 1810; John Keats at thirty-six in 1831; Emily Bronte at twenty-two in 1840 and Anne Bronte at twenty-nine in 1849; Heinrich Heine at fifty-nine in 1856; D. H. Lawrence at forty-five in 1930; and George Orwell at forty-seven in 1950.

40. Wainwright 1991; Feldman 2000.

41. WHO 2004.

42. Xu, Jin, and Zhang 2000.

43. WHO 2003. Some low-grade infections can be missed by sputum smear microscopy, which only detects bacterial concentrations above one-thousand bacteria per milliliter. More sensitive tests, including culture, enzyme-linked immunosorbent assays

(ELISA), and PCR, have been advocated, but implementation is difficult in rudimentary laboratories. Culture traditionally requires at least eight weeks and a Biosafety Level 3 laboratory. PCR has been successfully used at a research institute in Ghana but, like ELISA, it is presently too expensive for routine use (Wilson et al. 2003).

44. Yimer, Bjune, and Alene 2005.

45. Lawn, Afful, and Acheampong 1998; Steen and Mazonde 1998; Needham et al. 2001; Lienhardt et al. 2001.

46. Nicholls 2005.

47. WHO 2006b; Singh, Upshur, and Padayatchi 2007.

48. Basu et al. 2009; Dowdy et al. 2008; Basu et al. 2007. The inception of the epidemic is reviewed by Singh, Upshur, and Padayatchi 2007.

49. Smolinski et al. 2003.

50. Cox et al. 2006.

51. Gandhi et al. 2006; Basu et al. 2007; Singh, Upshur, and Padayatchi 2007; Jones, Hesketh, and Yudkin 2008.

52. STOP-TB 2006.

53. Johnson et al. 2008; Pai, Ramsay, and O'Brien 2008.

54. Pai et al. 2009; Pai and O'Brien 2008; Perkins, Roscigno, and Zumla 2006.

55. Paramasivan et al. 2010.

56. Institute of Medicine (U.S.) Committee for the Study on Malaria Prevention and Control: Status Review and Alternative Strategies and Oaks 1991; Carson 2002; Needham and Canning 2003.

57. The intense endemicity in Africa, the hypervirulence of the parasite *P. falciparum*, and the resilience of its vector *Anopheles gambiae* were important roadblocks to eradication and still present serious challenges to malaria control on the continent: "British Contributions to Medical Research and Education in Africa after the Second World War" (1999); Gallup and Sachs 2001; Arrow, Panosian, and Gelband 2004.

58. Bill and Melinda Gates Foundation 2007; Roberts and Enserink 2007.

59. Roberts and Enserink 2007, 1544.

60. Hoffman 2000, 1509.

61. Aylward et al. 2000.

CHAPTER 8

1. Nuland 1989, 420.

2. Tornheim et al. 2007, 541. The Yambuku investigation is documented in "Ebola Haemorrhagic Fever in Zaire, 1976" (1978).

3. Garrett 1994, 197.

4. For example, see Blair 1956, 258. Meredith Turshen (1984) acknowledges that diagnostic precision and medical record-keeping showed gradual improvement late in the colonial period, but they never reached optimal standards and have declined considerably in many African countries from the 1970s.

5. Mandomando et al. 2007.

6. Lamikanra, Okeke, et al., unpublished data in preparation for scholarly publication; Mandomando et al. 2007.

7. Feierman, Janzen, and Joint Committee on African Studies 1992, 18.

8. Curtin 1990; Addae 1997.

9. Curtin 1990.

10. Mortality rates for European civilians in Cameroon declined from 69 per 1,000 in the period 1893–1901 to 31 per 1,000 in 1903–12 (Curtin 1990).

11. Addae 1997; Packard 2000; Vaughan 1991.

12. Curtin 1990; Addae 1997.

13. Addae 1997, 185.

14. Ibid., 189.

15. Cited in ibid., 87–88. In 2004, most countries in sub-Saharan Africa had between <1 and 2 laboratory health workers per 10,000 population while in the Middle East and North Africa, the range was 2–7 (in 2001/2002, New Zealand, Finland and the United States respectively had 10, 20, and 23). Data from the WHO statistics database www.who.int/whosis.

16. Through their explorations, and by linking isolated areas by road and rail, colonialists facilitated the rapid spread of previously localized infectious conditions among previously nonimmune populations. Europeans imported tuberculosis and may have brought other diseases to Africa (Kiple 1993). Colonialists contributed less directly to the infectious disease burden by lowering nutritional status, first by substituting cash crops for food crops and later by introducing infant formula.

17. Vaughan 1991; Worboys 2000.

18. Dispensaries mostly served Africans. Europeans were discouraged from residing too far from towns with European quarters that were equipped with hospitals (Addae 1997, 30–31).

19. Schram 1971, 349. In contrast, both Western and indigenous doctors receive at least eighteen years of formal education and apprenticeship.

20. Colonial Office 1948; Brieger et al. 2004.

21. Ferguson 2007.

22. Packard 2000; Prins 1989.

23. "British Contributions to Medical Research and Education in Africa after the Second World War" (1999).

24. Zahra 1956, 931.

25. Oshinsky 2005, 71; emphasis added.

26. Suit No NIC/8/2006 (2008).

27. Twumasi 1975. See also Turshen 1984 for a critique of the emphasis on curative medicine in Tanzania.

28. Twumasi 1975, plate 20.

29. Ibid., 85.

30. Ibid.

31. Twumasi 1975; Turshen 1984; Addae 1997.

32. Quoted in Porter 1998, 679.

33. Nkrumah 1963, 163. The section title is an adaptation of a more popular Nkrumah quote made in response to a question about his allegiance to the United States or the Soviet Union: "We face neither East nor West; we face Forward."

34. Verhoef and Fluit 2006.

35. Barker et al. 1986; Gicquelais et al. 1990.

36. Barker et al. 1986, 231; Pettersson, Wigzell, and Perlman 1987.

37. Although almost a third of these people are mortuary staff, this includes pathologists and a large number of technicians, scientists, and consultants who work at the bench.

38. Kim 2005, 545.

39. PATH 2008; UNICEF and WHO 2009.

40. Kebede and Polderman 2004.

41. Vaughan 1991, 155.

42. Dineva et al. 2005; Panhotra et al. 2005; Prati 2006.

43. This system already operates for vaccines and drugs. For example, ivermectin, a potent, broad-spectrum antiparasitic and antihelminthic (deworming) drug, has a considerable veterinary market. Ivermectin has earned so much income from veterinary use

in the West—an estimated US$1 billion annually—that its innovator company, Merck Sharp and Dome, has been able to donate the drug to control programs in Africa and South America (Omura and Crump 2004; Geary 2005).

44. Malaria (Usdin, Guillerm, and Chirac 2006); meningococcal meningitis (Djibo et al. 2006; Chanteau et al. 2006); leishmaniasis (Diane et al. 2006); and plague (Chanteau et al. 2003).

45. Bosompem et al. 1997.

46. Usdin, Guillerm, and Chirac 2006.

CONCLUSION

1. Ishengoma et al. 2009.

2. Newman et al. 2004.

3. Polage et al. 2006.

4. Guyon et al. 1994; Reyburn et al. 2008.

5. Reyburn et al. 2008.

6. Megan Vaughan (1991) describes the layout of a yaws eradication clinic to illustrate what I call the conveyor belt mode. The author of the paper describing this system, which was built for mass health care delivery, stated that "the system has been aptly described as a 'sausage machine'" (Zahra 1956, 932). The description could not have originated in Nsukka, Nigeria, where the clinic was located, since sausages were unknown there. Vaughan concludes: "Though colonial biomedicine, and colonial states more generally, 'unitized' their subjects, they did not 'individualize' them for...there was a strong strand of thinking which held that Africans were, by definition, hardly capable of being individuals at all" (Vaughan 1991, 202–3).

7. See Turshen 1984; Twumasi 1975; and Obadare 2005.

8. Phillips, Van Bebber, and Issa 2006.

9. Shillcutt et al. 2008 modeled the cost-effectiveness of malaria diagnostics. They find that at low to medium prevalence, diagnostics are cost effective and cost-saving. At very high prevalences, using diagnostics does incur marginal additional costs in their model. However, they acknowledge that the model assumes that diagnostics are *only* used for malaria and that costing parameters used are conservative. Additionally, they do not include the cost of selective pressure, which promotes costly resistance in their analysis. Other studies illustrating the cost-effectiveness of malaria testing are detailed in chapter 2.

10. Garrett 1994, 198. Procuring anything in Africa today can be difficult, and diagnostic reagents present a particularly formidable challenge, since many are heat labile and need a cold chain for shipment. If routine diagnostic laboratories were dotted around the countries in which they exist, the most basic and bulky materials could be obtained from local suppliers and distributors. Interventions that focus on eradicating delays mediated by local customs officials could also be implemented specifically for diagnostics, analogous to expedited clearance for vaccine shipments.

11. The chairman of the Medical Laboratory Science Council of Nigeria, Professor Dennis Agbonlahor, remarked: "In University College Hospital (UCH), Ibadan, grouping antisera were produced in large quantities in the 1970s and 1980s by Medical Laboratory Scientists. Similarly, in the National Veterinary Research Institute, VOM, various culture media for the multiplication and maintenance of bacterial organisms were produced by Medical Laboratory Scientists. All these have been abandoned today in preference for imported ones, which are not necessarily better than locally produced ones" (quoted by Ukwuoma 2006).

12. Farmer 2004; Farmer et al. 1999; Scrimshaw 1974.

13. See Wolman et al.'s (2000) review of diagnostic test development. In 2008, the Quidel Corporation of San Diego manufactured rapid point-of-care diagnostics for influenza, respiratory syncytial virus, *Helicobacter pylori*, and Group A streptococci. See http://www/quidel.com/products/product_list.php?cat=1&by+state_disease&group=1. Following the 2002 anthrax spore attacks, scientists designed a rapid test to allow U.S. postal workers, who are not scientists, to screen mail for *Bacillus anthracis*. Similar methodology was subsequently used to rapidly identify Marburg-infected patients in Angola and patients with Rift Valley fever in Kenya (Ulrich et al. 2006; Duse 2008).

14. Maryke Henton, personal communication. See also http://en.bvt.fr/p-bvtfrpuben/display.aspx?srv=p-bvtfr&typ=pub&lang=en&cmd=view&style=styles/specie.xsl&select=PRODUCT[@IDeqPRODUCT_108].

15. Nwaka 2005; Commission for Africa 2005.

16. WHO 2006a.

17. For example, see the molecular lab-in-a-case marketed by Smith diagnostics, http://www.smithsdetection.com/eng/veterinary_diagnostics.php. For reviews that outline how new technologies can advance the development of appropriate diagnostics, see Perkins and Bell 2008 and Mabey et al. 2004.

18. Mtove et al. 2010. The test employed at the rural Tanzanian hospital is described at the manufacturer's website, http://www.hemocue.com/index.php?page=3002.

19. Michel et al. 2006; Boehme et al. 2007.

20. Peeling et al. 2006.

21. Okeke and Wain 2008.

22. Masum et al. 2007; Singer et al. 2008; Bosompem et al. 1997; Koukounari et al. 2009; Mathebula et al. 2009.

23. In addition to facilities, African scientists require funding to procure and maintain consumables, equipment, and services necessary for their research as well as networking, grant writing, and publication assistance (Okeke and Wain 2008; Mboya-Okeyo, Ridley, and Nwaka 2009; Kwabena Bosompem, personal communication).

24. Kennedy 2003.

25. Schram 1971; Addae 1997; Ojo 2004; Muula and Maseko 2006.

26. Breslauer et al. 2009; Bellina and Missoni 2009; Zimic et al. 2009.

27. Ihekweazu, Anya, and Anosike 2005; Berhan 2008; Larsen 2008.

28. Packard 2000, 106.

29. van den Brandhof et al. 2006.

30. Hampton et al. 1975.

31. Wolman et al. 2000.

32. van den Brandhof et al. 2006.

33. IID 2000; Hennessy et al. 2004.

34. van den Brandhof et al. 2006.

35. Bello et al. 2004; Andre et al. 2005; and personal communication from staff at Obafemi Awolowo University Teaching Hospital, Ile-Ife.

36. Million 2006.

37. Acute respiratory infections, AIDS, diarrhea, malaria, sexually transmitted infections, and tuberculosis ("The Right Tools Can Aave Lives" 2006).

38. Okeke et al. 2007.

39. Gillis 2005. Schistosomiasis (Kwabena Bosompem, personal communication); typhoid (Baker, Favorov, and Dougan 2010); *Haemophilus influenzae* type B (Shearer et al. 2010).

40. Jones et al. 2008.

41. Paramasivan et al. 2010.

42. Severe acute pneumonitis among deployed U.S. military personnel—Southwest Asia, 2003. This outbreak turned out to be noninfectious; however, justification for a

diagnostic facility was maintained because diagnostic support was needed for treatment and there was a potential threat of biological attack.

43. Craft and Riddell 2005. The labs were set up at locations as diverse as a makeshift building at the hospital that had served the Iraqi elite prior to the overthrow of Saddam Hussein. Before the establishment of these facilities, available diagnostic capabilities at the best sites were limited to blood smears for malaria, other slide parasitology, and Gram stain to visualize some bacteria. These facilities were inadequate but were equivalent to or better than those available in most sub-Saharan African countries. The U.S. military deemed it essential to provide on-site facilities for the culture and susceptibility testing of bacteria commonly implicated in community- and hospital-acquired infections and for serological tests for common viruses. A diagnostic laboratory entirely dependent on continuous supply and support from abroad is efficient over a short period of time, with assured procurement of supplies. Over the long term, this setup is expensive, impracticable, and typically unsustainable.

44. Barrett 2006, 181.

45. Jones et al. 2008.

46. Articulated by Michael Kazatchkine (2007) of the Global Fund in an interview published in the Bulletin of the World Health Organization.

47. In 1998, a £1 million grant from the British Department for International Development to the Malawi health services to support development of medical laboratory services was equivalent to 40% of the country's health budget for 2005–06. This sum was very useful, but still too small to alleviate diagnostic insufficiency at the grassroots (Muula and Maseko 2006).

48. WHO Regional Office for Africa 2008, 1.

49. Attaran 2005.

50. Mabey et al. 2004.

51. Data presented by Ishengoma et al. 2009, citing documents from the Tanzanian Ministry of Health.

52. Declaration of Alma-Ata 1978.

53. Ohrt et al. 2007.

54. Larsen 2008; Cohen 2007; Paramasivan et al. 2010.

55. The declaration states that "in order to improve and sustain access to laboratory services, there must be an integration of laboratory support for tuberculosis, malaria and HIV disease programs" (WHO Regional Office for Africa 2008, 2). It does, however, go on to define this as "part of the greater health system."

56. A century ago, medical research institutions provided clinical diagnostic services and produced biomedical reagents and vaccines. The Accra research laboratory was renowned for its work on plague following a 1908 epidemic, but also produced smallpox vaccine and provided clinical diagnostic services (Addae 1997, 183). Two decades later, laboratory services in Ghana were restructured so that diagnostic services were separated from research centers (Addae 1997, 188). Although the research institution continued to provide expertise and support for diagnostic services, diagnostic laboratory staffing was always poor, and patient-centered labs were gradually eroded. Today, the Noguchi Medical Research Institute is an international center of excellence for tropical disease research, while the Korle Bu teaching hospital laboratory struggles to maintain its uncharacteristically broad offerings of diagnostic services for its patients. The vast majority of patients who do not access tertiary care have few options for diagnostic support.

57. Feary et al. 2005.

58. Newman et al. 2004; Mutanda, Omari, and Wamola 1989; Ukwuoma 2004.

59. Hopkins, Asiimwe, and Bell 2009.

60. Laboratory safety must also be stepped up to assure the well-being of workers, patients, and the wider community.

61. Polage et al. 2006, 529.

62. Rather than the pain from the needle, patients are reluctant to undergo blood tests because of the loss of blood, which has spiritual as well as physiological significance in many cultures. The motives for drawing blood are often considered sinister, and include international blood trafficking conspiracy theories (Geissler et al. 2008; Masiye et al. 2008; Mfutso-Bengo et al. 2008).

63. Masiye et al. 2008; Mfutso-Bengo et al. 2008.

64. Many successful African biomedical science programs are initiated and sustained from the outside. However, Africa-led programs have great potential for sustainability, growth, and translational impact ("Science and Africa: A Message to the G8 Summit" 2005; Okeke and Wain 2008; Zumla et al. 2010).

65. African Network for Drugs and Diagnostic Innovation (Mboya-Okeyo, Ridley, and Nwaka 2009). Wellcome Trust African Institutions Initiative website, http://www.well come.ac.uk/Funding/Biomedical-science/International-funding/Global-health-research/ WTX055734.htm.

Works Cited

Abalaka, J. O. 2004. Attempts to cure and prevent HIV/AIDS in central Nigeria between 1997 and 2002: Opening a way to a vaccine-based solution to the problem? *Vaccine* 22 (29–30):3819–28.
———. 2005. [Design, development, and successful application of safe and effective HIV
therapeutic and prophylactic vaccines]. *Zhonghua Nan Ke Xue* 11 (1):8–16. Ab-
stracted by Medline.
Abrams, M. E. 1979. Costs of tests. *J R Coll Physicians Lond* 13 (4):217–18.
The Abuja Declaration and the Plan of Action. 2000.
Acholonu, Catherine Obianuju. 1999. *The Igbo roots of Olaudah Equiano: An anthropo-
logical research.* Owerri, Nigeria: Afa Publications.
Addae, Stephen. 1997. *The evolution of modern medicine in a developing country:
Ghana 1880–1960.* Edinburgh: Durham Academic Press.
Adegbola, R. A., P. C. Hill, O. Secka, et al. 2006. Serotype and antimicrobial susceptibil-
ity patterns of isolates of *Streptococcus pneumoniae* causing invasive disease in
The Gambia 1996–2003. *Trop Med Int Health* 11 (7):1128–35.
Adegbola, R. A., O. Secka, G. Lahai, et al. 2005. Elimination of *Haemophilus influ-
enzae* type b (Hib) disease from The Gambia after the introduction of rou-
tine immunisation with a Hib conjugate vaccine: A prospective study. *Lancet*
366 (9480):144–50.
Adio, Waziri. 2004. Between AIDS and development. *ThisDay,* 9 December.
Agadzi, V. K., Y. Aboagye-Atta, J. W. Nelson, D. R. Hopkins, and P. L. Perine. 1985. Yaws
in Ghana. *Rev Infect Dis* 7 Suppl 2:S233–36.
Agadzi, V. K., Y. Aboagye-Atta, J. W. Nelson, P. L. Perine, and D. R. Hopkins. 1983. Resurgence of yaws in Ghana. *Lancet* 2 (8346):389–90.
Aledort, J. E., A. Ronald, M. E. Rafael, et al. 2006. Reducing the burden of sexually
transmitted infections in resource-limited settings: The role of improved diagnostics. *Nature* 444 Suppl 1:59–72.
Alibek, Ken, and Stephen Handelman. 1999. *Biohazard: The chilling true story of the
largest covert biological weapons program in the world, told from the inside by the
man who ran it.* New York: Random House.
Alikor, D. E., and N. O. Erhabor. 2006. Trend of HIV-seropositivity among children in
a tertiary health institution in the Niger Delta Region of Nigeria. *Afr J Health
Sci* 13 (1–2):80–85.
Alsop Z. 2007. Ebola outbreak in Uganda "atypical," say experts. *Lancet* 370 (9605):2085.
Alubo, O. 2001. The promise and limits of private medicine: Health policy dilemmas
in Nigeria. *Health Policy Plan* 16 (3):313–21.
AMFm, Task Force. 2007. Affordable Medicines Facility—Malaria: Technical design.
Roll Back Malaria partnership.
Amin, A. A., D. Zurovac, B. B. Kangwana, et al. 2007. The challenges of changing national
malaria drug policy to artemisinin-based combinations in Kenya. *Malar J* 6:72.
Amirali, W., C. Moshiro, and K. Ramaiya. 2004. Assessment of clinical case-definition
for HIV/AIDS in Tanzania. *East Afr Med J* 81 (1):226–29.

Andre, M., M. Eriksson, S. Molstad, C. Stalsbylundborg, A. Jacobsson, and I. Odenholt. 2005. The management of infections in children in general practice in Sweden: A repeated 1-week diagnosis-prescribing study in 5 counties in 2000 and 2002. *Scand J Infect Dis* 37 (11–12):863–69.

Antonio, M., H. Dada-Adegbola, E. Biney, et al. 2008. Molecular epidemiology of pneumococci obtained from Gambian children aged 2–29 months with invasive pneumococcal disease during a trial of a 9-valent pneumococcal conjugate vaccine. *BMC Infect Dis* 8:81.

APUA, Alliance for the Prudent Use of Antibiotics. 2001. Antibiotic resistance: Synthesis of recommendations by expert policy groups. Geneva: Alliance for the Prudent Use of Antibiotics, World Health Organization.

Araya, T., G. Reniers, A. Schaap, et al. 2004. Lay diagnosis of causes of death for monitoring AIDS mortality in Addis Ababa, Ethiopia. *Trop Med Int Health* 9 (1):178–86.

Arrow, K. J., C. B. Panosian, and H. Gelband, eds. 2004. *Saving lives, buying time: Economics of malaria drugs in an age of resistance.* Washington, D.C.: National Academies Press.

Arthur, R. R. 2002. Ebola in Africa—discoveries in the past decade. *Euro Surveill* 7 (3):33–6.

Atta, Sefi. 2005. *Everything good will come: A novel.* Northampton, Mass.: Interlink Books.

Attaran, A. 2005. An immeasurable crisis? A criticism of the Millennium Development Goals and why they cannot be measured. *PLoS Med* 2 (10):318.

Attaran, A., K. I. Barnes, C. Curtis, et al. 2004. WHO, the Global Fund, and medical malpractice in malaria treatment. *Lancet* 363 (9404):237–40.

Aylward, B., K. A. Hennessey, N. Zagaria, J. M. Olive, and S. Cochi. 2000. When is a disease eradicable? 100 years of lessons learned. *Am J Public Health* 90 (10):1515–20.

Aylward, R. B. 2006. Eradicating polio: Today's challenges and tomorrow's legacy. *Ann Trop Med Parasitol* 100 (5–6):401–13.

Aylward, R. B., and M. Birmingham. 2005. The human story. *Br Med J* 331 (7527):1261–62.

Baker, S., M. Favorov, and G. Dougan. 2010. Searching for the elusive typhoid diagnostic. *BMC Infect Dis* 10 (1):45.

Balter, M. 2000. Malaria: Can WHO roll back malaria? *Science* 290 (5491):430.

Baquero, F., and J. Campos. 2003. The tragedy of the commons in antimicrobial chemotherapy. *Rev Esp Quimioter* 16 (1):11–13.Barker, R. H., Jr., L. Suebsaeng, W. Rooney, G. C. Alecrim, H. V. Dourado, and D. F. Wirth. 1986. Specific DNA probe for the diagnosis of *Plasmodium falciparum* malaria. *Science* 231 (4744):1434–46.

Barrett, S. 2004. Eradication versus control: The economics of global infectious disease policies. *Bull World Health Organ* 82 (9):683–88.

——. 2006. The smallpox eradication game. *Public Choice* 130:179–207.

Basnyat, B. 2005. Typhoid and paratyphoid fever. *Lancet* 366 (9497):1603.

Basnyat, B., A. P. Maskey, M. D. Zimmerman, and D. R. Murdoch. 2005. Enteric (typhoid) fever in travelers. *Clin Infect Dis* 41 (10):1467–72.

Basu, S., J. R. Andrews, E. M. Poolman, et al. 2007. Prevention of nosocomial transmission of extensively drug-resistant tuberculosis in rural South African district hospitals: An epidemiological modelling study. *Lancet* 370 (9597):1500.

Basu, S., G. H. Friedland, J. Medlock, et al. 2009. Averting epidemics of extensively drug-resistant tuberculosis. *Proc Natl Acad Sci* 106 (18):7672–77.

Bateman, C. 2006. Taking uBhejane by the horn(s). *S Afr Med J* 96 (5):382–86.

Bausch, D. G., M. Borchert, T. Grein, et al. 2003. Risk factors for Marburg hemorrhagic fever, Democratic Republic of the Congo. *Emerg Infect Dis* 9 (12):1531–37.

Bausch, D. G., A. H. Demby, M. Coulibaly, et al. 2001. Lassa fever in Guinea: I. Epidemiology of human disease and clinical observations. *Vector Borne Zoonotic Dis* 1 (4):269–81.

Bausch, D. G., S. T. Nichol, J. J. Muyembe-Tamfum, et al. 2006. Marburg hemorrhagic fever associated with multiple genetic lineages of virus. *N Engl J Med* 355 (9):909–19.

Bausch, D. G., P. E. Rollin, A. H. Demby, et al. 2000. Diagnosis and clinical virology of Lassa fever as evaluated by enzyme-linked immunosorbent assay, indirect fluorescent-antibody test, and virus isolation. *J Clin Microbiol* 38 (7):2670–77.

Bausch, D. G., S. S. Sesay, and B. Oshin. 2004. On the front lines of Lassa fever. *Emerg Infect Dis* 10 (10):1889–90.

Beatty, Alexandra S., Kimberly A. Scott, Peggy Tsai, Institute of Medicine (U.S.). Committee on Achieving Sustainable Global Capacity for Surveillance and Response to Emerging Diseases of Zoonotic Origin, Institute of Medicine (U.S.). Board on Global Health, and National Research Council (U.S.). Board on Agriculture and Natural Resources. 2008. *Achieving sustainable global capacity for surveillance and response to emerging diseases of zoonotic origin: Workshop report.* Washington, D.C.: National Academies Press.

Behets, F., A. Disasi, R. W. Ryder, et al. 1991. Comparison of five commercial enzyme-linked immunosorbent assays and Western immunoblotting for human immunodeficiency virus antibody detection in serum samples from Central Africa. *J. Clin. Microbiol.* 29 (10):2280–84.

Bell, D. R., P. Jorgensen, E. M. Christophel, and K. L. Palmer. 2005. Malaria risk: Estimation of the malaria burden. *Nature* 437 (7056):E3–4; discussion, E4–5.

Bell, D., and M. D. Perkins. 2008. Making malaria testing relevant: Beyond test purchase. *Trans R Soc Trop Med Hyg* 102 (11):1064–66.

Bell, D., C. Wongsrichanalai, and J. W. Barnwell. 2006. Ensuring quality and access for malaria diagnosis: How can it be achieved? *Nat Rev Microbiol* 4 (9):682–95.

Bellina, L., and E. Missoni. 2009. Mobile cell-phones (M-phones) in telemicroscopy: Increasing connectivity of isolated laboratories. *Diagn Pathol* 4:19.

Bello, I. S., F. A. Arogundade, A. A. Sanusi, I. T. Ezeoma, E. A. Abioye-Kuteyi, and A. Akinsola. 2004. Knowledge and utilization of Information Technology among health care professionals and students in Ile-Ife, Nigeria: A case study of a university teaching hospital. *J Med Internet Res* 6 (4):e45.

Berhan, Y. 2008. Medical doctors profile in Ethiopia: Production, attrition and retention. In memory of 100-years Ethiopian modern medicine & the new Ethiopian millennium. *Ethiop Med J* 46 Suppl 1:1–77.

Berhane, Y. 2004. Challenges in advancing public health. *Ethiop J Health Dev* 18 (1):1.

Berkelman, R., G. Cassell, S. Specter, M. Hamburg, and K. Klugman. 2006. The "Achilles Heel" of global efforts to combat infectious diseases. *Clin Infect Dis* 42 (10):1503–4.

Berkley, J. A., B. S. Lowe, I. Mwangi, et al. 2005. Bacteremia among children admitted to a rural hospital in Kenya. *N Engl J Med* 352 (1):39–47.

Bertherat, E., S. Bekhoucha, S. Chougrani, et al. 2007. Plague reappearance in Algeria after 50 years, 2003. *Emerg Infect Dis* 13 (10):1459–62.

Biggar, R. J., P. L. Gigase, M. Melbye, et al. 1985. ELISA HTLV retrovirus antibody reactivity associated with malaria and immune complexes in healthy Africans. *Lancet* 2 (8454):520–53.

Bill and Melinda Gates Foundation. 2007. Bill and Melinda Gates call for new global commitment to chart a course for malaria eradication. http://www.

gatesfoundation.org/press-releases/Pages/course-for-malaria-eradication-071017-2.aspx.

Bizuwork, T., S. D. Makombe, K. Kamoto, and A. D. Harries. 2007. WHO stage 3 disease conditions and outcomes in patients started on antiretroviral therapy in Malawi. *J Infect Devel Ctries* 1 (2):118–22.

Blair, D. M. 1956. Bilharziasis survey in British West and East Africa, Nyasaland and the Rhodesias. *Bull World Health Organ* 15:203–73.

Blomberg, B., K. P. Manji, W. K. Urassa, et al. 2007. Antimicrobial resistance predicts death in Tanzanian children with bloodstream infections: A prospective cohort study. *BMC Infect Dis* 7:43.

Boehme, C. C., P. Nabeta, G. Henostroza, et al. 2007. Operational feasibility of using loop-mediated isothermal amplification for diagnosis of pulmonary tuberculosis in microscopy centers of developing countries. *J Clin Microbiol* 45 (6):1936–40.

Bohannon, J. 2006. Arata Kochi profile: Fighting words from WHO's new malaria chief. *Science* 311 (5761):599.

Bonnet, M. J., P. Akamituna, and A. Mazaya. 1998. Unrecognized Ebola hemorrhagic fever at Mosango Hospital during the 1995 epidemic in Kikwit, Democratic Republic of the Congo. *Emerg Infect Dis* 4 (3):508–10.

Bosompem, K. M., I. Ayi, W. K. Anyan, T. Arishima, F. K. Nkrumah, and S. Kojima. 1997. A monoclonal antibody-based dipstick assay for diagnosis of urinary schistosomiasis. *Trans R Soc Trop Med Hyg* 91 (5):554–56.

Breman, J. G., and C. N. Holloway. 2007. Malaria surveillance counts. *Am J Trop Med Hyg* 77 (6 Suppl):36–47.

Breman, J. G., P. Piot, K. M. Johnson, et al. 1977. The epidemiology of Ebola haemorrhagic fever in Zaire, 1976. Paper read at Ebola Virus Haemorrhagic Fever conference, Antwerp, Belgium.

Breslauer, D. N., R. N. Maamari, N. A. Switz, W. A. Lam, and D. A. Fletcher. 2009. Mobile phone based clinical microscopy for global health applications. *PLoS One* 4 (7):e6320.

Brieger, W. R., P. E. Osamor, K. K. Salami, O. Oladepo, and S. A. Otusanya. 2004. Interactions between patent medicine vendors and customers in urban and rural Nigeria. *Health Policy Plan* 19 (3):177–82.

Briese, Thomas, Janusz T. Paweska, Laura K. McMullan, et al. 2009. Genetic detection and characterization of Lujo virus, a new hemorrhagic fever-associated arenavirus from Southern Africa. *PLoS Pathog* 4 (5):e1000455.

British contributions to medical research and education in Africa after the Second World War. 2001. Wellcome Witness Seminar 10: British contributions to medical research and education in Africa after the Second World War, Wellcome Trust, London.

Brock, Thomas D. 1999. *Milestones in microbiology 1546 to 1940*. Washington, D.C.: ASM Press.

Brown, R. C. 1996. Antibiotic sensitivity testing for infections in developing countries: Lacking the basics. *JAMA* 276 (12):952–53.

Bryce, J., C. Boschi-Pinto, K. Shibuya, and R. E. Black. 2005. WHO estimates of the causes of death in children. *Lancet* 365 (9465):1147–52.

Burnum, J. F. 1986. Medical vampires. *N Engl J Med* 314 (19):1250–51.

Campbell, C. C. 2008. Halting the toll of malaria in Africa. *Am J Trop Med Hyg* 78 (6):851–53.

Carson, Rachel. 2002. *Silent spring*. 40th anniversary ed. Boston: Houghton Mifflin.

Carter, K. Codell. 2003. *The rise of causal concepts of disease: Case histories, the history of medicine in context*. Burlington, Vt.: Ashgate.

CBoH, Central Board of Health 2003. Guidelines for the diagnosis and treatment of malaria in Zambia. Lusaka, Zambia: Central Board of Health.

———. 2006. A roadmap for impact on malaria in Zambia. Lusaka, Zambia: Ministry of Health.

CDC, Centers for Disease Control and Prevention. 2010. Nigeria won: Guinea worms zero. In *Guinea worm wrap-up #194*. WHO Collaborating Center for Research, Training and Eradication of Dracunculiasis.

Chain, E., H. W. Florey, A. D. Gardner, et al. 1940. Penicillin as a chemotherapeutic agent. *Lancet* ii, 226–28.

Chambers, R. 1989. Vulnerability: How the poor cope. *Institute of Development Studies Bulletin*, April 2.

Chandler, C. I., R. Mwangi, H. Mbakilwa, R. Olomi, C. J. Whitty, and H. Reyburn. 2008. Malaria overdiagnosis: Is patient pressure the problem? *Health Policy Plan* 23 (3):170–78.

Chanteau, S., S. Dartevelle, A. E. Mahamane, S. Djibo, P. Boisier, and F. Nato. 2006. New rapid diagnostic tests for *Neisseria meningitidis* serogroups A, W135, C, and Y. *PLoS Med* 3 (9):e337.

Chanteau, S., L. Rahalison, L. Ralafiarisoa, et al. 2003. Development and testing of a rapid diagnostic test for bubonic and pneumonic plague. *Lancet* 361 (9353):211–16.

Chappuis, F., S. Sundar, A. Hailu, et al. 2007. Visceral leishmaniasis: What are the needs for diagnosis, treatment and control? *Nat Rev Microbiol* 5 (11):873–82.

Cheesebrough, M. 1984. *Medical laboratory manual for tropical countries*. Vol. 2 of 2 vols.Oxford: Butterworth-Heinemann.

Chigwedere, P., and M. Essex. 2010. AIDS denialism and public health practice. *AIDS Behav.* 14(2):237–47.

Chigwedere, P., G. R. Seage, S. Gruskin, T. H. Lee, and M. Essex. 2008. Estimating the lost benefits of antiretroviral drug use in South Africa. *J Acquir Immune Defic Syndr.* 49(4):410–15.

Close, William T. 1995. *Ebola: A documentary novel of its first explosion*. New York: Ivy Books.

Cohen, G. M. 2007. Access to diagnostics in support of HIV/AIDS and tuberculosis treatment in developing countries. *AIDS* 21 Suppl 4:S81–87.

Cohen, J. 2004. Containing the threat—don't forget Ebola. *PLoS Med* 1 (3):e59.

Colonial Office, U.K. 1948. *A doctor in Nigeria*. Wellcome Film.

Commission for Africa. 2005. *Our common interest*. London: Penguin Books.

Cooper, C. B., W. R. Gransden, M. Webster, et al. 1982. A case of Lassa fever: Experience at St Thomas's Hospital. *Br Med J (Clin Res Ed)* 285 (6347):1003–5.

Cox, F. E. G., ed. 1996. *Illustrated history of tropical diseases*. Wellcome Trust.

Cox, H., Y. Kebede, S. Allamuratova, et al. 2006. Tuberculosis recurrence and mortality after successful treatment: Impact of drug resistance. *PLoS Med* 3 (10):e384.

Craft, D. W., and S. W. Riddell. 2005. Deployed clinical microbiology support to a developing country. Sunrise symposium at the American Society for Microbiology 105th general meeting, Atlanta, Georgia.

Creager, Angela N. H., and Hannah Landecker. 2009. Technical matters: Method, knowledge and infrastructure in twentieth-century life science. *Nat Methods* 6 (10):701.

Cunningham, Andrew. 1992. Transforming plague: The laboratory and the identity of infectious disease. In *The laboratory revolution in medicine*, edited by A. Cunningham and P. Williams. Cambridge: Cambridge University Press.

Curtin, Philip, D. 1990. The end of the "white man's grave"? Nineteenth-century mortality in West Africa. *Journal of Interdisciplinary History* 21 (1):63–88.

D'Acremont, V., C. Lengeler, H. Mshinda, D. Mtasiwa, M. Tanner, and B. Genton. 2009. Time to move from presumptive malaria treatment to laboratory-confirmed diagnosis and treatment in African children with fever. *PLoS Med* 6 (1):e252.

D'Alessandro, U., A. Talisuna, and M. Boelaert. 2005. Editorial: Should artemisinin-based combination treatment be used in the home-based management of malaria? *Trop Med Int Health* 10 (1):1–2.

Daly, C. C., I. Hoffman, M. Hobbs, et al. 1997. Development of an antimicrobial susceptibility surveillance system for Neisseria gonorrhoeae in Malawi: Comparison of methods. *J Clin Microbiol* 35 (11):2985–88.

Davies, J. N. 1956. The history of syphilis in Uganda. *Bull World Health Organ* 15 (6):1041–55.

Declaration of Alma-Ata. 1978. International Conference on Primary Health Care, 6–12 September, Alma-Ata, USSR.

de Oliveira, A. M., J. Skarbinski, P. O. Ouma, et al. 2009. Performance of malaria rapid diagnostic tests as part of routine malaria case management in Kenya. *Am J Trop Med Hyg* 80 (3):470–74.

de Vries, P. J., P. A. Kager, and M. W. Borgdorff. 2004. WHO, the Global Fund, and medical malpractice in malaria treatment. *Lancet* 363 (9415):1161.

Diamond, J. 2002. Evolution, consequences and future of plant and animal domestication. *Nature* 418 (6898):700–707.

Dineva, M. A., D. Candotti, F. Fletcher-Brown, J. P. Allain, and H. Lee. 2005. Simultaneous visual detection of multiple viral amplicons by dipstick assay. *J Clin Microbiol* 43 (8):4015–21.

Djibo, S., B. M. Njanpop Lafourcade, P. Boisier, et al. 2006. Evaluation of the Pastorex meningitis kit for the rapid identification of Neisseria meningitidis serogroups A and W135. *Trans R Soc Trop Med Hyg* 100 (6):573–78.

Djimde, A., C. V. Plowe, S. Diop, A. Dicko, T. E. Wellems, and O. Doumbo. 1998. Use of antimalarial drugs in Mali: Policy versus reality. *Am J Trop Med Hyg* 59 (3):376–79.

Dodd, R. 1996. Patients sue "AIDS-cure" Kenyan scientist. *Lancet* 347 (9016):1688.

Domagk, G. 1935. Ein beitrag zur chemotherapie du bakteriellen infektionen. *Deutsche medizinische Wochenschrift* 61:250–53.

Dowdy, D. W., R. E. Chaisson, G. Maartens, E. L. Corbett, and S. E. Dorman. 2008. Impact of enhanced tuberculosis diagnosis in South Africa: A mathematical model of expanded culture and drug susceptibility testing. *Proc Natl Acad Sci* 105 (32):11293–98.

Drakeley, C., R. Gosling, and H. Reyburn. 2005. Malaria diagnosis and treatment: One size does not fit all. *PLoS Med* 2 (6):e156; author reply, e165.

Drosten, C., S. Gottig, S. Schilling, et al. 2002. Rapid detection and quantification of RNA of Ebola and Marburg viruses, Lassa virus, Crimean-Congo hemorrhagic fever virus, Rift Valley fever virus, dengue virus, and yellow fever virus by real-time reverse transcription-PCR. *J. Clin. Microbiol.* 40 (7):2323–30.

Durrhelm, D. N., P. J. Becker, K. Billinghurst, and A. Brink. 1997. Diagnostic disagreement—the lessons learnt from malaria diagnosis in Mpumalanga. *S Afr Med J* 87 (5):609–11.

Duse, A. G. 2008. Taking molecular and other diagnostic platforms into Africa. Presented at *American Society for Microbiology 108th general meeting*. Session 203: Special interest symposium. Infectious diseases in the developing world: Fostering international scientific exchange.

Ebola haemorrhagic fever in Zaire, 1976. 1978. *Bull World Health Organ* 56 (2):271–93.

Ebola—the plague fighters. 1996. NOVA documentary film, PBS.

Editors, PLoS Medicine. 2006. What are the priorities in malaria research? *PLoS Med* 3 (1):e83.

Ehrlich, Paul. 1908. Modern chemotherapy. (Ueber moderne chemoterapie: Vortrag gehalten in der X; Tagung der Deutschen Dermatologischen Gesellschaft). In *Milestones in microbiology,* edited by T. D. Brock. Washington, D.C.: ASM Press.

———. 1909. Ueber moderne chemoterapie: Vortrag gehalten in der X; Tagung der Deutschen Dermatologischen Gesellschaft. In *Beitrage zur experimentellen pathologie und chemoterapie.* Leipzig: Akademische Verlagsgesellschaft.

El Tahir, B. M. 1977. The haemorrhagic fever outbreak in Maridi, western equatoria, southern Sudan. Paper read at Ebola Virus Haemorrhagic Fever conference, Antwerp, Belgium.

Elujoba, A. A., O. Fadairo, and O. O. Irinoye. 2002. Sexually transmitted diseases (STD) and HIV/AIDS in the hands of traditional medicine practitioners in Ile-Ife: Diagnoses and treatment modalities. *Ife: Journal of the Insititute of Cultural Studies* (8):40–54.

English, M., H. Reyburn, C. Goodman, and R. W. Snow. 2009. Abandoning presumptive antimalarial treatment for febrile children aged less than five years—a case of running before we can walk? *PLoS Med* 6 (1):e1000015.

Enwere, G., E. Biney, Y. B. Cheung, et al. 2006. Epidemiologic and clinical characteristics of community-acquired invasive bacterial infections in children aged 2–29 months in The Gambia. *Pediatr Infect Dis J* 25 (8):700–705.

Ericsson, H. M., and J. C. Sherris. 1971. Antibiotic sensitivity testing: Report of an international collaborative study. *Acta Pathol Microbiol Scand [B] Microbiol Immunol* 217:Suppl 217.

Etuk, S. J., I. H. Itam, and E. E. Asuquo. 1999. Role of the spiritual churches in antenatal clinic default in Calabar, Nigeria. *East Afr Med J* 76 (11):639–43.

Evans, J. A., A. Adusei, C. Timmann, et al. 2004. High mortality of infant bacteraemia clinically indistinguishable from severe malaria. *Quart J Med* 97 (9):591–97.

Everett, D. B., K. J. Baisely, R. McNerney, et al. 2010. Association of schistosomiasis with false positive HIV test results in an African adolescent population. *J. Clin. Microbiol* 48 (5):1570–77.

Ewald, P. 2007. A new golden age of medicine. In *What is your dangerous idea? Today's leading thinkers on the unthinkable,* ed. J. Brockman, 84–89. New York: HarperCollins.

Fadeel, M. A., J. A. Crump, F. J. Mahoney, et al. 2004. Rapid diagnosis of typhoid fever by enzyme-linked immunosorbent assay detection of *Salmonella* serotype Typhi antigens in urine. *Am J Trop Med Hyg* 70 (3):323–28.

Farcas, G. A., R. Soeller, K. Zhong, A. Zahirieh, and K. C. Kain. 2006. Real-time polymerase chain reaction assay for the rapid detection and characterization of chloroquine-resistant *Plasmodium falciparum* malaria in returned travelers. *Clin Infect Dis* 42 (5):622–67.

Farmer, P., J. Furin, J. Bayona, et al. 1999. Management of MDR-TB in resource-poor countries. *Int J Tuberc Lung Dis* 3 (8):643–45.

Farmer, Paul. 1999. *Infections and inequalities: The modern plagues.* Berkeley: University of California Press.

———. 2004. *Pathologies of power: Health, human rights, and the new war on the poor.* With a new preface by the author, California series in public anthropology 4. Berkeley: University of California Press.

Feary, D. J., D. Hyatt, J. Traub-Dargatz, et al. 2005. Investigation of falsely reported resistance of *Streptococcus equi* subsp. zooepidemicus isolates from horses to trimethoprim-sulfamethoxazole. *J Vet Diagn Invest* 17 (5):483–86.

Feglo, P. K., E. H. Frimpong, and M. Essel-Ahun. 2004. Salmonellae carrier status of food vendors in Kumasi, Ghana. *East Afr Med J* 81 (7):358–61.

Feierman, Steven, John M. Janzen, and Joint Committee on African Studies. 1992. *The social basis of health and healing in Africa*. Comparative studies of health systems and medical care no. 30. Berkeley: University of California Press.

Feldman, Burton. 2000. *The Nobel Prize: A history of genius, controversy, and prestige*. New York: Arcade.

Ferguson, Niall. 2007. Independence? Try "aid-dependence." Colonialism didn't cause Africa's problems, and aid alone won't fix them. *L.A. Times*, March 11.

Fichet-Calvet, E., and D. J. Rogers. 2009. Risk maps of Lassa fever in West Africa. *PLoS Negl Trop Dis* 3 (3):e388.

Fisher-Hoch, S. P., O. Tomori, A. Nasidi, et al. 1995. Review of cases of nosocomial Lassa fever in Nigeria: The high price of poor medical practice. *Brit Med J* 311 (7009):857–59.

Fleming, A. 1929. On the antibacterial action of cultures of a Penicillium, with a special reference to their use in the isolation of *B. influenzae. Brit. J. Exp. Path.* 10:226–36.

Foege, W. H. 2002. Infectious diseases. In *Critical issues in global health*, edited by C. Koop, C. Pearson, and M. Schwarz. San Francisco: Jossey-Bass.

Ford, N., E. Mills, and A. Calmy. 2009. Rationing antiretroviral therapy in Africa—treating too few, too late. *N Engl J Med* 360 (18):1808–10.

Foster, K. R., and H. Grundmann. 2006. Do we need to put society first? The potential for tragedy in antimicrobial resistance. *PLoS Med* 3 (2):e29.

Frame, J. D., J. M. Baldwin, Jr., D. J. Gocke, and J. M. Troup. 1970. Lassa fever, a new virus disease of man from West Africa: I. Clinical description and pathological findings. *Am J Trop Med Hyg* 19 (4):670–76.

Francesconi, P., Z. Yoti, S. Declich, et al. 2003. Ebola hemorrhagic fever transmission and risk factors of contacts, Uganda. *Emerg Infect Dis* 9 (11):1430–37.

Frege, G. 1980. *The foundations of arithmetic: A logico-mathematical enquiry into the concept of number*. Evanston, Ill.: Northwestern University Press. Fuller, John Grant. 1974. *Fever: The hunt for a new killer virus*. London: Hart-Davis MacGibbon.

Gallup, J. L., and J. D. Sachs. 2001. The economic burden of malaria. *Am J Trop Med Hyg* 64 (1–2 Suppl):85–96.

Gandhi, N. R., A. Moll, A. W. Sturm, et al. 2006. Extensively drug-resistant tuberculosis as a cause of death in patients co-infected with tuberculosis and HIV in a rural area of South Africa. *Lancet* 368 (9547):1575–80.

Garrett, L. 2001. Understanding media's response to epidemics. *Public Health Rep* 116 Suppl 2:87–91.

Garrett, Laurie. 1994. *The coming plague: Newly emerging diseases in a world out of balance*. New York: Farrar, Straus and Giroux.

Gaskell, Elizabeth Cleghorn. 1866. *Wives and daughters: A novel*. New York: Harper & brothers.

Geary, T. G. 2005. Ivermectin 20 years on: Maturation of a wonder drug. *Trends Parasitol* 21 (11):530–32.

Geissler, P. W., A. Kelly, B. Imoukhuede, and R. Pool. 2008. "He is now like a brother, I can even give him some blood"—relational ethics and material exchanges in a malaria vaccine "trial community" in The Gambia. *Soc Sci Med* 67 (5):696–707.

Gicquelais, K. G., M. M. Baldini, J. Martinez, et al. 1990. Practical and economical method for using biotinylated DNA probes with bacterial colony blots to identify diarrhea-causing *Escherichia coli. J Clin Microbiol* 28 (11):2485–90.

Gillis, Justin. 2005. Lives lost as vaccine programs face delays, efforts to get medicine to poor children falter. *Washington Post*, A01.

Gisselquist, D., J. J. Potterat, S. Brody, and S. F. Minkin. 2004. Does selected ecological evidence give a true picture of HIV transmission in Africa? *Int J STD AIDS*
15 (7):434–39.

Gisselquist, D., R. Rothenberg, J. Potterat, and E. Drucker. 2002. HIV infections in
sub-Saharan Africa not explained by sexual or vertical transmission. *Int J STD
AIDS* 13 (10):657–66.

Goodman, C., W. Brieger, A. Unwin, A. Mills, S. Meek, and G. Greer. 2007. Medicine
sellers and malaria treatment in sub-Saharan Africa: What do they do and how
can their practice be improved? *Am J Trop Med Hyg* 77 (6 Suppl):203–18.

Gordon, S. B., S. Kanyanda, A. L. Walsh, et al. 2003. Poor potential coverage for 7-valent
pneumococcal conjugate vaccine, Malawi. *Emerg Infect Dis* 9 (6):747–49.

Grabowsky, M. 2008. The billion-dollar malaria moment. *Nature* 451 (7182):1051–52.

Graham, S. M., and M. English. 2009. Non-typhoidal salmonellae: A management challenge for children with community-acquired invasive disease in tropical African
countries. *Lancet* 373 (9659):267–69.

Granich, R. M., C. F. Gilks, C. Dye, K. M. De Cock, and B. G. Williams. 2008. Universal voluntary HIV testing with immediate antiretroviral therapy as a strategy for elimination of HIV transmission: A mathematical model. *Lancet* 373
(9657):48–57.Griner, P. F., and R. J. Glaser. 1982. Sounding boards: Misuse of
laboratory tests and diagnostic procedures. *N Engl J Med* 307 (21):1336–39.

Groopman, Jerome E. 2007. *How doctors think.* Boston: Houghton Mifflin.

Guerrant, R. L., R. Oria, O. Y. Bushen, P. D. Patrick, E. Houpt, and A. A. Lima. 2005.
Global impact of diarrheal diseases that are sampled by travelers: The rest of the
hippopotamus. *Clin Infect Dis* 41 Suppl 8:S524–30.

Guimard, Y., M. A. Bwaka, R. Colebunders, et al. 1999. Organization of patient care
during the Ebola hemorrhagic fever epidemic in Kikwit, Democratic Republic
of the Congo, 1995. *J Infect Dis* 179 Suppl 1:S268–73.

Guyon, A. B., A. Barman, J. U. Ahmed, A. U. Ahmed, and M. S. Alam. 1994. A baseline
survey on the use of drugs at the primary health care level in Bangladesh. *Bulletin WHO* 72:265–71.

Gwer, S., C. R. Newton, and J. A. Berkley. 2007. Over-diagnosis and co-morbidity of
severe malaria in African children: A guide for clinicians. *Am J Trop Med Hyg* 77
(6 Suppl):6–13.

Hamer, D. H., M. Ndhlovu, D. Zurovac, et al. 2007. Improved diagnostic testing and
malaria treatment practices in Zambia. *JAMA* 297 (20):2227–31.

Hampton, J. R., M. J. Harrison, J. R. Mitchell, J. S. Prichard, and C. Seymour. 1975.
Relative contributions of history-taking, physical examination, and laboratory
investigation to diagnosis and management of medical outpatients. *Br Med J* 2
(5969):486–89.

Harrison, L. H., V. Simonsen, and E. A. Waldman. 2008. Emergence and disappearance
of a virulent clone of *Haemophilus influenzae* biogroup aegyptius, cause of Brazilian purpuric fever. *Clin Microbiol Rev.* 21(4):594–605.

Hatta, Mochammad, and Henk L. Smits. 2007. Detection of Salmonella Typhi by
nested polymerase chain reaction in blood, urine, and stool samples. *Am J Trop
Med Hyg* 76 (1):139–43.

Helfand, R. F., W. J. Moss, R. Harpaz, S. Scott, and F. Cutts. 2005. Evaluating the impact
of the HIV pandemic on measles control and elimination. *Bull World Health
Organ* 83 (5):329–37.

Hennessy, T. W., R. Marcus, V. Deneen, et al. 2004. Survey of physician diagnostic
practices for patients with acute diarrhea: Clinical and public health implications. *Clin Infect Dis* 38 Suppl 3:S203–11.

Hill, P. C., C. O. Onyeama, U. N. Ikumapayi, et al. 2007. Bacteraemia in patients admitted to an urban hospital in West Africa. *BMC Infect Dis* 7:2.

Hoffman, S. L. 2000. Infectious disease: Research (genomics) is crucial to attacking malaria. *Science* 290 (5496):1509.

Holmes, E. C. 1998. Molecular epidemiology and evolution of emerging infectious diseases. *Br Med Bull* 54 (3):533–43.

Holmes, G. P., J. B. McCormick, S. C. Trock, et al. 1990. Lassa fever in the United States: Investigation of a case and new guidelines for management. *N Engl J Med* 323 (16):1120–23.

Hopkins, D. R. 1976. After smallpox eradication: Yaws? *Am J Trop Med Hyg* 25 (6):860–65.

Hopkins, H., C. Asiimwe, and D. Bell. 2009. Access to antimalarial therapy: Accurate diagnosis is essential to achieving long term goals. *Br Med J* 339:b2606.

Howie, S. R., M. Antonio, A. Akisanya, et al. 2007. Re-emergence of *Haemophilus influenzae* type b (Hib) disease in The Gambia following successful elimination with conjugate Hib vaccine. *Vaccine* 25 (34):6305–09.

Huang, Y. F., and N. Q. Lu. 2005. [Jeremiah Abalaka and his HIV vaccine]. *Zhonghua Nan Ke Xue* 11 (1):7–8.

Hughes, J. M., C. J. Peters, M. L. Cohen, and B. W. Mahy. 1993. Hantavirus pulmonary syndrome: An emerging infectious disease. *Science* 262 (5135):850–51.

Hull, H. F., and R. B. Aylward. 1999. The scientific basis for stopping polio immunization. *Am J Epidemiol* 150 (10):1022–1025.

Hunt, Nancy Rose. 1999. *A colonial lexicon of birth ritual, medicalization, and mobility in the Congo*. Durham, N.C.: Duke University Press.

Ibadin, M. O., and A. Ogbimi. 2004. Antityphoid agglutinins in African school aged children with malaria. *West Afr J Med* 23 (4):276–79.

Idris, A. A., and N. Idris. 2006. Personal experience: Overview of Sudan's experience with Ebola hemorhagic fever (1976). *Sudanese Journal of Public Health* 1 (1):49–55.

Ihekweazu, C., I. Anya, and E. Anosike. 2005. Nigerian medical graduates: Where are they now? *Lancet* 365 (9474):1847–48.

IID (Intestinal Infectious Disease), Study Team. 2000. A report of the study of infectious intestinal disease in England. London: Foodstandards Agency.

Iliffe, John. 2006. *The African AIDS epidemic: A history*. Oxford: James Currey; Athens: Ohio University Press.

Inegbenebor, U., J. Okosun, and J. Inegbenebor. 2010. Prevention of Lassa fever in Nigeria. *Trans R Soc Trop Med Hyg* 104 (1):51–54.

Institute of Medicine (U.S.), Committee for the Study on Malaria Prevention and Control: Status Review and Alternative Strategies, and S. C. Oaks. 1991. *Malaria: Obstacles and opportunities; a report of the Committee for the Study on Malaria Prevention and Control; Status Review and Alternative Strategies, Division of International Health, Institute of Medicine*. Washington, D.C.: National Academy Press.

Iriemenam, N. C., W. A. Oyibo, and A. F. Fagbenro-Beyioku. 2008. Dracunculiasis— the saddle is virtually ended. *Parasitol Res* 102 (3):343–47.

Ishengoma, D. R., R. T. Rwegoshora, K. Y. Mdira, et al. 2009. Health laboratories in the Tanga region of Tanzania: The quality of diagnostic services for malaria and other communicable diseases. *Ann Trop Med Parasitol* 103 (5):441–53.

Izugbara, C. O., and A. I. Afangideh. 2005. Urban< women's use of rural-based health care services: The case of Igbo women in Aba City, Nigeria. *J Urban Health* 82 (1):111–21.

Jacquet, D, M. Boelaert, J. Seaman, et al. 2006. Comparative evaluation of freeze-dried and liquid antigens in the direct agglutination test for serodiagnosis of visceral leishmaniasis (ITMA-DAT/VL). *Trop Med Int Health* 11 (12):1777–84.

Jelinek, T., M. P. Grobusch, and G. Harms. 2001. Evaluation of a dipstick test for the rapid diagnosis of imported malaria among patients presenting within the network TropNetEurop. *Scand J Infect Dis* 33 (10):752–54.

Jelinek, T., M. P. Grobusch, S. Schwenke, et al. 1999. Sensitivity and specificity of dipstick tests for rapid diagnosis of malaria in nonimmune travelers. *J Clin Microbiol* 37 (3):721–23.

Jenner, Edward. 1798. An inquiry into the causes and effects of the variolae vaccinae, a disease discovered in some western counties of England, particularly Gloucestershire, and known by the name of The Cow Pox. Reprinted in *Milestones in Microbiology 1546–1940*, edited by T. D. Brock, 121–25. Washington, D.C.: ASM Press, 1999.

Johnson, K. M., P. A. Webb, and D. L. Heymann. 1978. Evaluation of the plasmapheresis program in Zaire. In *Ebola virus hemorrhagic fever*, edited by S. R. Pattyn. Amsterdam: Elsevier/North-Holland Biomedical Press.

Johnson, R., A. M. Jordaan, R. Warren, et al. 2008. Drug susceptibility testing using molecular techniques can enhance tuberculosis diagnosis. *J Infect Dev Ctries* 2 (1):40–45.

Jones, K. D., T. Hesketh, and J. Yudkin. 2008. Extensively drug-resistant tuberculosis in sub-Saharan Africa: An emerging public-health concern. *Trans R Soc Trop Med Hyg* 102 (3):219–24.

Jones, K. E., N. G. Patel, M. A. Levy, et al. 2008. Global trends in emerging infectious diseases. *Nature* 451 (7181):990–93.

Jordan, T. 2001. British contributions to medical research and education in Africa after the Second World War. In Wellcome Witness Seminar 10: British contributions to medical research and education in Africa after the Second World War. L. Reynolds and E. Tansey, eds. London: The Wellcome Trust.

Kariuki, S., G. Revathi, N. Kariuki, J. Kiiru, J. Mwituria, and C. A. Hart. 2006. Characterisation of community acquired non-typhoidal Salmonella from bacteraemia and diarrhoeal infections in children admitted to hospital in Nairobi, Kenya. *BMC Microbiol* 6:101.

Kazatchkine, M. 2007. The Global Fund expands its role: Interview by the Bulletin. *Bull World Health Organ* 85 (10):742–43.

Kebede, A., and A. M. Polderman. 2004. Etiology of acute diarrhea in adults in southwestern Nigeria. *J Clin Microbiol* 42 (8):3909; author reply, 3909–10.

Kennedy, Pagan. 2003. Necessity is the mother of invention. *New York Times*, November 30.

Kernéis, Solen, Lamine Koivogui, N'Faly Magassouba, et al. 2009. Prevalence and risk factors of Lassa seropositivity in inhabitants of the forest region of Guinea: A cross-sectional study. *PLoS Negl Trop Dis* 3 (11):e548.

Khan, A. S., A. Sanchez, and A. K. Pflieger. 1998. Filoviral haemorrhagic fevers. *Br Med Bull* 54 (3):675–92.

Khan, A. S., F. K. Tshioko, D. L. Heymann, et al. 1999. The reemergence of Ebola hemorrhagic fever, Democratic Republic of the Congo, 1995: Commission de Lutte contre les Epidemies a Kikwit. *J Infect Dis* 179 Suppl 1:S76–86.

Khan, S. H., A. Goba, M. Chu, et al. 2008. New opportunities for field research on the pathogenesis and treatment of Lassa fever. *Antiviral Res* 78 (1):103–15.

Kim, J. Y. 2005. Jim Yong Kim—WHO HIV/AIDS director: Interviewed by Pam Das. *Lancet Infect Dis* 5 (9):544–47.

Kim, J. Y., and C. Gilks. 2005. Scaling up treatment—why we can't wait. *N Engl J Med* 353 (22):2392–94.

Kiple, Kenneth F. 1993. *The Cambridge world history of human disease.* Cambridge: Cambridge University Press.

Kirkland, D. 2003. Preliminary findings on the socio-economic impact of Lassa fever in Sierra Leone. *Lassa Fever Update* (February), 16.

Koch, Robert. 1876. Die Aetiologie der Mizbrand-Krakheit, begründet auf die Entwicklungsgeschichte des Bacillus Anthracis. *Beiträge zur Biologie der Pflanzen* 2 (2):277–310.

——. 1880. Investigations into the etiology of traumatic infective diseases. In *Milestones in Microbiology 1546–1940,* edited by T. D. Brock. Washington, D.C.: ASM Press.

——. 1881. Zur Untersuchung von Pathogenen Organismen. *Mittheilungen aus dem Kaiserlichen Gesundheitsamte* 1:1–48.

——. 1882. Die Ätiologie der tuberkulose. *Berliner Klinischen Wochenschrift* 15:221–30.

——. 1884. Die Aetiologie der tuberculose. *Mittheilungen aus dem Kaiserlichen Gesundheitsamte* 2:1–88.

Korenromp, E. L., J. Miller, R. E. Cibulskis, M. Kabir Cham, D. Alnwick, and C. Dye. 2003. Monitoring mosquito net coverage for malaria control in Africa: Possession vs. use by children under 5 years. *Trop Med Int Health* 8 (8): 693–703.

Koukounari, A., J. P. Webster, C. A. Donnelly, et al. 2009. Sensitivities and specificities of diagnostic tests and infection prevalence of *Schistosoma haematobium* estimated from data on adults in villages northwest of Accra, Ghana. *Am J Trop Med Hyg* 80 (3):435–41.

Kvalsund, M. P., A. Haworth, D. L. Murman, E. Velie, and G. L. Birbeck. 2009. Closing gaps in antiretroviral therapy access: Human immunodeficiency virus–associated dementia screening instruments for non-physician healthcare workers. *Am J Trop Med Hyg* 80 (6):1054–59.

Kwena, Z. A. 2004. Politics, etiquette and the fight against HIV/AIDS in Kenya: Negotiating a common front. *Africa Development* 29 (4):113–31.

Laboratory support for poliomyelitis eradication: Memorandum from a WHO meeting. 1989. *Bull World Health Organ* 67 (4):365–67.

Lamunu, M., J. J. Lutwama, J. Kamugisha, A. Opio, and J. Nambooze. 2002. Containing hemorrhagic fever epidemic, the Ebola experience in Uganda (October 2000–January 2001). Paper read at 10th International Congress on Infectious Disease, Singapore.

Lantin, J. P., R. Peitrequin, and P. C. Frei. 1987. Screening for anti-HTLV-III/LAV antibody in high-risk subjects: Sensitivity and specificity of commercial tests. *Int Arch Allergy Appl Immunol* 82 (3–4):487–89.

Larsen, C. H. 2008. The fragile environments of inexpensive CD4$^+$ T-cell enumeration in the least developed countries: Strategies for accessible support. *Cytometry B Clin Cytom* 74 Suppl 1:S107–16.

Lassa Fever—Nigeria (05). 2009. *Promed,* 5 March.

Lawn, J. E., S. Cousens, and J. Zupan. 2005. 4 million neonatal deaths: When? Where? Why? *Lancet* 365 (9462):891–900.

Lawn, S. D., B. Afful, and J. W. Acheampong. 1998. Pulmonary tuberculosis: Diagnostic delay in Ghanaian adults. *Int J Tuberc Lung Dis* 2 (8):635–40.

Leach, A., T. F. McArdle, W. A. Banya, et al. 1999. Neonatal mortality in a rural area of The Gambia. *Ann Trop Paediatr* 19 (1):33–43.

Leader, A., and A. Snyder. 2006. Essays in public health and preventive medicine: History and health care in Angola. *Mt Sinai J Med* 73 (2):567–68.

Leavitt, Judith Walzer. 1996. *Typhoid Mary: Captive to the public's health*. Boston: Beacon Press.

Le Fanu, James. 2000. *The rise and fall of modern medicine*. New York: Carroll and Graf.

Leroy, E. M., S. Baize, C. Y. Lu, et al. 2000. Diagnosis of Ebola haemorrhagic fever by RT-PCR in an epidemic setting. *J Med Virol* 60 (4):463–67.

Leroy, E. M., A. Epelboin, V. Mondonge, et al. 2009. Human Ebola outbreak resulting from direct exposure to fruit bats in Luebo, Democratic Republic of Congo, 2007. *Vector Borne Zoonotic Dis* 9 (6):723–28.

Leroy, E. M., B. Kumulungui, X. Pourrut, et al. 2005. Fruit bats as reservoirs of Ebola virus. *Nature* 438 (7068):575–76.

Leroy, E. M., P. Rouquet, P. Formenty, et al. 2004. Multiple Ebola virus transmission events and rapid decline of central African wildlife. *Science* 303 (5656):387–90.

Leroy, E. M., P. Telfer, B. Kumulungui, et al. 2004. A serological survey of Ebola virus infection in central African nonhuman primates. *J Infect Dis* 190 (11):1895–99.

Levine, Ruth. 2004. *Millions saved: Proven successes in global health*. Washington, D.C.: Center for Global Development.

Levy, S. B. 2002. *The antibiotic paradox: How the misuse of antibiotics destroys their curative power*. Cambridge: Perseus.

Lienhardt, C., J. Rowley, K. Manneh, et al. 2001. Factors affecting time delay to treatment in a tuberculosis control programme in a sub-Saharan African country: The experience of The Gambia. *Int J Tuberc Lung Dis* 5 (3):233–39.

Lin, M., B. Dong, Z. Tang, et al. Analysis of data on surveillance of typhoid and paratyphoid fever in Guangxi 2000–2004. Paper read at 6th International Conference on Typhoid Fever and Other Salmonelloses, Guilin, China.

Lister, Joseph. 1878. On the lactic fermentation and its bearings on pathology. *Transactions of the Pathological Society of London* 29:425–67.

Lubell, Y., H. Reyburn, H. Mbakilwa, et al. 2007. The cost-effectiveness of parasitologic diagnosis for malaria-suspected patients in an era of combination therapy. *Am J Trop Med Hyg* 77 (6 Suppl):128–32.

———. 2008. The impact of response to the results of diagnostic tests for malaria: Cost-benefit analysis. *Br Med J* 336 (7637):202–5.

Luchavez, J., M. E. Lintag, M. Coll-Black, F. Baik, and D. Bell. 2007. An assessment of various blood collection and transfer methods used for malaria rapid diagnostic tests. *Malaria J* 6 (1):149.

Lundqvist, T., S. L. Fisher, G. Kern, et al. 2007. Exploitation of structural and regulatory diversity in glutamate racemases. *Nature* 447 (7146):817–22.

Mabey, D., R. W. Peeling, A. Ustianowski, and M. D. Perkins. 2004. Diagnostics for the developing world. *Nat Rev Microbiol* 2 (3):231–40.

Magnaval, J. F., A. Berry, R. Fabre, and S. Cassaing. 2006. Plasmodium falciparum chloroquine-resistance transporter gene detection in imported Plasmodium falciparum malaria cases. *Clin Infect Dis* 42 (12):1806–7.

Makler, M. T., C. J. Palmer, and A. L. Ager. 1998. A review of practical techniques for the diagnosis of malaria. *Ann Trop Med Parasitol* 92 (4):419–33.

Makundi, E. A., L. E. Mboera, H. M. Malebo, and A. Y. Kitua. 2007. Priority setting on malaria interventions in Tanzania: Strategies and challenges to mitigate against the intolerable burden. *Am J Trop Med Hyg* 77 (6 Suppl):106–11.

Mandomando, I. M., E. V. Macete, J. Ruiz, et al. 2007. Etiology of diarrhea in children younger than 5 years of age admitted in a rural hospital of southern Mozambique. *Am J Trop Med Hyg* 76 (3):522–27.

Marburg hemorrhagic fever—Angola (46). 2005. *Promed*, 30 May.

Marx, A., J. D. Glass, and R. W. Sutter. 2000. Differential diagnosis of acute flaccid paralysis and its role in poliomyelitis surveillance. *Epidemiol Rev* 22 (2):298–316.

Masiye, F., N. Kass, A. Hyder, P. Ndebele, and J. Mfutso-Bengo. 2008. Why mothers choose to enroll their children in malaria clinical studies and the involvement of relatives in decision making: Evidence from Malawi. *Malawi Med J* 20 (2):50–56.

Masiye, F., and C. Rehnberg. 2005. The economic value of an improved malaria treatment programme in Zambia: Results from a contingent valuation survey. *Malar J* 4:60.

Mason, C. 2008. The strains of Ebola. *Canad Med Assoc J* 178 (10):1266–67.

Masum, H., A. S. Daar, S. Al-Bader, R. Shah, and P. A. Singer. 2007. Accelerating health product innovation in sub-Saharan Africa. *Innovations* 2 (4):129–49.

Mathebula, Nsovo S., Jeseelan Pillay, Gianna Toschi, Jan A. Verschoor, and Kenneth I. Ozoemena. 2009. Recognition of anti-mycolic acid antibody at self-assembled mycolic acid antigens on a gold electrode: A potential impedimetric immuno-sensing platform for active tuberculosis. *Chem Commun* (23):3345–47.

Mboera, L. E., E. A. Makundi, and A. Y. Kitua. 2007. Uncertainty in malaria control in Tanzania: Crossroads and challenges for future interventions. *Am J Trop Med Hyg* 77 (6 Suppl):112–18.

Mboya-Okeyo, T., R. G. Ridley, and S. Nwaka. 2009. The African Network for Drugs and Diagnostics Innovation. *Lancet* 373 (9674):1507–8.

McCormick, J. B., I. J. King, P. A. Webb, et al. 1987. A case-control study of the clinical diagnosis and course of Lassa fever. *J Infect Dis* 155 (3):445–55.

McElroy, P. D., A. A. Lal, W. A. Hawley, et al. 1999. Analysis of repeated hemoglobin measures in full-term, normal birth weight Kenyan children between birth and four years of age. III. The Asemobo Bay Cohort Project. *Am J Trop Med Hyg* 61 (6):932–40.

McLean, A. R. 1998. Vaccines and their impact on the control of disease. *Br Med Bull* 54 (3):545–56.

Mda, Z. 2007. *Cion: A novel.* New York: Picador.

Meda, N., I. Ndoye, S. M'Boup, et al. 1999. Low and stable HIV infection rates in Senegal: Natural course of the epidemic or evidence for success of prevention? *AIDS* 13 (11):1397–405.

Mellor, Nicholas. 2004. Obituary: Dr Aniru Conteh—Lassa fever specialist who became an icon to relief workers. *Independent,* 9 April.

Mengara, Daniel. 2005. Contagion and containment in the African mind: A cultural approach to disease in Africa. Paper read at Africa Conference 2005: African Health and Illness, Austin, Texas.

Mensah, P., R. Noora, J. Welbeck, and P. K. Nyame. 2000. Laboratory diagnosis of typhoid fever in Accra. *Ghana Med J* 34 (2):67–70.

Mfutso-Bengo, J., F. Masiye, M. Molyneux, P. Ndebele, and A. Chilungo. 2008. Why do people refuse to take part in biomedical research studies? Evidence from a resource-poor area. *Malawi Med J* 20 (2):57–63.

Michel, C. E., A. W. Solomon, J. P. Magbanua, et al. 2006. Field evaluation of a rapid point-of-care assay for targeting antibiotic treatment for trachoma control: A comparative study. *Lancet* 367 (9522):1585–90.

Miles, S. H. 2003. HIV in insurgency forces in sub-Saharan Africa—a personal view of policies. *Int J STD AIDS* 14 (3):174–78.

Miller, P., and M. Bohnhoff. 1950. The development of bacterial resistance to chemo-therapeutic agents. *Ann Rev Microbiol* 4:201–22.

Million, R. P. 2006. Impact of genetic diagnostics on drug development strategy. *Nat Rev Drug Discov* 5 (6):459–62.

Minor, P. D. 2004. Polio eradication, cessation of vaccination and re-emergence of disease. *Nat Rev Microbiol* 2 (6):473–82.

Minot, G. R., and W. P. Murphy. 1926. Treatment of pernicious anemia by a special diet. JAMA 87:470–76.

Mirza, N. B. 1995. Diagnosis and over diagnosis of typhoid fever. *East Afr Med J* 72 (12):753–54.

Mitiku, K., G. Mengistu, and B. Gelaw. 2003. The reliability of blood film examination for malaria at the peripheral health unit. *Ethiop J Health Dev* 17 (3):197–204.

Molyneux, D. H., D. R. Hopkins, and N. Zagaria. 2004. Disease eradication, elimination and control: The need for accurate and consistent usage. *Trends Parasitol* 20 (8):347–51.

Monath, T. P. 1975. Lassa fever: Review of epidemiology and epizootiology. *Bull World Health Organ* 52 (4–6):577–92.

——. 1999. Ecology of Marburg and Ebola viruses: Speculations and directions for future research. *J Infect Dis* 179 Suppl 1:S127–38.

Moore, M. R., R. E. Gertz, Jr., R. L. Woodbury, et al. 2008. Population snapshot of emergent *Streptococcus pneumoniae* serotype 19A in the United States, 2005. *J Infect Dis* 197 (7):1016–27.

Msellem, M. I., A. Martensson, G. Rotllant, et al. 2009. Influence of rapid malaria diagnostic tests on treatment and health outcome in fever patients, Zanzibar: A crossover validation study. *PLoS Med* 6 (4):e1000070.

Mtove, G., B. Amos, L. von Seidlein, et al. 2010. Invasive salmonellosis among children admitted to a rural Tanzanian hospital and a comparison with previous studies. *PLoS One* 5 (2):e9244.

Mugyenyi, P., A. S. Walker, J. Hakim, et al. 2010. Routine versus clinically driven laboratory monitoring of HIV antiretroviral therapy in Africa (DART): A randomised non-inferiority trial. *Lancet* 375 (9709):123–31.

Mulholland, E. K., O. O. Ogunlesi, R. A. Adegbola, et al. 1999. Etiology of serious infections in young Gambian infants. *Pediatr Infect Dis J* 18 (10 Suppl):S35–41.

Murphy, S. C., and J. G. Breman. 2001. Gaps in the childhood malaria burden in Africa: Cerebral malaria, neurological sequelae, anemia, respiratory distress, hypoglycemia, and complications of pregnancy. *Am J Trop Med Hyg* 64 (1–2 Suppl):57–67.

Murray, C. J., and A. D. Lopez. 1997. Global mortality, disability, and the contribution of risk factors: Global Burden of Disease Study. *Lancet* 349 (9063):1436–42.

Murru, M. 2004. AIDS, primary health care and poverty. *Health Policy and Development* 2 (1):1–12.

Musher, D. M. 2006. Pneumococcal vaccine—direct and indirect ("herd") effects. *N Engl J Med* 354 (14):1522–24.

Mutanda, L. N., A. M. Omari, and I. A. Wamola. 1989. Adaptation of a method of measuring zone diameters of bacterial growth inhibition by antibiotics to suit developing countries. *East Afr Med J* 66 (7):441–47.

Muula, A. S., and F. C. Maseko. 2006. Medical laboratory services in Africa deserve more. *Clin Infect Dis* 42 (10):1503.

Muyembe-Tamfum, J. J., M. Kipasa, C. Kiyungu, and R. Colebunders. 1999. Ebola outbreak in Kikwit, Democratic Republic of the Congo: Discovery and control measures. *J Infect Dis* 179 Suppl 1:S259–62.

Mwanziva, C., S. Shekalaghe, A. Ndaro, et al. 2008. Overuse of artemisinin-combination therapy in Mto wa Mbu (river of mosquitoes), an area misinterpreted as high endemic for malaria. *Malar J* 7:232.

Nabarro, D. 1999. Roll Back Malaria. *Parassitologia* 41 (1–3):501–04.

Nabarro, D. N., and E. M. Tayler. 1998. The "roll back malaria" campaign. *Science* 280 (5372):2067–68.

Naheed, A., P. K. Ram, W. A. Brooks, et al. 2008. Clinical value of Tubex and Typhidot rapid diagnostic tests for typhoid fever in an urban community clinic in Bangladesh. *Diagn Microbiol Infect Dis* 61 (4):381–86.

Nahlen, B. L., E. L. Korenromp, J. M. Miller, and K. Shibuya. 2005. Malaria risk: Estimating clinical episodes of malaria. *Nature* 437 (7056):e3; discussion, e4–5.

NCCLS, National Committee on Clinical Laboratory Standards. 1990. Methods for dilution antimicrobial susceptibility tests for bacteria that grow aerobically, 2nd edition; Approved standard. Villanova, Penn.: National Committee for Clinical Laboratory Standards.

———. 2003. Performance standards for antimicrobial disk susceptibility tests, 8th edition; Approved standard. Villanova, Penn.: National Committee for Clinical Laboratory Standards.

Needham, Cynthia. 2000. *Intimate strangers: Unseen life on Earth*. Washington, D.C.: ASM Press.

Needham, Cynthia, and Richard Canning. 2003. *Global disease eradication: The race for the last child*. Washington, D.C.: ASM Press.

Needham, D. M., S. D. Foster, G. Tomlinson, and P. Godfrey-Faussett. 2001. Socio-economic, gender and health services factors affecting diagnostic delay for tuberculosis patients in urban Zambia. *Trop Med Int Health* 6 (4):256–59.

Neil, K., S. Sodha, L. Luswago, et al. 2009. Outbreak of typhoid fever with high rate of intestinal perforation, Kasese District, Uganda—2008–2009. *Am J Trop Med Hyg* 81 (5 Suppl 1):330S.

Newman, M. J., E. Frimpong, A. Asamoah-Adu, E. Sampane-Donkor, and J. A. Opintan. 2004. Resistance to antimicrobial drugs in Ghana. Ghanaian-Dutch Collaboration for Health Research and Development.

Nicholls, H. 2005. Combating tuberculosis. *Wellcome Focus: Antibiotic resistance—an unwinnable war?*, 31.

Nkrumah, Kwame. 1963. The Academy of Sciences dinner, after dinner speech. November 30, 1963, at Fourth Anniversary of the Academy of Sciences, Ghana. In *Selected speeches: Kwame Nkrumah*. Ghana: Afram Publishers, 1997.

Nordstrand, A., I. Bunikis, C. Larsson, et al. 2007. Tickborne relapsing fever diagnosis obscured by malaria, Togo. *Emerg Infect Dis* 13 (1):117–23.

Norrby, S. R. 2005. Infectious disease emergencies: Role of the infectious disease specialist. *Clin Microbiol Infect* 11 Suppl 1:9–11.

Norrby, S. R., C. E. Nord, and R. Finch. 2005. Lack of development of new antimicrobial drugs: A potential serious threat to public health. *Lancet Infect Dis* 5 (2):115–19.

Nsubuga, P., S. McDonnell, B. Perkins, et al. 2002. Polio eradication initiative in Africa: Influence on other infectious disease surveillance development. *BMC Public Health* 2:27.

Nsutebu, E. F., P. Martins, and D. Adiogo. 2003. Prevalence of typhoid fever in febrile patients with symptoms clinically compatible with typhoid fever in Cameroon. *Trop Med Int Health* 8 (6):575–78.

Nsutebu, E. F., P. M. Ndumbe, and D. Adiogo. 2002. The distribution of anti-Salmonella antibodies in the sera of blood donors in Yaounde, Cameroon. *Trans R Soc Trop Med Hyg* 96 (1):68–69.

Nsutebu, E. F., P. M. Ndumbe, and S. Koulla. 2002. The increase in occurrence of typhoid fever in Cameroon: Overdiagnosis due to misuse of the Widal test? *Trans R Soc Trop Med Hyg* 96 (1):64–67.

Nuland, Sherwin B. 1989. *Doctor: The biography of medicine*. New York: Vintage Books.

Nwaka, S. 2005. Drug discovery and beyond: The role of public-private partnerships in improving access to new malaria medicines. *Trans R Soc Trop Med Hyg* 99 Suppl 1:S20–9.

Nwapa, Flora. 1966. *Efuru*. [London]: Heinemann.

Obadare, E. 2005. A crisis of trust: History, politics, religion and the polio controversy in northern Nigeria. *Patterns of Prejudice* 39 (3):265–66.

Ogunbodede, E. O., M. O. Folayan, and M. A. Adedigba. 2005. Oral health-care workers and HIV infection control practices in Nigeria. *Trop Doct* 35 (3):147–150.

Ogungbamila, F. O., and A. O. Ogundaini, eds. 1993. *Traditional healing methods in the control and treatment of infectious diseases*. Ile-Ife, Nigeria: Antimicrobial Plant Research Group, Obafemi Awolowo Univerisity.

Ohrt, C., P. Obare, A. Nanakorn, et al. 2007. Establishing a malaria diagnostics centre of excellence in Kisumu, Kenya. *Malar J* 6:79.

Ojo, O. S. 2004. *"...To judge the living and the dead..." The pathologist, the misery, the mystery and the final diagnosis: An interminable quest for excellence*. Inaugural Lecture Series 172. Ile-Ife, Nigeria: Obafemi Awolowo University Press.

Okeke, I. N. 2006. Diagnostic insufficiency in Africa. *Clin Infect Dis* 42 (10):1501–53.

———. 2009. The tragedy of antimicrobial resistance: Achieving a recognition of necessity. *Current Science* 97 (11):1564–72.

Okeke, I. N., A. O. Aboderin, D. K. Byarugaba, O. Ojo, and J. A. Opintan. 2007. Growing problem of multidrug-resistant enteric pathogens in Africa. *Emerg Infect Dis* 13 (11):1640–46.

Okeke, I. N., and A. Lamikanra. 1995. Quality and bioavailability of tetracycline capsules in a Nigerian semi-urban community. *Int J Antimicrob Ag* 5:245–50.

———. 2001. Quality and bioavailability of ampicillin capsules dispensed in a Nigerian semi-urban community. *Afr J Med Med Sci* 30 (1–2):47–51.

Okeke, I. N., and J. Wain. 2008. Post-genomic challenges for collaborative research in infectious diseases. *Nat Rev Microbiol* 6 (11):858–64.

Okiro, E. A., S. I. Hay, P. W. Gikandi, et al. 2007. The decline in paediatric malaria admissions on the coast of Kenya. *Malar J* 6:151.

Oldstone, Michael B. A. 1998. *Viruses, plagues, and history*. New York: Oxford University Press.

Olopoenia, L. A., and A. L. King. 2000. Widal agglutination test—100 years later: Still plagued by controversy. *Postgrad Med J* 76 (892):80–84.

Olukoya, P., and J. Ferguson. 2003. Olikoye Ransome-Kuti. *Lancet* 362:175.

Omura, S., and A. Crump. 2004. The life and times of ivermectin—a success story. *Nat Rev Microbiol* 2 (12):984–89.

Opintan, J. A., and M. J. Newman. 2007. Distribution of serogroups and serotypes of multiple drug resistant *Shigella* isolates. *Ghana Med J* 41 (1):4–8.

Orji, J. N. 1982. A re-assessment of the organisation and benefits of the slave and palm produce trade amongst the Ngwa-Igbo. *Canadian Journal of African Studies* 16 (3):523–48.

Oshinsky, David M. 2005. *Polio: An American story*. Oxford: Oxford University Press.

Oshisada, Victor. 2006. The HIV-baby controversy. Editorial opinion, *Guardian* (Lagos), 29 June.

Osler, William. 1892. *The principles and practice of medicine: Designed for the use of practitioners and students of medicine*. New York: D. Appleton and Company.

O-tipo, S., K. Neil, S. Sodha, et al. 2009. Typhoid fever outbreak in Kasese District, Uganda: 103 cases with intestinal perforation. *Am J Trop Med Hyg* 81 (5 Suppl 1):330.

Outbreak news: Ebola haemorrhagic fever, Uganda—end of the outbreak. 2008. *Wkly Epidemiol Rec* 83 (10):89–90.

Outbreak of Ebola haemorrhagic fever in Yambio, south Sudan, April—June 2004. 2005. *Wkly Epidemiol Rec* 80 (43):370–75.

Packard, Randall M. 2000. Post-colonial medicine. In *Medicine in the 20th century,* edited by R. Cooter and J. Pickstone. Amsterdam: Harwood Academic.

Pai, M., J. Minion, H. Sohn, A. Zwerling, and M. D. Perkins. 2009. Novel and improved technologies for tuberculosis diagnosis: Progress and challenges. *Clin Chest Med* 30 (4):701–16.

Pai, M., and R. O'Brien. 2008. New diagnostics for latent and active tuberculosis: State of the art and future prospects. *Semin Respir Crit Care Med* 29 (5):560–68.

Pai, Madhukar, Andrew Ramsay, and Richard O'Brien. 2008. Evidence-based tuberculosis diagnosis. *PLoS Med* 5 (7):e156.

Palmer, A., M. Weber, K. Bojang, T. McKay, and R. Adegbola. 1999. Acute bacterial meningitis in The Gambia: A four-year review of paediatric hospital admissions. *J Trop Pediatr* 45 (1):51–53.

Palumbi, S. R. 2001. Humans as the world's greatest evolutionary force. *Science* 293 (5536):1786–90.

Panhotra, B. R., Z. U. Hassan, C. S. Joshi, and A. Bahrani. 2005. Visual detection of multiple viral amplicons by dipstick assay: Its application in screening of blood donors a welcome tool for limited resource settings. *J Clin Microbiol* 43 (12):6218; author reply, 6218–19.

Paramasivan, C. N., E. Lee, K. Kao, et al. 2010. Experience establishing tuberculosis laboratory capacity in a developing country setting. *Int J Tuberc Lung Dis* 14 (1):59–64.

PATH, Program for Appropriate Technology in Health. 2008. Diarrheal disease advocacy: Findings from a scan of the global funding and policy landscape. Seattle: Program for Appropriate Technology in Health.

Paweska, J. T. 2007. *Lassa fever—South Africa ex Nigeria* [Promed-MAIL] 2007 [cited 14 March].

Payne, D. J., M. N. Gwynn, D. J. Holmes, and D. L. Pompliano. 2007. Drugs for bad bugs: Confronting the challenges of antibacterial discovery. *Nat Rev Drug Discov* 6 (1):29–40.

Peeling, R. W. 2007. Diagnostics for sexually transmitted infections. Presented in *Diagnostics in the tropics—time to take the guesswork out of clinical practice.* Symposium 33 in the 56th Annual meeting of the American Society for Tropical Medicine and Hygiene. Philadelphia.

Peeling, R. W., D. Mabey, A. Herring, and E. W. Hook. 2006. Why do we need quality-assured diagnostic tests for sexually transmitted infections? *Nat Rev Microbiol* 4 (12 Suppl):S7–19.

Pelton, S. I., A. M. Loughlin, and C. D. Marchant. 2004. Seven valent pneumococcal conjugate vaccine immunization in two Boston communities: Changes in serotypes and antimicrobial susceptibility among Streptococcus pneumoniae isolates. *Pediatr Infect Dis J* 23 (11):1015–22.

Perkins, M. D., G. Roscigno, and A. Zumla. 2006. Progress towards improved tuberculosis diagnostics for developing countries. *Lancet* 367 (9514):942–43.

Perkins, M., and D. Bell. 2008. Working without a blindfold: The critical role of diagnostics in malaria control. *Malaria Journal* 7 (Suppl 1):S5.

Peters, R. P., E. E. Zijlstra, M. J. Schijffelen, et al. 2004. A prospective study of bloodstream infections as cause of fever in Malawi: Clinical predictors and implications for management. *Trop Med Int Health* 9 (8):928–34.

Peterson, A. T., D. S. Carroll, J. N. Mills, and K. M. Johnson. 2004. Potential mamma-lian filovirus reservoirs. *Emerg Infect Dis* 10 (12):2073–81.

Petri, R. J. 1887. Eine kleine modification des Koch'schen plattenverfahrens. *Centralb-latt für Bacteriologie und Parasitenkunde* 1:279–80.

Pettersson, U., H. Wigzell, and P. Perlman. 1987. Malaria diagnosis. *Science* 236 (4797):11–12.

Petti, C. A., C. R. Polage, and D. R. Hillyard. 2006. Screening laboratory requests. *Emerg Infect Dis* 12 (11):1792–93.

Phillips, K. A., S. Van Bebber, and A. M. Issa. 2006. Diagnostics and biomarker devel-opment: Priming the pipeline. *Nat Rev Drug Discov* 5 (6):463–69.

Phillips, M., J. Kumate-Rodriguez, and F. Mota-Hernández. 1989. Costs of treating diarrhoea in a children's hospital in Mexico City. *Bull World Health Organ* 67 (3):273–80.

Phillips, R. S. 2001. Current status of malaria and potential for control. *Clin. Microbiol. Rev.* 14 (1):208–26.

Pincock, S. 2006. Bekololari Ransome-Kuti. *Lancet* 367:810.

Planche, T., and S. Krishna. 2005. The relevance of malaria pathophysiology to strate-gies of clinical management. *Curr Opin Infect Dis* 18 (5):369–75.

Plowe, C. V., and T. E. Wellems. 1995. Molecular approaches to the spreading problem of drug resistant malaria. *Adv Exp Med Biol* 390:197–209.

Polage, C. R., G. Bedu-Addo, A. Owusu-Ofori, et al. 2006. Laboratory use in Ghana: Physician perception and practice. *Am J Trop Med Hyg* 75 (3):526–31.

Porter, Roy. 1998. *The greatest benefit to mankind: A medical history of humanity.* New York: W. W. Norton.

Poupard, J. A., S. F. Rittenhouse, and L. R. Walsh. 1994. The evolution of antimicrobial susceptibility testing methods. In *Antimicrobial susceptibility testing—critical issues for the '90s,* edited by J. Poupard, L. Walsh, and B. Kleger. New York: Ple-num Press.

Prati, Daniele. 2006. Non-sterile injections, contaminated blood, and the spread of HIV. *Lancet* 368 (9541):1064.

Preston, Richard. 1995. *The hot zone.* Rockland, Mass.: Wheeler Pub.

Priddy, F., F. Tesfaye, Y. Mengistu, et al. 2005. Potential for medical transmission of HIV in Ethiopia. *AIDS* 19 (3):348–50.

Prins, Gwyn. 1989. But what was the disease? The present state of health and healing in African studies. *Past and Present* 124:159–79.

Progress in reducing global measles deaths, 1999–2004. 2006. *MMWR Morb Mortal Wkly Rep* 55 (9):247–49.

Progress toward strengthening blood transfusion services—14 countries, 2003–2007. 2008. *MMWR Morb Mortal Wkly Rep* 57 (47):1273–77.

Rapatski, B. L., F. Suppe, and J. A. Yorke. 2005. HIV epidemics driven by late disease stage transmission. *J Acquir Immune Defic Syndr* 38 (3):241–53.

Reducing tests. 1981. *Lancet* 1 (8219):539–40.

Reyburn, H., H. Mbakilwa, R. Mwangi, et al. 2007. Rapid diagnostic tests compared with malaria microscopy for guiding outpatient treatment of febrile illness in Tanzania: Randomised trial. *Br Med J* 334 (7590):403.

Reyburn, H., R. Mbatia, C. Drakeley, et al. 2004. Overdiagnosis of malaria in pa-tients with severe febrile illness in Tanzania: A prospective study. *Br Med J* 329 (7476):1212.

Reyburn, H., E. Mwakasungula, S. Chonya, et al. 2008. Clinical assessment and treat-ment in paediatric wards in the north-east of the United Republic of Tanzania. *Bull World Health Organ* 86 (2):132–39.

Reyburn, H., J. Ruanda, O. Mwerinde, and C. Drakeley. 2006. The contribution of microscopy to targeting antimalarial treatment in a low transmission area of Tanzania. *Malar J* 5:4.

Richmond, J. K., and D. J. Baglole. 2003. Lassa fever: Epidemiology, clinical features, and social consequences. *Br Med J* 327 (7426):1271–75.

The right tools can save lives. 2006. *Nature* 444 (7120):681.

Roberts, L. 2009a. Polio eradication: Looking for a little luck. *Science* 323 (5915):702–5.

———. 2009b. Public health: Type 2 poliovirus back from the dead in Nigeria. *Science* 325 (5941):660–61.

Roberts, L., and M. Enserink. 2007. Malaria. Did they really say... eradication? *Science* 318 (5856):1544–45.

Robottom, John. 1991. *Health and Medicine 1750–1900*. London: Longman.

Roels, T. H., A. S. Bloom, J. Buffington, et al. 1999. Ebola hemorrhagic fever, Kikwit, Democratic Republic of the Congo, 1995: Risk factors for patients without a reported exposure. *J Infect Dis* 179 Suppl 1:S92–7.

Roper, C., R. Pearce, S. Nair, B. Sharp, F. Nosten, and T. Anderson. 2004. Intercontinental spread of pyrimethamine-resistant malaria. *Science* 305 (5687):1124.

Ross, Ronald. 1905. The progress of tropical medicine. *Journal of the African Society* 4 (15): 271–89.

Rouquet, P., J. M. Froment, M. Bermejo, et al. 2005. Wild animal mortality monitoring and human Ebola outbreaks, Gabon and Republic of Congo, 2001–2003. *Emerg Infect Dis* 11 (2):283–90.

Sachs, J. D. 2005. Achieving the Millennium Development Goals—the case of malaria. *N Engl J Med* 352 (2):115–17.

Sachs, Jeffrey. 2005. *The end of poverty: Economic possibilities for our time*. New York: Penguin.

Salmon, D. E. 1881. Investigations of swine plague and fowl cholera. In *Contagious diseases of domesticated animals*. Washington: U.S. Department of Agriculture.

Sam-Abbenyi, A., M. Dama, S. Graham, and Z. Obate. 1999. Dracunculiasis in Cameroon at the threshold of elimination. *Int J Epidemiol* 28 (1):163–68.

Santer, M. 2009. Richard Bradley: A unified, living agent theory of the cause of infectious diseases of plants, animals, and humans in the first decades of the 18th century. *Perspect Biol Med* 52 (4):566–78.

Schapira, A. 1994. A standard protocol for assessing the proportion of children presenting with febrile disease who suffer from malarial disease. World Health Organization.

Schmid, G. P., A. Buve, P. Mugyenyi, et al. 2004. Transmission of HIV-1 infection in sub-Saharan Africa and effect of elimination of unsafe injections. *Lancet* 363 (9407):482–88.

Schoofs, M. 1999. AIDS: The agony of Africa. Part Two: A tale of two brothers. *Village Voice* 44 (45):47–48, 51–52.

Schram, Ralph. 1971. *A history of the Nigerian health services. With an introd. by Sir Samuel Manuwa*. [Ibadan]: Ibadan University Press.

Schroeter, J. 1875. Uber einige durch bacterien gebildete pigmente (Concering a few pigments generated by bacteria). Beiträge zur Biologie der Pflanzen 1(2):109–26.

Science and Africa: A message to the G8 summit. 2005. *Nature* 435 (7046):1146–49.

Scott, S., W. J. Moss, S. Cousens, et al. 2007. The influence of HIV-1 exposure and infection on levels of passively acquired antibodies to measles virus in Zambian infants. *Clin Infect Dis* 45 (11):1417–24.

Scrimshaw, N. S. 1974. Myths and realities in international health planning. *Am J Public Health* 64 (8):792–98.

Severe acute pneumonitis among deployed U.S. military personnel—Southwest Asia. 2003. *MMWR Morb Mortal Wkly Rep* 52 (36):857–59.

Shearer, Jessica C., Meghan L. Stack, Marcie R. Richmond, Allyson P. Bear, Rana A. Hajjeh, and David M. Bishai. 2010. Accelerating policy decisions to adopt *Haemophilus influenzae* Type b vaccine: A global, multivariable analysis. *PLoS Med* 7 (3):e1000249.

Shillcutt, S., C. Morel, C. Goodman, et al. 2008. Cost-effectiveness of malaria diagnostic methods in sub-Saharan Africa in an era of combination therapy. *Bull World Health Organ* 86 (2):101–10.

Shilts, Randy. 1988. *And the band played on: Politics, people, and the AIDS epidemic.* New York: Penguin Books.

Showstack, J. A., S. A. Schroeder, and M. F. Matsumoto. 1982. Changes in the use of medical technologies, 1972–1977: A study of 10 inpatient diagnoses. *N Engl J Med* 306 (12):706–12.

Singer, E. 2005. International partnership launches malaria model in Zambia. *Nat Med* 11 (7):695.

Singer, P. A., A. S. Daar, S. Al-Bader, et al. 2008. Commercializing African health research: Building life science convergence platforms. In Gehner, M., S. Jupp and S. A. Matlin, *Global forum update on research for health volume 5: Fostering innovation for global health.* Woodbridge, UK: Pro-Book Publishing.Singh, J. A., R. Upshur, and N. Padayatchi. 2007. XDR-TB in South Africa: No time for denial or complacency. *PLoS Med* 4 (1):e50.

Smolinski, Mark S., Margaret A. Hamburg, Joshua Lederberg, and Institute of Medicine (U.S.). Committee on Emerging Microbial Threats to Health in the 21st Century. 2003. *Microbial threats to health: Emergence, detection, and response.* Washington, D.C.: National Academies Press.

Snow, R. W., M. H. Craig, C. R. J. C. Newton, and R. W. Steketee. 2003. The public health burden of *Plasmodium falciparum* malaria in Africa: Deriving the numbers. *Disease Control Priorities Project Working Paper No 11. Bethesda, Maryland: Fogarty International Center, National Institutes of Health.*Snow, R. W., C. A. Guerra, A. M. Noor, H. Y. Myint, and S. I. Hay. 2005. The global distribution of clinical episodes of *Plasmodium falciparum* malaria. *Nature* 434 (7030):214–17.

Snow, R. W., E. L. Korenromp, and E. Gouws. 2004. Pediatric mortality in Africa: *Plasmodium falciparum* malaria as a cause or risk? *Am J Trop Med Hyg* 71 (2 Suppl): 16–24.

Sofowora, A. 1982. *Medicinal plants and traditional medicine in Africa.* Chichester, West Sussex: John Wiley.

Sokoloff, Boris. 1954. *The miracle drugs.* 3rd ed. New York: Prentice-Hall.

Sosa, A., D. K. Byarugaba, C. F. Amábile-Cuevas, P-R Hseuh, and I. N. Okeke, eds. 2009. *Antimicrobial resistance in developing countries.* New York: Springer.

Sow, S. O., S. Diallo, J. D. Campbell, et al. 2005. Burden of invasive disease caused by *Haemophilus influenzae* type b in Bamako, Mali: Impetus for routine infant immunization with conjugate vaccine. *Pediatr Infect Dis J* 24 (6):533–37.

Steen, T. W., and G. N. Mazonde. 1998. Pulmonary tuberculosis in Kweneng District, Botswana: Delays in diagnosis in 212 smear-positive patients. *Int J Tuberc Lung Dis* 2 (8):627–34.

Steketee, Richard W., Naawa Sipilanyambe, John Chimumbwa, et al. 2008. National malaria control and scaling up for impact: The Zambia experience through 2006. *Am J Trop Med Hyg* 79 (1):45–52.

Stetten, D. 1978. Victory over Variola. *ASM News* 44 (12):639.

STOP-TB, Partnership. 2006. Actions for life: Towards a world free of tuberculosis. The global plan to stop tuberculosis 2006–2015.

Suit No NIC/8/2006 2008. National Industrial Court, Abuja, Nigeria.

Suzuki, Y., and T. Gojobori. 1997. The origin and evolution of Ebola and Marburg viruses. *Mol Biol Evol* 14 (8):800–806.

Talbot, George H., John Bradley, John E. Edwards, Jr., David Gilbert, Michael Scheld, and John G. Bartlett. 2006. Bad bugs need drugs: An update on the development pipeline from the Antimicrobial Availability Task Force of the Infectious Diseases Society of America. *Clin Infect Dis* 42 (5):657–68.

Tan, T. Q. 2003. Antibiotic resistant infections due to *Streptococcus pneumoniae:* Impact on therapeutic options and clinical outcome. *Curr Opin Infect Dis* 16 (3):271–77.

Tankhiwale, S. S., G. Agrawal, and S. V. Jalgaonkar. 2003. An unusually high occurrence of *Salmonella enterica* serotype paratyphi A in patients with enteric fever. *Indian J Med Res* 117:10–12.

Tapia, M. D., S. O. Sow, S. Medina-Moreno, et al. 2005. A serosurvey to identify the window of vulnerability to wild-type measles among infants in rural Mali. *Am J Trop Med Hyg* 73 (1):26–31.

Teepe, R. G., B. K. Johnson, D. Ocheng, et al. 1983. A probable case of Ebola virus haemorrhagic fever in Kenya. *East Afr Med J* 60 (10):718–22.

Tegbaru, B., H. Meless, A. Kassu, D. Tesema, N. Gezahegn, W. Tamene, E. Hailu, H. Birhanu, and T. Messele. 2004. Laboratory services in hospitals and regional laboratories in Ethiopia. *Ethiop J Health Dev* 18 (1):43–47.

Terris-Prestholt, F., D. Watson-Jones, K. Mugeye, et al. 2003. Is antenatal syphilis screening still cost effective in sub-Saharan Africa? *Sex Transm Infect* 79 (5):375–81.

Thomas, Lewis. 1978. *The lives of a cell: Notes of a biology watcher.* New York: Penguin Books.

Thompson, L. J., S. J. Dunstan, C. Dolecek, et al. 2009. Transcriptional response in the peripheral blood of patients infected with *Salmonella enterica* serovar Typhi. *Proc Natl Acad Sci U S A* 106 (52):22433–38.

Thwing, J. I., J. Mihigo, A. P. Fernandes, et al. 2009. How much malaria occurs in urban Luanda, Angola? A health facility-based assessment. *Am J Trop Med Hyg* 80 (3):487–91.

Tornheim, J. A., A. S. Manya, N. Oyando, S. Kabaka, R. F. Breiman, and D. R. Feikin. 2007. The epidemiology of hospitalized pneumonia in rural Kenya: The potential of surveillance data in setting public health priorities. *Int J Infect Dis* 11 (6):536–43.

Towner, K. J., N. J. Pearson, F. S. Mhalu, and F. O'Grady. 1980. Resistance to antimicrobial agents of Vibrio cholerae El Tor strains isolated during the fourth cholera epidemic in the United Republic of Tanzania. *Bull World Health Organ* 58 (5):747–51.

Towner, J. S., X. Pourrut, C. G. Albarino, et al. 2007. Marburg virus infection detected in a common African bat. *PLoS ONE* 2 (1):e764.

Towner, J. S., P. E. Rollin, D. G. Bausch, et al. 2004. Rapid diagnosis of Ebola hemorrhagic fever by reverse transcription-PCR in an outbreak setting and assessment of patient viral load as a predictor of outcome. *J Virol* 78 (8):4330–41.

Towner, J. S., T. K. Sealy, M. L. Khristova, et al. 2008. Newly discovered Ebola virus associated with hemorrhagic fever outbreak in Uganda. *PLoS Pathog* 4(11):e1000212.Trape, J. F. 2001. The public health impact of chloroquine resistance in Africa. *Am J Trop Med Hyg* 64 (1–2 Suppl):12–17.

Troup, J. M., H. A. White, A. L. Fom, and D. E. Carey. 1970. An outbreak of Lassa fever on the Jos plateau, Nigeria, in January–February 1970. A preliminary report. *Am J Trop Med Hyg* 19 (4):695–96.

Turshen, Meredeth. 1984. *The political ecology of disease in Tanzania.* New Brunswick, N.J.: Rutgers University Press.

Two accused over "fake" HIV tests. 2006. *BBC News online,* 30 October.

Twumasi, P. A. 1975. *Medical systems in Ghana: A study in medical sociology.* Accra: Ghana Publishing Corporation.

Ukwuoma, Ben. 2004. Medical lab scientists suggest measures to curb microbial drug resistance. *Guardian,* 11 December.

———. 2006. Council shuts 50 medical labs in Abuja, Benin. *Guardian,* 1 July.

Ulrich, M. P., D. R. Christensen, S. R. Coyne, et al. 2006. Evaluation of the Cepheid GeneXpert system for detecting Bacillus anthracis. *J Appl Microbiol* 100 (5):1011–16.

UNICEF and WHO. 2009. Diarrhoea: Why children are still dying and what can be done. UNICEF and WHO.

Update: International Task Force for Disease Eradication, 1990 and 1991. 1992. *MMWR Morb Mortal Wkly Rep* 41 (3):40–42.

Usdin, M., M. Guillerm, and P. Chirac. 2006. Neglected tests for neglected patients. *Nature* 441 (7091):283–84.

Uzochukwu, Benjamin, Eric Obikeze, Obinna Onwujekwe, Chima Onoka, and Ulla Griffiths. 2009. Cost-effectiveness analysis of rapid diagnostic test, microscopy and syndromic approach in the diagnosis of malaria in Nigeria: Implications for scaling-up deployment of ACT. *Malar J* 8 (1):265.

van den Brandhof, W. E., A. I. Bartelds, M. P. Koopmans, and Y. T. van Duynhoven. 2006. General practitioner practices in requesting laboratory tests for patients with gastroenteritis in the Netherlands, 2001–2002. *BMC Fam Pract* 7:56.

van Riet, E., A. A. Adegnika, K. Retra, et al. 2007. Cellular and humoral responses to influenza in Gabonese children living in rural and semi-urban areas. *J Infect Dis* 196 (11):1671–1678.

Vaughan, Megan. 1991. *Curing their ills: Colonial power and African illness.* Cambridge: Polity Press.

Verhoef, J., and A. Fluit. 2006. Surveillance uncovers the smoking gun for resistance emergence. *Biochem Pharmacol* 71 (7):1036–41.

Vila, J., J. Gascon, S. Abdalla, et al. 1994. Antimicrobial resistance of Shigella isolates causing traveler's diarrhea. *Antimicrob Agents Chemother* 38 (11):2668–70.

Wainwright, M. 1991. Streptomycin: Discovery and resultant controversy. *Hist Philos Life Sci* 13 (1):97–124.

Walsh, P. D., K. A. Abernethy, M. Bermejo, et al. 2003. Catastrophic ape decline in western equatorial Africa. *Nature* 422 (6932):611–14.

Walsh, P. D., R. Biek, and L. A. Real. 2005. Wave-like spread of Ebola Zaire. *PLoS Biol* 3 (11):e371.

Wammanda, R., and S. Onazi. 2009. Ability of mothers to assess the presence of fever in their children: Implication for the treatment of fever under the IMCI guidelines. *Ann Afr Med* 8 (3):173–76.

Watson-Jones, D., M. Oliff, F. Terris-Prestholt, et al. 2005. Antenatal syphilis screening in sub-Saharan Africa: Lessons learned from Tanzania. *Trop Med Int Health* 10 (9):934–43.

White, R. G., K. K. Orroth, J. R. Glynn, et al. 2008. Treating curable sexually transmitted infections to prevent HIV in Africa: Still an effective control strategy? *J Acquir Immune Defic Syndr* 47 (3):346–53.

WHO, World Health Organization. 1948. Constitution of the World Health Organization. Official Record of the World Health Organization. Geneva.

——. 1973. Chemotherapy of malaria and resistance to antimalarials: Report of a WHO Scientific Group. *WHO Technical Report Series* 529:1–21.

——. 1988. Aquired immune deficiency syndrome (AIDS), 1987 case definition for the CDC/WHO case definition for AIDS. *Weekly Epidemiological Record* 63:1–8.

——. 1996. Assessment of therapeutic efficacy of antimalarial drugs for uncomplicated falciparum malaria in areas with intense transmission. Geneva: World Health Organization.

——. 2001a. Interventions and strategies to improve the use of antimicrobials in developing countries. Geneva: World Health Organization.

——. 2001b. WHO global strategy for containment of antibiotic resistance. Geneva: World Health Organization.

——. 2003. Treatment of tuberculosis: Guidelines for national programmes. Geneva: World Health Organization.

——. 2004. Global tuberculosis control—surveillance, planning, financing. Geneva: World Health Organization.

——. 2005. Revision of the International Health Regulations. Geneva: World Health Organization.

——. 2006a. Diagnostics for tuberculosis: Global demand and market potential. Geneva: World Health Organization.

——. 2006b. Extensively drug-resistant tuberculosis (XDR-TB): Recommendations for prevention and control. *Weekly Epidemiological Record* 81:430–32.

——. 2006c. Guidelines for the treatment of malaria.

——. 2006d. The role of laboratory diagnosis to support malaria disease management: Focus on the use of rapid diagnostic tests in areas of high transmission.

——. 2008. World malaria report.

——. 2009a. Malaria Rapid Diagnostic Test Performance—results of WHO product testing of malaria RDTs: Round 1 (2008).

——. 2009b. World malaria report.

WHO and CDC. 1998. Infection control for viral haemorrhagic fevers in the African health care setting.

WHO and UNICEF. 2003. The Africa Malaria Report. Geneva: World Health Organization and UNICEF.

WHO Regional Office for Africa. 2008. The Maputo Declaration on Strengthening Laboratory Systems. Maputo, Mozambique, 24 January. http://www.finddiagnostics.org/export/sites/default/programs/scaling_up/lab_preparedness/docs/Maputo-Declaration_2008.pdf.

Wilson, I. K., D. G. Achel, M. D. Wilson, et al. 2003. The detection of tuberculosis in paucibacillary sputum samples in Ghana using PCR. *Ghana Med J* 37 (3):117–21.

Wilson, P. E., W. Kazadi, D. D. Kamwendo, V. Mwapasa, A. Purfield, and S. R. Meshnick. 2005. Prevalence of pfcrt mutations in Congolese and Malawian *Plasmodium falciparum* isolates as determined by a new Taqman assay. *Acta Trop* 93 (1):97–106.

Wolman, Dianne Miller, Andrea L. Kalfoglou, Lauren LeRoy, and Institute of Medicine (U.S.). Committee on Medicare Payment Methodology for Clinical Laboratory Services. 2000. *Medicare laboratory payment policy: Now and in the future.* Washington, D.C.: National Academy Press.

Wongsrichanalai, C., M. J. Barcus, S. Muth, A. Sutamihardja, and W. H. Wernsdorfer. 2007. A review of malaria diagnostic tools: Microscopy and rapid diagnostic test (RDT). *Am J Trop Med Hyg* 77 (6 Suppl):119–27.

Wongsrichanalai, C., A. L. Pickard, W. H. Wernsdorfer, and S. R. Meshnick. 2002. Epidemiology of drug-resistant malaria. *Lancet Infect Dis* 2 (4):209–18.

Woolhouse, M. E. 2002. Population biology of emerging and re-emerging pathogens. *Trends Microbiol* 10 (10 Suppl):S3–7.

Woolhouse, M. E., and S. Gowtage-Sequeria. 2005. Host range and emerging and re-emerging pathogens. *Emerg Infect Dis* 11 (12):1842–47.

Wootton, David. 2006. *Bad medicine: Doctors doing harm since Hippocrates.* Oxford: Oxford University Press.

Worboys, Micheal. 2000. Colonial medicine. In *Medicine in the 20th century,* edited by R. Cooter and J. Pickstone. Amsterdam: Harwood Academic Publishers.

Wright, P. 2004. Aniru Conteh. *Lancet* 363 (9423):1831.

Xu, Q., S. G. Jin, and L. X. Zhang. 2000. Cost effectiveness of DOTS and non-DOTS strategies for smear-positive pulmonary tuberculosis in Beijing. *Biomed Environ Sci* 13 (4):307–13.

Yimer, S., G. Bjune, and G. Alene. 2005. Diagnostic and treatment delay among pulmonary tuberculosis patients in Ethiopia: A cross-sectional study. *BMC Infect Dis* 5 (1):112.

Zahra, A. 1956. Yaws eradication campaign in Nsukka division, Eastern Nigeria: A preliminary review. *Bull World Health Organ* 15:911–35.

Zhong, Nan Shan, and Guang Qiao Zeng. 2003. Our strategies for fighting Severe Acute Respiratory Syndrome (SARS). *Am. J. Respir. Crit. Care Med.* 168 (1):7–9.

Zimic, M., J. Coronel, R. H. Gilman, C. G. Luna, W. H. Curioso, and D. A. Moore. 2009. Can the power of mobile phones be used to improve tuberculosis diagnosis in developing countries? *Trans R Soc Trop Med Hyg* 103 (6):638–40.

Zumla, A., J. Huggett, K. Dheda, C. Green, N. Kapata, and P. Mwaba. 2010. Trials and tribulations of an African-led research and capacity development programme: The case for EDCTP investments. *Trop Med Int Health* 15 (4):489–94.

Zurovac, D., B. A. Larson, W. Akhwale, and R. W. Snow. 2006. The financial and clinical implications of adult malaria diagnosis using microscopy in Kenya. *Trop Med Int Health* 11 (8):1185–94.

Zurovac, D., B. Midia, S. A. Ochola, M. English, and R. W. Snow. 2006. Microscopy and outpatient malaria case management among older children and adults in Kenya. *Trop Med Int Health* 11 (4):432–40.

Zurovac, D., J. Njogu, W. Akhwale, D. H. Hamer, B. A. Larson, and R. W. Snow. 2008. Effects of revised diagnostic recommendations on malaria treatment practices across age groups in Kenya. *Trop Med Int Health* 13 (6):784–87.

Index

Note: Italic page numbers refer to tables.

Abalaka, Jeremiah, 102
Affordable Medicines Facility for Malaria, 33
Africa: infectious disease burden of, 6, 18;
    malaria as endemic to, 27, 38, 122, 167n13,
    181n57; and smallpox, 107; stereotype as
    infectious continent, 78, 95, 106; and stereo-
    types of HIV infection, 93–94, 95. *See also
    specific countries*
African Institutions Initiative, 161
African medical systems: and clinical record-
    keeping, 65, 125–26, 181n4; colonial model
    of health care system as template for, 131,
    132–33, 135; development of, 142; and
    health care access, 18, 24, 28, 45, 155; imper-
    sonal nature of, 65–66, 143–44; inadequacy
    of, 5, 6, 20, 35; medical pluralism in, 25,
    135; and medical research, 158, 185n56; in
    modern environment, 4, 19; role of, 163n2;
    successful programs of, 106; Western models
    for, 18, 149–50. *See also* diagnostic develop-
    ment; diagnostic insufficiency; indigenous
    medicine; laboratory diagnostics
African Network for Drugs and Diagnostic
    Innovation, 161
AIDS (acquired immune deficiency syn-
    drome): AIDs-related syndromes, 179n34;
    clinical case definition for, 105; and di-
    agnostic insufficiency, 96, 102, 178n24;
    etiologic agents of, 93, 96, 97; and intestinal
    parasite infection rates, 138; myths sur-
    rounding, 178n14; and Nigeria, 67–68, 94,
    100–102; prevalence of, 98, 100–101; skepti-
    cism about, 94, 95–96, 98, 177n4; stigma
    associated with, 97, 99; treatment for, 101–2,
    178n24, 178n25; vaccines for, 102, 103–4;
    and vulnerability to diseases resembling ty-
    phoid, 49; and Western medicine, 103
American Society for Clinical Pathology, 154
American Society for Microbiology, 149, 154
American Society of Tropical Medicine and
    Hygiene, 122–23
Angola, 34, 69, 72, 170n58, 184n13
Anikulapo-Kuti, Fela, 98–99

anthrax, 16, 127, 184n13
antimicrobials: appropriate application of, 7,
    127; and drug resistance, 44, 50–51, 54, 57,
    62, 63, 115, 150, 155; lack of profitability in
    development of, 53, 63; narrow-spectrum,
    57; overprescribing of, 53, 115, 131; selective
    pressure from drug use, 51, 62, 114, 124,
    126, 183n9; and susceptibility testing, 58, 59,
    60, 156; types of, 171n4
antiretroviral drugs, 97, 98, 101, 102, 103–5
Aro confederation, 21–22, 166n2
Aro-Ndizuogu, Nigeria, 21–24
artemether-lumefantrine, 33, 169n37
artemisinin, 171n4
artemisinin-based combination therapies
    (ACTs), 33, 34, 62, 123, 159, 168n32
Asia: and malaria, 27, 36, 50; and smallpox,
    107; and typhoid fever, 46, 48, 170n3
Attah, Sefi, 11

BACTEC instrumentation, 121
bacteremia, 41, 42
bacterial infections: and child mortality, 41, 54,
    55, 56; clinical diagnosis of, 127; diagnos-
    tic tests for, 46–48, 57, 145, 148, 155, 156,
    161; and fevers, 37; identifying, 44; malaria
    confused with, 29, 40, 41, 43, 47; and sus-
    ceptibility testing, 59; treatment of, 56–57;
    vaccines for, 115
bacteriology, 15, 16, 56, 164n12, 164–65n13,
    165n18
Bank-Anthony, Mobolaji, 66, 173n3
Banu, Rahima, 109
Barker, Robert H., 136
Bassi, Agostino, 14
Bill and Melinda Gates Foundation, 123–24
Biosafety Level 4, 76, 156
Bosompem, Kwabena, 140
Botswana, 94, 100, 119, 120, 149, 177n4
Böttger, Eric, 46
Brazil, 88
Brefeld, Julius Oscar, 15
Brock, Thomas, 7, 166n19